Understanding Brain Damage
A primer of neuropsychological evaluation

D1558953

To My Students

He most honors my style who learns under it to destroy the teacher.

Walt Whitman, Song of Myself, 47.

For Churchill Livingstone:

Publisher: Mike Parkinson
Editorial Co-ordination: Editorial Resources Unit
Production Controller: Mrs Niall G. C. Small
Design: Design Resources Unit
Sales Production Executive: Marion Pollock

Understanding Brain Damage

A PRIMER OF NEUROPSYCHOLOGICAL EVALUATION

Kevin W. Walsh BA, MBBS, MSc., FACRM, FBPsS, FAPsS
Formerly Reader in Psychology, University of Melbourne;
Honorary Senior Neuropsychologist, Austin Hospital, Melbourne,
Australia

SECOND EDITION

CHURCHILL LIVINGSTONE
EDINBURGH LONDON MELBOURNE NEW YORK AND TOKYO 1991

CHURCHILL LIVINGSTONE
Medical Division of Longman Group UK Limited

Distributed in the United States of America by
Churchill Livingstone Inc., 1560 Broadway, New York,
N.Y. 10036, and by associated companies, branches and
representatives throughout the world.

First edition 1985
Second edition 1991

ISBN   0-443-04320-5

British Library Cataloguing in Publication Data
Walsh, Kevin W.
    Understanding brain damage.—2nd ed.
    1. Medicine. Neuropsychology
    I. Title
    616.8

Library of Congress Cataloguing in Publication Data
Walsh, Kevin W.
    Understanding brain damage: a primer of neuropsychological
    evaluation/Kevin W. Walsh.—2nd ed.
        p. cm.
    Includes bibliographical references and index.
    ISBN 0 443 04320 5
    1. Brain damage—Diagnosis.   2. Neuropsychological tests.
I. Title
    [DNLM: 1. Brain Diseases—diagnosis—case studies. 2. Brain
Injuries—diagnosis—case studies. Neuropsychological Tests.
4. Neuropsychology—case studies. 5. Organic Mental Disorders—
diagnosis—case studies. WL 141 W225u]
    RC387.5.W35 1991
    616.8'0475—dc20
    DNLM/DLC
    for Library of Congress   90-15094
                                                          CIP

Produced by Longman Singapore Publishers (Pte) Ltd.
Printed in Singapore

iv

Preface to the Second Edition

Since the first edition has proved useful particularly in training programmes and in helping psychologists isolated from specialist centres in gaining some appreciation of neuropsychological evaluation, the present version has remained essentially the same but has been updated with material from the recent literature and explanatory comment arising from readers' and users' comments. It should be stressed that the presentation of only a small number of well-known psychometric tests was utilized for the primary purpose of the text as a teaching vehicle with the assumption that developing neuropsychologists would add to their repertoire the many and varied tests which would be appropriate for different cases in line with the hypothesis testing model outlined. Much more detail was available and expounded when many of the illustrative cases were used in the author's teaching sessions but it was not possible to present much of this in a small text. A good deal of this information was related to 'medical' findings, in particular the clinical neurological examination and the result of investigative procedures such as neuro-imaging and pathological studies. The next stage of development of the neuropsychologist involves the incorporation of this neurological side of the *neuro-psychology* equation and will be included in the more advanced volume in preparation. However, it was felt that much of the present approach could be used by clinical psychologists faced with common neuropsychological problems to allow them to deal with those within their level of expertise and to make appropriate referrals to specialist neuropsychologists in much the same way as general practitioners operate in regard to medical specialities.

My particular thanks goes to those psychologists who have welcomed me to their countries to expand and clarify the basic philosophy.

Melbourne, 1991   K.W.

Preface to the First Edition

The concept of neuropsychological evaluation presented in this primer assumes a reciprocal relationship between the growth of neuropsychological knowledge and the effectiveness of clinical practice. On the one hand increasing sophistication of our knowledge of brain—behaviour relationships derived from research studies should contribute to our understanding of the nature of the difficulties encountered by the individual patient. On the other hand neuropsychological examinations should provide numerous instances in which emerging neuropsychological notions can be confirmed, disconfirmed or modified since the biological factor analysis provided by unique pathological situations in individual cases is constantly available to the practising clinician. The stand taken is that the clinical neuropsychologist can adopt the role of applied scientist. The author makes no claim to present anything new apart from emphasis on the need for a thorough grounding in major features of the clinical neurosciences before embarking on specialist practice in neuropsychology. Discussion with colleagues in many countries has shown that the type of clinical approach advocated here is carried out in one form or another in numerous centres. However, it also became obvious that despite their widespread use such clinical approaches were grossly underrepresented in the literature. This was not the case for the other major approach, namely the actuarial approach represented by the use of sundry test batteries. Here the documentation is more than adequate for those wishing to acquire a basis of information for practising in this way.

The reasons for the discrepancy between the common usage of a clinical, problem-oriented, individualized methodology and the dearth of published material are many. On one hand, informative single case histories are unlikely to find a ready outlet in the psychological journals. This is quite unlike the situation in medicine where such cases turn up in a wide variety of periodicals. On the other, an individual or group needs extensive and varied clinical practice to make the publication of a collection of cases worthwhile.

The present introductory work arose from many requests to provide some illustrative cases for those wishing to use or expand a problem-oriented methodology. The commencement of a two-year postgraduate course in clinical neuropsychology in Melbourne in 1978 offered the opportunity to make a modest reply to those requests. With only one or two exceptions the cases which follow have been selected from those seen by graduate students and their supervisors since that time. A more extensive case study collection from the case books presented by graduates as part of their final examination is currently being compiled as a reference source.

The uniqueness of each case further complicated the arrangement of this primer. The present format is an attempt to convey some of the range of problems met with in our teaching clinics and each largely reflects a referral source, e.g. neurological service, neurovascular unit, psychiatry and neurosurgery though there is obvious overlap. With the limited scope of the work no attempt has been made to cover all areas of practice nor was it possible to cover each selected area systematically with relevant cases. Thus, while the cases in each chapter illustrate some of the points made in the preceding summary, not all points covered in each summary are illustrated in what follows. It is to be hoped that the present series of cases will provide a number of lessons which might be generalized to other situations. In other words the primer should not be looked on as a cook-book.

The inclusion of certain cases might puzzle some readers. While the bulk of the cases are those to be met in a broad neuropsychological practice, less commonly encountered problems are included if they can teach something of value. In other instances the selection of the cases has been based on situations where graduate students have been seduced into making an incorrect inference through lack of experience or failure to apply the principles outlined in Chapter 1.

The author has also avoided presenting only cases in which the examination has been optimal both in completeness and rigour of pursuing the proposed model. The exigencies of practice often mean that testing has, for practical reasons, to be terminated in an inconclusive state.

The limited scope of the book has also meant a good deal of condensation of the case material particularly of the arguments in favour of what may appear to some to be equally attractive differential diagnoses. In this regard the author is acutely aware that the interpretation presented in some cases may not always be the 'correct one'. More likely hypotheses may occur to readers. This is inherent in the nature of the material but again the author seeks refuge in the excuse that some of this is imposed by the scope of the book as a primer. Obviously if it generates argument about preferable differential diagnoses it will have served a useful purpose.

The condensation should not leave the impression that the 'contextual' factors stressed so validly by Lezak (1980) have been overlooked. It can be assumed that no personal, social, educational, occupational or other factors of relevance were known to be present unless mentioned.

In some ways the unsatisfactory brevity of the cases has been the result of an attempt to convey the variety of questions which might be tackled by this method. It is hoped that this has not been at the expense of understanding. Readers may also be surprised that a relatively small number of tests has been included since it is argued that familiarity with a considerable test arsenal is vital to effective practice in clinical neuropsychology. Once again the addition of too many unfamiliar tests would have expanded the text beyond its modest expectations. It was felt that if the general conception or philosophy could be conveyed using a small number of well-known tests then clinicians could turn to such excellent sources as Lezak (1983) to check which other relevant tests might be available for a particular problem. It is assumed that most psychologists will be familiar with this material while non-psychologists may find useful the brief test descriptions given in the Appendix.

In the case examples all the initials and, where necessary, some biographical details not essential to the interpretation of the case have been changed to preserve anonymity of the patients.

Finally, it should be stressed that this is not intended to be a textbook of clinical neuropsychology. It does, however, make a basic assumption that the most effective management, treatment and rehabilitation is most likely to arise out of evaluation against a background of knowledge of neuropsychological syndromes. Its intent is to form some part of the bridge between the many textbooks of human neuropsychology and the emerging manuals of treatment and rehabilitation.

Melbourne, 1984   K.W.

Acknowledgements

My thanks go to the members of the Departments of Neurology and Neuropsychology of the Austin Hospital for their continuing support and a particular vote of thanks to Dr David Darby who taught me the skills of word-processing which facilitated this edition.

K.W.

Contents

1. **Methodological considerations   1**

    Types of neuropsychological assessment   1
    Early approaches   1
    Current methods of neuropsychological assessment   2
    Test battery definitions   3

    Problems of interpretation   10
    Insensitivity of certain quantitative data   10
    Complex tests and inference making   14
    Face validity and incorrect inference   16

    Concept of the neuropsychological syndrome   18
    The syndrome as concordance   19
    Monothetic and polythetic descriptions   19
    The syndrome as probability   20
    Neuropsychological dissection of sub-syndromes   21
    The method of extreme cases   22
    Double dissociation of function   23
    Dangers of the syndrome method   27
    Clinical practice and theoretical development   27

    Incorporating neuropsychological knowledge   28
    The psycho-anatomical model   28

    References   33

2. **Alcohol related brain damage   37**

    The Wernicke–Korsakoff syndrome   37
    History   37
    Neuropathology   38
    Clinical features   38
    Psychometric features   40
    Forms of axial amnesia   41

Chronic alcoholism without amnesia 41
  Neuropathology of chronic alcoholism 42
  Psychosocial deficit in chronic alcoholism 44
  Social drinking and cognition 46
  Evolution of cognitive change 47
  The right hemisphere hypothesis 49
  The anterior or frontal hypothesis 50
  Implications of psychological deficit 52
  Premature ageing 52
  Reversibility, recovery and prognosis 53

Case examples 53
  Korsakoff psychosis 53
  Borderline Korsakoff psychosis 58
  A Korsakoff variant 61
  Borderline Korsakoff syndrome 64
  A non-alcoholic memory disorder in a heavy drinker 66
  A non-amnesic intellectual disorder 69

References 73

3. Intellectual decline 79

Diagnosis of dementia 79
  Alzheimer's disease 80
  Non-Alzheimer primary dementia 83
  Dementia and cerebrovascular disease 84
  Normal pressure hydrocephalus 86
  Other forms of dementia 87

Pseudodementia 87
  Depression, dementia and pseudodementia 88

Cerebral pathology and behavioural change 94
  CT scan, atrophy and cognitive loss 94
  Cognitive testing 96
  Premorbid ability 98
  Rating scales 99

Case examples 99

References 113

4. Pseudoneurological disorders 119

Conversion reactions 119
  Hysterical symptoms versus hysterical personality 120
  Psychoanalytic theory of hysteria 120
  Hysteria as communication 121
  Hysteria versus malingering 121
  Role theory as a unifying framework 125
  Expression of the role 125

Hysterical pseudodementia 127

Circumscribed pseudoneurological disorders 127

Psychogenic amnesia 128
  Theory and practice 128
  'Hysterical' amnesia 129

Neuropsychological assessment 130
  Nonspecific test effects 130
  Enactment in the test situation 130
  Symptom and syndrome validity 131

Case examples 133
  Possible organic confusional state 133
  An unusual case of dyslexia and dysgraphia 136
  Post-traumatic neurosis 139
  Neurological lesion with functional overlay 145
  Non-organic amnesic syndrome 148
  Post-traumatic neurosis 152

The other side of the coin 156
  Query functional or organic 157

References 159

5. Adaptive behaviour and head injury 163

Outcome of severe head injury 163
  Measures of severity 163
  Psychological deficit 164
  Intellectual recovery 166
  Outcome scales 167

Pathology of head injury 168

Adaptive behaviour and the frontal lobes 170
  Dorsolateral frontal cortex 170
  Basal and basomedial frontal cortex 176
  Medial cortex 179

Laterality and the frontal lobes   179

Amnesia   181

Case examples   182

References   201

6. **Cerebrovascular disorders   207**

   Pathological conditions   208

   Cerebral infarction   208
      Anatomy of the cerebral arteries   208
      Major arteries of the brain and associated disorders   210
      Lacunar state   218
      Transient ischaemic attacks   219
      Surgical treatment   220

   Cerebral haemorrhage   221

   Glossary   222

   Case examples   223
      Transient ischaemic attacks   223
      Cerebral infarction   225
      Aneurysmal amnesia   228
      Transient global amnesia   232
      Thalamic amnesia   235
      Non-invasive monitoring   242
      Intracerebral haemorrhage   243

   References   248

7. **Epilogue: roles for the neuropsychologist   253**

   The evaluative role   253
      The fallacious inference   254
      Sharing of variance   255
      Experimental investigation   255

   The educational role   255

   The rehabilitative role   257
      Summarizing measures   258
      Individualized treatment   258
      Prognostic and outcome studies   259

The medico-legal role 259
  Who is an expert? 259
  Faults in conducting the examination 260
  Faults in reporting the examination 261
  Cross-examination 265

Case examples 265
  Whiplash 265
  Carbon monoxide poisoning 274
  Conclusion 277

References 277

Appendix 279

1. Methodological considerations

TYPES OF NEUROPSYCHOLOGICAL ASSESSMENT

Early approaches

Single tests of brain damage and 'organicity'; screening procedures

One of the earliest applications of psychological testing in the area of neuropsychology was the attempt to identify those suffering organically based disturbances from those whose deficits were caused by other than organic factors. The approach had its historical antecedents in the relation of clinical psychology to psychiatric hospital practice where the question organic versus functional had (and still has) some significance. Unfortunately this question was often accompanied by an assumption that there existed some functional deficit which was a concomitant of any and every form of organic cerebral impairment. With this philosophy it was thus possible to conceive of 'a test for brain damage.'

In the light of the growing knowledge of specific brain–behaviour relationships over recent decades it is surprising to find that single tests of brain damage such as the Bender Gestalt and Memory for Designs tests continued to be used for a long time in this way; indeed, new tests have been put forward on the basis of this assumption (Visser 1980). However, the literature has shown many negative examples of the use of tests for this purpose (e.g. Rosen 1971). Bruell & Albee (1962) have even demonstrated negative findings for the Memory for Designs Test (Graham & Kendall 1960) in a case of right hemispherectomy. Such a striking finding should remind us that it is all too easy to make a false assumption about the nature of the process involved in the successful accomplishment of a test, and the areas of the brain deemed to be of paramount importance in its performance. It has become obvious from such negative findings in patients who have had supposedly necessary parts of the brain removed, that many complex tasks can still be carried out successfully in different ways. However, the fact that the task can still be carried out successfully after removal of a vital part of the brain in no way signifies that this part does not normally form a vital part of the organic substrate for the performance.

Although the use of single tests of brain damage has declined, the basic notion of a 'cutting point' between brain damaged and non brain damaged scores is still inherent in the derivation of impairment indices from an aggregation or 'battery' of apparently unrelated tests. The foremost index of this type has been that derived from the Halstead–Reitan Neuropsychological Test Battery in its various forms. The

1

debate about the usefulness of such estimates of 'brain damage' is by no means over. Mapou (1988) has argued that such methods are no longer appropriate, while the counter argument has been put strongly by Kane et al (1989).

A notion that has been accepted uncritically in much of this work is the assumption that a test which has been validated on clearly defined brain damaged groups may be useful for the day to day business of clinical assessment. As long ago as 1966 Yates pointed out that the predictive validity of tests derived in this way might be quite low. Yates (1954) also reminded us that many forget that even where a test shows a highly significant group difference it may still be of little clinical use because of an unacceptable level of misclassification.

The criticism of single tests of brain damage does not mean that individual tests which are performed poorly by a high proportion of patients with cerebral impairment cannot be used in situations where screening procedures might be useful. It does imply, however, that negative instances should be given careful consideration. An analogous situation in medicine would apply to a symptom such as a rise in temperature, viz many illnesses are accompanied by fever yet a normal temperature does not preclude illness, even very serious illness. Busy practitioners in psychology might well resort to the early administration of several such tests which are poorly performed in a high proportion of cases with proven brain impairment. It will still be the case that even the exhibition of a large collection of such tests will prove negative in individual cases *unless the impaired function is tapped in the process.*

The extensive work of McFie (1969 and 1975) demonstrated that the Digit–Symbol subtest of the Wechsler scales shows impairment with lesions in virtually any location in a high proportion of cases. The Symbol–Digit Modalities Test (Smith 1973, 1975) has added to the substitution test an opportunity to compare the patient's performance utilizing two forms of response: oral and manual. Though false positives rule out the use of these tests in isolation, the small proportion of false negatives supports their use for those interested in screening methods.

Another test of flexible mental operations which has proved useful is the Trail Making Test (see Appendix). It has the advantage of brevity and also yields a high proportion of correct identification (Korman & Blomberg 1963).

The rationale of screening procedures might be that good performance renders the presence of brain damage less likely but does not preclude it, while a poor performance should call for further investigation.

An alternative method of screening might be focused on areas of cognitive functioning rather than on individually sensitive tests. In those situations where specific hypotheses are not apparent at the outset we have found it useful to begin with a careful examination of two areas: (1) memory in its various aspects; and (2) adaptive, problem-solving behaviour.

Current methods of neuropsychological assessment

A major divergence

With the rapid growth of clinical neuropsychology in the past three decades there has been diversification of methods employed by individual neuropsychologists. An adequate summary is beyond the scope of the present work. However, the number of features on which approaches differ is small enough for a brief comparison to be attempted.

Lezak (1980) in common with other authors points to the degree to which quantification is employed as one such major distinction. The pioneering work of Reitan has been followed by an immense accumulation of data from various groups of brain impaired individuals and remains a rich source of data for research and clinical evaluation in neuropsychology. The method 'is based upon (a) a systematic application of the same task in much the same manner as possible to every candidate for neuropsychological assessment; and (b) diagnostic impressions generated from frequency studies relating best score patterns to diagnostic categories' (Lezak 1980). It is essentially an actuarial approach largely, if not solely, concerned with quantitative data. A review of the theoretical and methodological bases of the most extensively used battery employed over many years, namely the Halstead-Reitan Neuropsychological Test Battery, is provided by Reitan (1986).

At the other end of the continuum are those methods in which quantification is given a lesser consideration, particular emphasis being placed on qualitative observations in what are considered to be unique cases. This, as Lezak points out, is the method of Luria and his followers but is by no means restricted to such a theoretical position.

The arguments in favour of each method follow the earlier debate on clinical versus statistical prediction so ably outlined by Meehl and others from the 1950s (e.g. Meehl 1954, 1960, 1961, 1972). This literature is worth examination particularly by those who have commenced neuropsychological practice recently.

Lezak (1980) has also pointed out that neuropsychologists brought up essentially with one model may subsequently incorporate features from another although, as in other spheres of training, early introduced biases tend to be resistant to change.

What is a neuropsychological battery?

Much of the difference between individuals and 'schools' of neuropsychological practice can be discussed in relation to the term 'battery of tests'.

Test battery definitions
   '(1) A group of related tests combined to yield a single total score that is of maximal efficiency in measuring for a specified purpose or ability or trait. (2) a group of related tests to be administered at one time' (English & English 1958)
'a group of tests whose results are combined into a single score' (Chaplin 1968)
'a group of tests used in combination into a single score' (Freeman 1962)
'a group of different tests designed to test a broad ability. The intercorrelations between the individual tests should not be too high, but the correlation between the overall result and the criteria should be higher than that of the individual test' (Eysenck et al 1972)
'a diagnostic battery is a set of tests having comparable norms and usually organized in an easily administered series with uniform style' (Cronbach 1949)

The term 'battery'is also used somewhat loosely to refer to the collection of tests from which a particular neuropsychologist may draw the measures to be used in an individual case. According to the knowledge and experience of the practitioner this may range from the whole armamentarium of published tests and experimental procedures to a very small group of tests most of which are used by a particular psychologist on most occasions.

In answer to the question as to which test battery they favour, many neuropsychologists will reply that the tests selected will depend on the nature of the presenting problem. Quite simply, a major distinction exists between the use of a set or predetermined battery of tests and an individualized or flexible selection from a larger range of measures. The latter method 'adapts tests to the referral problem and to particular disabilities' (Russell 1982).

The selection of tests may entail a one step process, i.e. a group of tests is chosen in the belief that these will provide the information needed to answer the questions. Sometimes the issues will remain unresolved but observations derived from the primary set of tests may suggest that further specific tests may provide the answer, i.e. a stepwise approach, as used by many. Much of the efficacy of this method turns on the selection of the primary group of tests since the use of tests which do not touch the problem at all will give apparently negative results. In reporting such negative results it is important to inform the referral agency that 'nothing abnormal was detected with the tests used'. It is of help to colleagues familiar with psychological tests to specify in detail which particular tests *were* used. They should certainly be documented in hospital practice and in medico-legal cases. Unfortunately, negative reports are often written which contain the implication that no impairment is present. We should bear in mind Teuber's dictum 'absence of evidence is not evidence of absence' (of impairment). Russell (1982) points out that the entire controversy between fixed versus flexible test use 'hinges on a single rather obvious principle that is axiomatic to neuropsychology: *one cannot determine whether a certain function of the brain is impaired unless that function is tested.*'

As mentioned above, the stepwise method may commence with a fixed set of tests which might be termed a screening battery. It suffers from the shortcomings inherent in all fixed methods. However, many find the method useful in situations where referral questions are too general and background information on the patient is minimal. Such occasions have become increasingly less frequent with the transmission of knowledge of neuropsychology and behaviourial neurology to the various professions dealing with brain impaired individuals. One of the chief roles for the neuropsychologist is to educate referral agencies as to the nature and form of questions which might reasonably be asked. An excellent medium for this educative role is a well written neuropsychological report.

Advantages and disadvantages of fixed and flexible testing

Even a preliminary consideration suggests that advantages of one method over another will depend on the purpose for which the examination is being carried out, and because of the frequency of approaches which partake of either the fixed or flexible approach the dichotomous comparison which follows is somewhat artificial. Its purpose is to throw into relief differences in the philosophy of assessment which may help a choice to be made in a particular situation.

'Probably the major advantage of a well constructed set battery is that tests can be compared to each other in order to obtain reliable and valid patterns. That is, if the tests in a battery are standardized together so that a score on one test can be directly compared with scores on another test, then a meaningful pattern of results may be obtained' (Russell 1982). In this way the battery method lends itself to the application of sophisticated statistical techniques such as cluster analysis. Examples of such applications have appeared from time to time in the literature.

Pattern analysis is also a feature of flexible systems,where it takes a number of forms. Some would claim that, since scores from different tests are not strictly comparable, valid patterns cannot be derived. Moreover, not only are non-comparable scores used but qualitative features are combined with quantitative scores. In some instances both types of test-derived data are combined with information from the patient's history and a consideration of his subjective complaints. This combination of different sorts of data reaches one extreme form in the concept of the 'clinical syndrome' described below. To claim that this is invalid is to deny in this situation a method which has continually proved to be of use in clinical medicine. The following vignette typifies the situation.

A previously well patient complains of abdominal pain which has moved over several hours from the upper central region to become fixed in the right lower quadrant. Questioning reveals that he has lost his appetite and is constipated. Examination demonstrates tenderness over a particular point in the right lower abdominal quadrant. There is a mild degree of fever and the white cell count is moderately elevated.

In considering the differential diagnosis of the above case, there is no doubt that acute appendicitis is the most likely pathology to be revealed at operation, despite the fact that the diagnosis derives from a pattern which combines different classes of information.

The importance of qualitative data.   To play down the value of qualitative data seems almost to imply that only that which is quantitative is truly objective. The use of quantitative data omits much behaviour observed in the test situation. 'A test response is not a score; scores, where applicable, are abstractions designed to facilitate intra-individual and inter-individual comparisons, and as such they are extremely useful in clinical testing. However to reason or to do research only in terms of scores or score patterns is to do violence to the nature of the raw material. *'The scores do not communicate the responses in full'* [my italic]. (Schafer quoted in Shapiro 1951). While it may be possible, and advantageous, to introduce quantification where possible, much useful information in clinical neuropsychology does not lend itself readily to such quantification.

Efficiency and relevance.   With a fixed battery there may be a danger of omitting coverage of a vital area of psychological function. For example, considering the frequency of memory disorders in neurological populations, it is surprising to see no explicit examination of memory in some set batteries. Lezak (1976) believes 'that "ready-made" batteries are inefficient and often do not adequately answer the questions that are specific to the patient's referral problems.' On the other hand they may also be uneconomic because of the necessary application of tests which are irrelevant to the problem at hand.

Individual differences in premorbid ability.   Another major point of division between the extremes of fixed versus flexible methods is the concept of deficit measurement. Several fixed batteries, particularly the Halstead–Reitan battery now possess a large, well researched body of information about the performance of large samples of several target populations against which to compare the current performance of individuals. The difficulty lies in knowing what the individual premorbid level might have been. This difficulty is shared by other methods including the individualized approach. Many of these attempt to overcome the problem by making a 'best estimate' of past level from present performances. Several measures are in use, singly or in combination. The most common is to compare the patient's relative performance on separate measures. Within certain limits individuals will perform most tests at about the same level. The degree of variation between subtests of the WAIS, for example, is often used as a starting point, and direct or indirect use is made of normative data available for the tests. This gives a probability as to how extreme a difference between two scores might be in order to be considered significant. This method has the limitation that, where only quantitative measures are used, 'real' differences which lie within an acceptable range may be discounted, resulting in the failure to diagnose latent or early neurological disorders.

There is a further danger in combining two or more better performances to use as a comparison for the significance of the scatter of scores: the averaging process may lose further information. Lezak (1988) has reasoned cogently against the misleading use of summarizing or superscores, e.g. the IQ measures of the Wechsler Scales, and argues that the patient's highest current level of achievement may form the best estimate of premorbid ability. These points and others are supported later in this chapter by the data in Case BC.

One recent attempt to handle the problem of regression from present to past performance has been the derivation of the New Adult Reading Test (Nelson & O'Connell 1978, Nelson 1982). Our clinical experience supports the authors' claim that the ability to perform this task holds up well in the face of most forms of cerebral impairment. (See Appendix and Ch. 3).

Estimates of premorbid level are also made from biographical data such as highest level of educational or occupational achievement. This estimate may work well in one direction, e.g. it may be assumed with safety that a university graduate would be able to perform at a generally high level on certain tests. However, the fact that an individual does not have a high level of education cannot be taken to mean that he does not have a high level of ability or intelligence.

The cut-off score.   The method of deficit measurement by group comparison also has its difficulties. Most of these are related to the use of cutting points or scores and are discussed in psychological texts. 'The rigorous application of cut-off scores in clinical work may be criticized in so far as it involves needless loss of information concerning severity of deficit, etc., but there are situations in which a cut-off score can serve as a useful guide. The actual cut-off score chosen will depend not only on the nature of the population for which it is intended (in particular the base-rate of the 'target' population) but also on the purpose for which the test is being used since this latter affects the types and proportions of misclassifications which are acceptable.' (Nelson 1976). In the common situation where neuropsychological assessment forms only part of the total examination, more leeway may be accepted in the direction of too many false positives since these may be checked for concordance with other findings.

The context of the examination. It is implicit in what has been said that a set battery method of the extreme sort may fail to take account of what Lezak (1980) has nicely termed contextual factors. She highlights the necessity for taking into account the patient's situation in the broadest sense of that term, e.g. social history, present life circumstances, medical history, and circumstances surrounding the examination. In the example of symptoms of appendicitis mentioned above it would be important to note the sex of the patient since a misdiagnosis of salpingitis would be a possibility. It is regrettable that these dimensions of what Lezak calls 'the multidimensional contextual framework' need explication, since they have generally received emphasis in clinical training but 'blind' interpretation of data from fixed collections of tests has had wide vogue and continues to be practised. Some have gone so far as to claim that knowledge of background factors may interfere with interpretation. Against this one may point to the superiority of clinical versus statistical prediction in situations such as that described by Reitan (1964) where the same data were examined by the two methods.

Training of neuropsychologists. An important practical issue of current concern is the training of neuropsychologists. Different methods demand different characteristics in both trainees and teachers, and the amount of effort necessary to acquire proficiency will vary according to the method being taught. One of the advantages of a set battery is that administration is readily taught because of the use of a fixed array of standard tests. Relatively stereotyped questions such as the laterality of the lesion can be answered with a fair degree of competence with only a short course at graduate level (Lewinsohn 1971). Whether such questions are any longer being asked of neuropsychologists is another matter. The training of technicians to administer the battery is also claimed to be an economy, leaving the more demanding process of interpretation to be done by the neuropsychologist.

At the other extreme the nature of an individualized approach requires more training if only for the reason that a wider knowledge of test procedures is needed. Substitution of tests may need to be made where motor, sensory or other deficits form a bar to the use of a frequently employed test, e.g. a motor difficulty may preclude the use of the Digit–Symbol Substitution Test of the WAIS. Part of the difficulty can be overcome by the use of the similar Symbol–Digit Modalities Test which permits an oral instead of a written response, or the Multiple Choice version of the Benton Visual Retention Test may be used where a motor difficulty impairs the subject's graphic ability.

Training with a flexible or individualized approach usually implies the application of theoretical knowledge, often of a particular kind. Speaking of the Luria type of examination as exemplified in the tests published by Christensen (1975), Golden notes that 'although the test offers potentially more information, the most valuable information requires that the user be aware of the theoretical system on which the test is based. This, indeed, is a drawback of almost all tests offering qualitative observations.' (Golden 1979) Thus, what is a fundamental strength for the proponents of one approach is a drawback for the other. Similarly, the largely atheoretical nature of many fixed systems is seen by some as a factor which seriously constrains the range of applicability and further development of such systems. At the present time there is little public knowledge on the efficacy of an individualized approach to place against the available information on the Halstead–Reitan and other test batteries, nor does a scientific comparison study appear feasible. The publication of case material has not yet found ready access in psychological as it has in medical journals, though this situation may change. Even the extensive writings of Luria provide only a small number of fully documented cases which would serve as models for developing clinicians. Many of the cases tend to be put forward as 'modal' or 'typical' but, however valuable they may be in providing knowledge of the function of regional systems, they fail to give a realistic appreciation of the range and complexity of symptomatology experienced in clinical practice. Without such a body of case material the trainee wishing to follow an individualized approach may be restricted by the availability of clinical supervision and a breadth of case material to use as a frame of reference. It is not surprising then that training courses in individualized methodology are few in number.

This does not exhaust a consideration of the strengths and weaknesses of fixed versus flexible approaches and there is little doubt that personality factors in the trainees, the effects of undergraduate training as well as practical considerations such as availability of training, the structure of professions in various countries and numerous other factors will influence the neuropsychologist's method of practice.

Hypothesis testing

The majority of practitioners of an individualized methodology appear to favour some form of hypothesis-testing model. They differ in the degree to which this is explicit rather than implicit, in the more or less systematic ways the hypotheses are examined, in the degree to which ongoing neuropsychological knowledge is incorporated into their system, and in a number of other important parameters. In its explicit form the hypothesis-testing method is epitomized by the experimental investigation of the single case advocated for so long by Shapiro (1951, 1973). After reminding us of the concept of error in measurement, this author argues that this should prevent us from making unwarranted generalizations from the data but should not prevent us from using observations in a systematic way to advance our understanding of the individual case.

The awareness of error makes us look upon any psychological observation not as something conclusive but as the basis of one or more hypotheses about the patient. One's degree of confidence in any hypothesis suggested by an observation would depend upon the established degree of validity of that observation and upon information about the patient concerned. If one or more hypotheses are suggested by an observation, then steps must be taken to test them. In this way further observations are accumulated in a systematic manner. It should then become possible to arrive at a psychological description in which we can have greater confidence. The additional observations may in turn suggest new hypotheses which have in turn to be tested. We are thus led to the method of the systematic investigation as a means of improving the validity of our conclusion about an individual patient. (Shapiro 1973)

Working hypotheses may arise from generalizations which have emerged from the research literature. Clinical neuropsychology is becoming very rich in this regard as evidenced by the proliferation of books and articles in the past decade. As this work grows, converging lines of evidence make the generalizations more secure and thus facilitate the development of crucial tests on the various hypotheses. It is the wealth of individual experience with the effectiveness of specific hypothesis-testing measures which is missing from the literature and this needs to be remedied for further development of the method. Otherwise clinicians have to go through the long, painful (and unnecessary) process of discovery for themselves.

The experimental method should reduce much of the error associated with the unsystematic use of psychological tests. As mentioned below many test responses have a complex determination and specific hypothesis testing should clarify the processes operating in a single case.

The length of the examination.   Shapiro considered that this process might lack appeal as, at the outset, it looks time consuming. In fact, in our experience, it is often more economical than the application of a routine battery of tests, many of which may be irrelevant to the questions being asked. Since in clinical practice certain questions tend to recur frequently, trainees quite soon recognize the most likely hypotheses and the most productive tests to be used in particular situations. Subsequent case evaluation in the light of neurological or neurosurgical knowledge continually improves the process.

In busy clinical practice, time is an expensive commodity and on some occasions the clinician has to tender an opinion after less than ideal examination of the patient. In this situation his report should make it clear to the referring source that the opinion consists 'of the hypotheses which the applied scientist thinks best account for the data at his disposal, and which he would choose to test next if he had sufficient time and suitable means' (Shapiro, 1973). The term 'suitable means' often takes the form of appropriate tests. In some cases these do not exist but this situation is becoming rare as neuropsychology develops and clinicians working in a particular field are likely to acquire the tests which prove useful in answering the most common hypotheses. Hopefully the present primer will add to the store of information.

The practical question of time taken for an examination must be seen in relation to the seriousness or importance of the questions being asked. In a situation where the neuropsychologist is in direct contact with the referring professional the stepwise procedure may be terminated or extended according to considered opinion after consultation, since converging information from other neurosciences is normally being accumulated.

The question of time has been partly answered in set battery methodology. This approach has been unpopular with many clinicians but there may be some situations, even in the single case method, where less experienced examiners could carry out much of the routine testing. In such situations an experienced neuropsychologist should control the decision-making or successive steps in the investigation and the examiners (e.g. psychology graduates in training) should be trained to record all the qualitative features of the patient's responses, so that the same interpretation would be made as that of an examination carried out by a more experienced clinician. If no significant information is lost in the process there can be little objection to a method which has worked so well in clinical medicine for so long. There is an added advantage in that it may force neuropsychologists to make explicit to themselves and others the nature of their decision-making processes.

PROBLEMS OF INTERPRETATION

Insensitivity of certain quantitative data

The following case illustrates the apparent lack of sensitivity of some tests to even quite major cerebral pathology. This seems to be most evident in highly intelligent subjects, though it may be seen at all levels of intelligence.

Case: BC

A 55-year-old university graduate employed as an applied scientist in a medical laboratory presented with the following history.

Some seventeen years before he had suffered a generalized epileptic seizure. At the time neurological investigation produced nothing of note. Further investigation after another seizure six years later was also unfruitful. On the current admission BC reported a third fit and, for the first time, he mentioned subjective difficulties . He described a memory problem and slight difficulty with word finding extending back several months but was still able to carry on his profession. Clinical neurological examination was again negative and neuropsychological examination was requested as part of the search for a possible localized lesion as the source of his disorder.

The psychologist felt that a preliminary examination with the Wechsler Intelligence and Memory scales would allow opportunity for observations which might suggest hypotheses for further examination. The scores were as follows:

Wechsler Adult Intelligence Scale

Information	17	Digit–Symbol	7
Comprehension	16	Picture Completion	11
Arithmetic	15	Block Design	12
Similarities	13	Picture Arrangement	11
Digit Span	11	Object Assembly	13
VIQ130		PIQ122	

Wechsler Memory Scale

Information	3
Orientation	5
Mental Control	9
Logical Memory	10
Digit Span	12
Visual Reproduction	13

Associate Learning   12 (4,0;5,3;5,2)
MQ122

(The designation 3,0 etc. on Associate Learning signifies that the patient was successful on 3 of the 6 'easy' or logically associated pairs, e.g. baby-cries, while learning none of the 'hard' or new associations such as 'crush-dark'. This designation will be used throughout.)

The summarizing or superscores, although in the superior range, are misleading for a number of reasons and, as Lezak (1988) has commented, may add nothing while they conceal a good deal if they are taken to mean a superior overall level of functioning thereby implying that no significant deficit is present. Contextual factors e.g. the late onset of epilepsy and the subjective complaints of higher intellectual decline, should warn that a neuropsychological disorder must be seriously considered in this case.

The subtest scores cover a wider range and if one takes the best estimate of premorbid ability from the best three subtests (again as suggested by Lezak) it is apparent that several subtests are considerably below this estimate. The higher estimate was further supported by the nature of the patient's research work.

The psychologist, a recent graduate in clinical psychology with only a short component in neuropsychology, noted that despite an 'adequate' score on Block Design, BC had much more difficulty with item no. 8 than might have been expected for such an intelligent person. Further, she noted that, despite an MQ of 122, his performances on Logical Memory and Associate Learning were clearly inferior to that expected of an educated man and, moreover, contrasted with a very good performance on Visual Reproduction. This raised not only the possibility of a memory disorder (in keeping with his subjective complaints) but also the possibility that such a memory difficulty, if present, might be verbal specific.

The presence of these observations coupled with his history suggested that a relatively silent lesion might be producing verbal memory, learning and problem solving difficulties. In the absence of neurological signs it was thought advisable to examine more closely verbal memory and adaptive functions served by frontal regions. The presence of a frontal lesion could also be consonant with the 'negative' clinical neurological examination which, at this stage, had not yet progressed to specialized neuroradiological investigations. These hypotheses led to the administration of further tests.

Rey Auditory Verbal Learning Test

Trial	1	2	3	4	5
Patient (BC)	5	7	7	10	11
Manual Labourers*	7.0	10.5	12.9	13.4	13.9
Professionals*	8.6	11.8	13.4	13.8	14.0

(*from Lezak 1976)

Not only was the patient's verbal acquisition well below expectation but he was able to recall only four words after interference from an interpolated list. This marked degree of proactive interference strongly suggests neurological impairment (Lezak 1976, p 354).

Associative verbal fluency (see Appendix). This test was chosen both because of the patient's subjective complaint of a word finding difficulty and because it is sensitive to left frontal lesions even in patients who are ostensibly non-aphasic (Walsh 1987). The mean score of only 8.7 on the three letters (F, A, S) indicated an exceedingly gross deficit in a man of such obvious intellectual ability. Testing then moved to other measures sensitive to frontal lobe involvement.

Wisconsin Card Sorting Test. This was given in the original form (Grant & Berg 1948). Having readily acquired the concept of colour, BC shifted without difficulty to the concept of shape but, after responding to several examples of this concept, he reverted to sorting by colour on four consecutive occasions, each time snapping his fingers and exclaiming in frustration. He clearly knew what the correct response was in these cases but was totally unable to inhibit his incorrect responses. Despite numerous trials he was unable to attain the remaining concept, namely number. The psychologist commented that this quality of performance had only been described with significant frontal lesions. It was all the more striking in a patient of such high intellectual ability. This pointer to the frontal lobe was confirmed by giving one of Luria's tasks of the 'verbal regulation of behaviour': 'If I say 'red' squeeze my hand, if I say 'green' do nothing'. Although he was able to retain and repeat the instructions, he was once again unable to inhibit responses which he clearly recognized as being at variance with the instructions.

Thus, two tests showed vividly some types of difficulty shown by patients with frontal lesions, particularly the pathognomonic sign of 'dissociation between knowing and doing'.

Further testing failed to elicit any signs of hemineglect, spatial disruption or other features associated with impairment in the right hemisphere. While realizing the incomplete nature of the examination, the opinion was given that there appeared to be considerable disruption of cerebral function and this had its maximum impact in the left frontotemporal area. A CT scan revealed a large left frontal glioma.

A limited amount of information is available from the post-operative examination of this case but repeat of the WAIS was very instructive. Preoperative levels are given in parentheses:

Verbal IQ	150	(130)
Performance IQ	123	(122)
Memory Quotient	143+	(122)

Several further points are worth making: (a) the presence of a marked improvement in BC's verbal IQ after resection of a major portion of his left frontal lobe reminds us that, in some instances at least, earlier writers such as Hebb (1949) were correct in asserting that the presence of pathological tissue may be more inimical to function than the removal of it. It also highlights earlier points on the estimate of prior ability; (b) despite a ceiling MQ of 143, BC still had objective evidence of a memory difficulty, e.g. his scores on the three trials of Associate Learning were 6,0; 6,1; 6,1. In view of his excellent performance on Logical Memory it was thought that this difficulty might represent a 'frontal amnesia' (Walsh 1987, p 144-147). However, further examination was not deemed desirable because of the serious nature of the lesion; (c) the frontal signs were still very much in evidence; and (d) the small difference pre-operatively between the WAIS Verbal and Performance summary scores with VIQ greater than PIQ reinforces the comments elsewhere in this text on the futility of utilizing such differences as an index of lateralization.

Succeeding chapters provide numerous examples of how adequate summary scores can conceal incapacitating deficits, particularly the adaptive behaviour syndrome discussed in Chapters 2 and 5.

A second case extract might reinforce at this juncture the striking lack of sensitivity of the summarizing Memory Quotient of Wechsler Memory Scale.

Case: RS

A 64-year-old man suffered a stroke as the result of rupture of a left posterior cerebral artery aneurysm (Fig. 1.1) which resulted in the not uncommon combination of loss of vision in the right half visual fields of each eye, i.e. a right homonymous hemianopia, together with a severe memory difficulty. There were no other neurological or neuropsychological signs or symptoms.

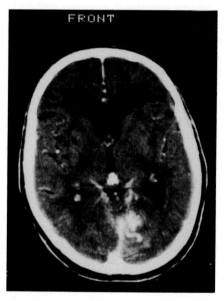

Fig. 1.1 Case RS. CT scan showing vascular malformation on the inner aspect of the left occipital region.

Eight months after the incident the Wechsler Memory scores were as follows:

WMS

Information	5	Digits Total	11(6,5)
Orientation	4	Visual Reproduction	11.5
Mental Control	9	Associate Learning	8 (5.0;6.0;6.0)
Memory Passages	12.5		
MQ 120			

Despite the most severe amnesic disorder that it is possible to imagine, whereby the patient forgot from one moment to the next what he had just been told or what had just occurred, he managed to produce a quotient of 120! Every other memory and learning task was performed abysmally. To argue, as one often hears in medico-legal cases that a person with superior scores or quotients cannot have serious deficits is to commit the gravest of errors.

Complex tests and inference making

Another shortcoming of psychological studies of brain impairment might be termed 'the principle of multiple determination'. Kinsbourne (1972) has used the term 'final common pathway' to express the idea: 'Behavioural deficits are defined in terms of impaired test performance. But impaired test performance may be a final common pathway for expression of quite diverse types of impairment.' Smith (1975) takes as an example what is probably the test most frequently reported as showing decrement with brain damage in various forms and locations, namely the Digit–Symbol Substitution Test: 'The responses are the end product of the integration of visual, perceptual, oculomotor, fine manual motor, and mental functions.' Among the mental functions we might mention attentional, planning and memory factors without exhausting all the contributing elements. It is therefore important to be aware that low scores on this or any other test may be due to disturbance in any of the functions involved or any combination of them. This highlights one of the shortcomings of methods which rely solely on quantitative information. Expressed simply this means that there may be different determinants of failure in individual cases even where there is a comparable level of score.

One of the few tests designed specifically to clarify the source of failure in this area of performance is the Symbol–Digit Modalities Test (Smith 1973, 1975). The test differs fundamentally from the Digit–Symbol Substitution Test as used in the Wechsler scales by requiring the subject to reproduce the digits rather than the symbols by inverting the usual form of the test. This allows the responses to be spoken as well as written and thus provides an opportunity to dissociate the manual expression from the other processes involved in this task. Poor performance on the Digit–Symbol Substitution Test is often ascribed to a slow rate of information processing. If the spoken version is performed well this can scarcely be the case.

The 2-4-6-8 phenomenon

An example of multiple determination of responses taken from our own practice involves the much used block design copying task. If we think of the major steps in its solution we see that visual, perceptual, spatial, planning and praxic elements are all necessary. These are no doubt supported by inner verbal symbolic and other processes in some individuals. Thus a test of block design copying entails the integrated action of widely dispersed brain systems and may therefore be disturbed by lesions in a variety of cortical and subcortical locations. How are we to determine which of the single or several determinants are operating in the individual case?

Among the more helpful factors in this elucidation is observation of qualitative features of the patient's behaviour.

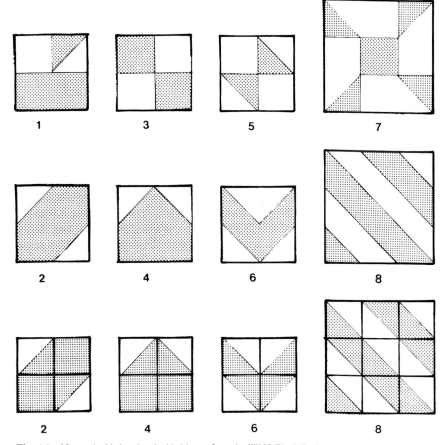

Fig. 1.2 Non-embedded and embedded items from the WAIS Block Design subtest.

Figure 1.2 shows eight of the items on the original WAIS Block Design subtest. We have noted along with many other workers that 'brain damaged' patients frequently fail badly on this task. However, we have noted that in a sizeable proportion of patients the difficulties are much greater on items 2, 4, 6 and 8 while items 1, 3, 5 and 7 present little difficulty. An examination of these two subsets of items reveals that they differ in one major regard. In items 1, 3, 5 and 7 the design may be copied readily by matching one obvious perceptual unit with one face of the block. In items 2, 4, 6 and 8 preliminary analysis of the given design must be made before it is possible to select the correct faces with which to reconstitute the design. This is necessary since these items are of the embedded type, i.e. their elements are not immediately obvious perceptually. Thus these items will prove differentially difficult for those with analytical or problem solving disorders. This observation can prove useful in detecting such deficits, e.g. in patients with suspected frontal lesions.

This consideration has led to a mini-test for the differentiation between patients whose block design failure is on an 'anterior' or problem solving basis and those with a 'posterior' or visuo-spatial basis, though, of course, yet other mechanisms may be at work. This subsidiary test consists of placing over the design a plastic sheet on which the dividing lines between the constituent blocks are drawn (Fig. 1.2). Provided with this partial programme for the solution, most patients with frontal lesions are greatly helped. On the other hand, patients with posterior lesions tend to have even more difficulty than before since further information is added to their already disrupted visuo-spatial world.

These two classes of patients also tend to behave differently in their execution of the task. Patients with problem solving difficulties resulting from anterior (frontal) lesions mostly tend to work within the square format of the designs, but have difficulty in selecting the correct block faces with which to work and in integrating the faces to complete the design. Unless the anterior lesions are gross, constructional deviations outside the square format are relatively uncommon. Ben-Yishay et al (1971) have described some constructional deviations as follows: 'broken squares; rectangles; linearly placed horizontally, vertically, diagonally; irregular shapes/patterns wherein the individual blocks are improperly aligned with respect to one another and with the horizontal and vertical planes'. Such constructional deviations appear most frequently and dramatically in posterior lesions, particularly in the right hemisphere.

Information of this kind is scattered throughout the literature, e.g. Matarazzo (1972) commented about the Block Design test:

> Oddly enough, individuals who do best on the tests are not necessarily those who see, or at least follow, the pattern as a whole, but often those who are able to break it up into small portions. In this connection, an early study by Nadel (1938) on intellectual disturbances following certain (frontal lobe) brain lesions is of interest. As between 'following the figure' and breaking up the design into its component parts, patients with frontal lobe lesions in contrast to the control group used the former method almost exclusively.

Many psychological reports tend to stop at the point where the patient is described as having difficulty with a particular task or set of tasks, e.g. the patient who fails on Block Design tests is said to have a 'visuospatial difficulty' without any attempt being made to specify further the nature of his difficulty. It is with such further specification, provided by qualitative features, that neuropsychology can provide added clinical information which will be of value in the management and rehabilitation of the patient. This makes important the publication of the rich store of qualitative observations, as stressed by Kaplan and other neuropsychologists worldwide.

Kaplan has termed the methodology of her group the 'Boston Process Approach' (Kaplan 1983). The method 'is based on a desire to understand the qualitative nature of the behaviour assessed by clinical psychometric instruments, a desire to reconcile descriptive richness with reliability and quantitative evidence of validity, and a desire to relate the behaviour assessed to the conceptual frame work of experimental neuropsychology' (Milberg et al 1986). They stress that theirs is not a 'battery approach' although they use a common core of tests together with several 'satellite tests' in order to 'clarify particular problem areas and *to confirm the clinical hypotheses developed from early observations of the patient'* (my italic). Detailed examples are given by Kaplan (1988).

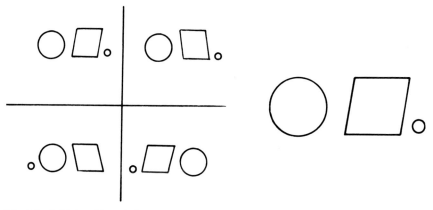

Fig. 1.3 A fabricated item similar to those of the multiple choice form of the Benton Visual Retention Test.

Face validity and incorrect inference

Inherent in what has been said is the danger in assuming that if a patient fails on a test, then that patient has a deficiency in the psychological function stated in the manual to be that measured by the test. In many uncritical psychological (including neuropsychological) reports this is apparent in the use of recognizable terminology from the manual and, in the poorest reports, the terminology changes as the writer describes the patient's performance on different tests.

Seductive or inadequate inferences

A simple example of making the wrong inference might be as follows: the patient produces a poor score on a memory for designs test, e.g. the Benton Visual Retention Test and this is reported as a 'visual memory deficit'. On occasion we have seen this extended to the further inference that 'the patient shows poor visual memory suggesting impairment of the right hemisphere' or even more specifically 'the patient shows differentially poor visual memory with normal verbal memory suggesting impairment of the right temporal region'. However, in the form given, the memory for designs test may have relied on the patient drawing the remembered stimulus. Thus one of the possible reasons for failure could be an executive, praxic or graphic difficulty, i.e. the reason for failure is the same as that which causes the patient to fail on other tasks with a constructional element. Awareness of such a possibility would prompt the use of a task where the constructional element has been removed, e.g. the Multiple Choice version of the BVRT (Fig. 1.3). Here the subject is shown a design and then must select it some time later from a multiple choice array which contains the item plus three distractors. The same logic applies, *mutatis mutandis*, to the examination of other possible causes for poor performance, e.g. perceptual difficulties.

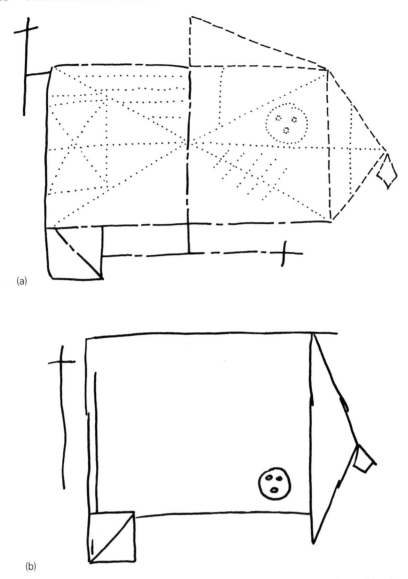

Fig. 1.4   Case AE. Rey Figure, Copy and Recall. The order of copying is shown from solid to dotted lines.

A less obvious example of an inadequate inference is given in the following case.

Case: AE

A 45-year-old housewife with a history of increasingly severe headaches was referred for examination. Her clinical neurological examination was unremarkable apart from a suspicious appearance of the optic fundi suggesting possible raised intracranial pressure. During a preliminary intellectual and memory examination the only depressed score was on the Visual Reproduction subtest of the Wechsler Memory Scale, Form I. To extend this area of examination the Rey Figure was given. A very good copy was made but the recall after three minutes was much impoverished (Fig. 1.4). The process of copying could be followed since the patient was given different coloured pencils as the copy proceeded. The rather unsystematic order of the copy followed by a much impoverished recall after three minutes suggested that the difficulty might be of the type termed 'frontal amnesia' (Barbizet 1970) and this was soon confirmed by a brain scan which revealed a large right frontal parasagittal meningioma.

After removal of the tumour the patient returned a maximum score on Visual Reproduction (WMS, Form II normal) but showed continuing difficulty with complex material such as the Rey Figure. That her poor recall was to a large degree the result of inadequate organization of her copy, as suggested by Lhermitte et al (1972), was confirmed when she retained complex visual material over a long period of time, as long as the examiner provided her with a systematic way of going about her preliminary drawing. Like most patients with frontal lesions she had to be provided with a strategy or programme for each separate complex item she was asked to recall. Left to her own devices she reverted to a poorly organized copy resulting in poor reproduction from memory. The distinction in this example is between a 'basic' visual memory disorder and an intellectual difficulty in organizing material for the process of committing it to memory. This type of distinction has important implications for the management of the patient as well as for regional diagnosis.

CONCEPT OF THE NEUROPSYCHOLOGICAL SYNDROME

The term syndrome is widely used in all areas of clinical endeavour. The word has had somewhat different connotations for different writers and this has led to confusion. Much of this confusion might be removed by agreement about a definition of the term or at least by a clarification of the way the term is used in different contexts.

The syndrome as concordance

Central to the concept is the sense of a unique constellation of signs and symptoms which occur together frequently enough to suggest an underlying disease process. The signs and symptoms, it is inferred, have a greater concordance among themselves than they each possess in relation to other signs and symptoms. Thus a true syndrome should be capable of being confirmed by appropriate statistical analysis of the strength of the mutual interrelationships. Though such testing has not been carried out very often, a case in point is the Gerstmann syndrome. Beginning with the study of Benton, several objective studies have discounted the validity of the four signs and symptoms (finger agnosia, acalculia, right-left disorientation, pure dysgraphia) as a unique set (Benton 1961, Heimburger et al 1964, Poeck & Orgass 1966). However, the term continues to be used in the neurological literature.

Much of the difficulty with the syndrome concept stems from the very complexity of symptomatology. Nevertheless, syndromes form useful working rules to deal with this complexity.

Furthermore, many widely accepted syndromes are marked by variability. They 'do not exist as fixed, consistent entities and as such they may be considered imaginary; however, when the presence of a particular grouping of findings indicates the underlying process with acceptable frequency the syndrome develops a meaning (reality) of its own' (Benson 1979). This is the syndrome as an abstraction.

Monothetic and polythetic descriptions

One of the major difficulties revolves around whether the term syndrome is intended to represent a fixed group of findings that is both sufficient and necessary for the ascription of a particular label, or that a common but not invariant set of findings defines the syndrome. A number of writers have pointed to the importance of this distinction in relation to taxonomy in neuropsychology (Russell et al 1970, Kertesz 1979, Walsh 1987). This reflects the distinction made between monothetic and polythetic classification in biological taxonomy. 'The ruling idea of monothetic groups is that they are formed by rigid and logical divisions so that the possession of a unique set of features is both sufficient and necessary for membership in the group thus defined.' (Sokal & Sneath 1963) With regard to the description of neurobehavioural syndromes, such a system does not seem appropriate in the light of our present knowledge. It is unable to deal with the aberrant case, e.g. Kertesz (1979) points out that the lack of a characteristic which forms one of the primary divisors will result in such an individual being 'moved to a taxon (group) away from its 'natural' position, *even though it is identical with its congeners in every way*.' [my italic].

Contrasted with the monothetic grouping is the polythetic or 'polytypic' (Beckner 1959). Here, all those cases which share a sufficient number of common characteristics are placed together in one group. However, 'no single feature is either essential to group membership or is sufficient to make an organism a member of the group' (Sokal & Sneath 1963). Beckner's (1959) definition is even more specific:

1. Each individual possesses a large number of characters in a certain set.
2. Each character in the set is possessed by a large number of individuals.
3. No character in the set is possessed by every individual.

Such an explicit formulation invites a number of questions or comments, e.g. in the individual case, how shall we decide what proportion of the characters constitutes 'a large number'? Moreover, practical experience in a number of fields of life has usually acquainted most of us with the fact that some characters are more important for group membership than others. This importance or weighting of individual characters varies from the pathognomonic to the less important. This weighting needs to be coupled with the measures of clustering or concordance before the full significance emerges. However, it is essential to stress that it is the total configuration in the Gestalt sense which imparts significance to the single attributes. A syndrome is, indeed, more than (or other than) the sum of its single constituents.

The absence of a 'usual' sign in a syndrome defined in a polythetic sense may be a function of the form of examination, e.g. a 'real' syndrome of appendicitis may lack the tenderness over McBurney's point because of the position of the appendix. However, a rectal examination may reveal just cause why the usual sign is apparently absent. Also, where two or more syndromes share several features in common, a distinction can only be made on the basis of a detailed knowledge of these syndromes and their variants. This process of differential diagnosis is discussed below.

Syndromes also vary in their degree of specificity or vagueness. The frontal lobe syndrome is a less well differentiated description than the general (or Korsakoff) amnesic syndrome. The reasons for this are partly historical.

A syndrome is thus a useful working fiction which allows us to create partial order out of the complexity of the patient's subjective complaints and the findings of our examinations. Those with a background in medicine are already familiar with the utility of the syndrome as a conceptual tool in everyday clinical practice. Most professional psychologists have been impressed by statistical comparisons of patients' performances with objectively studied performances of reference groups. The present approach accepts the importance of the data derived in this manner but considers that it should be supplemented by other methods, particularly the syndrome comparison approach. More and more psychologists have moved in the direction of syndrome analysis at least in clinical diagnostic practice. Piercy (1959) and McFie (1960) favoured this approach—'a patient's performance should be described not so much in terms of extent of deviation from statistical normality as in terms of approximation to an established syndrome or abnormality.' (McFie 1960)

The syndrome as probability

In discussing the objections to the syndrome method, Kinsbourne (1971) reminds us that the association between the constellation of signs and symptoms and the presence of a disease is probabilistic and not invariant: 'Partial syndromes abound, and it is often not clear how many ingredients have to be present to justify the diagnosis. This is particularly true since not all ingredients of a syndrome are of equal importance, their relative valuation being unformulated outcome of the interaction of medical instruction and clinical experience, and thus a somewhat individual process.' A fundamental question is whether the syndrome method rather than any other is likely to prove more effective 'in generating further scientific research questions, and contributions to the understanding of the functional organization of brain-behaviour activity' (Luria & Majovski 1977), and hence improve understanding of the individual patient, which is the principal role of clinical endeavour.

Kinsbourne (op.cit.) points out that correlative studies between lesion and syndrome need to employ valid experimental designs, and that appropriate statistical procedures such as cluster analysis should prove useful in the validation of clinical syndromes: 'Pending validation by appropriate testing, the clinically observed 'syndrome' represents an educated guess at a relationship which has value in generating hypotheses and experimentation.' One of the major tasks for neuropsychologists following this method is to increase the degree of confidence with which such probabilistic statements can be made, i.e. research support is needed to check the validity of the clinician's educated guesses so that they may be used by others. Although this task will often fall to full-time researchers, the clinician employing the experimental investigation of the single case is constantly generating data which could be used for this purpose.

Finally, experience teaches us that the definition of a syndrome may change over time. Such change may be in the direction of greater generality or specificity, and one syndrome may become subdivided into many. In some instances it might be possible and clinically advantageous to preserve both general and specific nomenclature. A case in point is provided by the study of memory disorders in the past three decades.

Neuropsychological dissection of sub-syndromes

One amnesic syndrome or several?

The amnesic disorder described originally by Korsakoff (see Ch. 2) presents certain characteristics, the chief among them being the presence of a general (nonspecific) failure of recent memory in the presence of preservation of immediate apprehension of stimuli and substantially preserved intellect. The syndrome appears to be strongly associated with damage in the mamillo-thalamic region caused by severe thiamine deprivation. The usual aetiology is malnutrition resulting from chronic alcoholism.

The term Korsakoff amnesia (general amnesic syndrome, or *the* amnesic syndrome) proved clinically useful for many years. However, two major sets of observations should lead to a revision of our use of the term:

Firstly, from the 1950s a good deal of information accumulated demonstrating that a markedly similar amnesic disorder arose whenever there was bilateral damage to the mesial aspects of the temporal lobes in the region of the hippocampus. Thus it appeared that a general amnesic syndrome arose whenever there was bilateral compromise of certain near-midline structures, irrespective of the nature of the aetiological agent. Some confusion arose over the use of the term Korsakoff amnesia, since the implication of alcoholism had been strongly reinforced by this time. Barbizet (1970) proposed the neutral term axial amnesia to cover the various cases.

Secondly, however, it was not very long before neuropsychological studies in France (Lhermitte & Signoret 1972) and America (Mattis et al 1978) demonstrated that while the mamillo-thalamic (Korsakoff) and hippocampal patients shared numerous amnestic features, they could also be discriminated on the basis of neuropsychological tests, i.e. there appeared to be two distinct subclasses of the one general amnesic syndrome. This differentiation of a broad syndrome into meaningful constituents is a common finding with the use of syndromes. A knowledge of the differentiating characteristics may well have diagnostic (and hence prognostic) significance and may also suggest appropriate methods of management or treatment.

In the French study cited, the alcoholic (mamillo-thalamic) patient showed improvement in recall when specific cues were provided while the post-encephalitic (hippocampal) patient did not. On the other hand, acquisition in the latter patient was greatly assisted by the provision of a logical relatedness between items to be teamed while this manoeuvre did not assist the alcoholic patient. (For further details see Ch. 2, Table.1)

Knowledge of a finding of this type should lead to questions of increasing specificity, e.g. the observation of a general amnesic syndrome should be followed by the question—which form of the syndrome? Such potentially fruitful questions depend on ever increasing knowledge, i.e. differential diagnosis does not take place in a vacuum. For a clinical method to be neuropsychological it should show a close relationship to the developing corpus of knowledge in neuropsychology.

This example of 'neuropsychological dissection' of the general amnesic syndrome not only provides useful clinical information but may further understanding of brain-behaviour relationships. One cannot fail to be impressed by the fact that the type of test on which the alcoholic patient has difficulty (the sundry Lhermitte & Signoret tasks) bears a striking resemblance to the difficulties described in patients with dorsolateral frontal lobe lesions. This may mean that the difference in performance of the two groups may depend as much on added lesions in the alcoholic group as the difference in location of lesions in the 'axial' region. Chapter 2 reviews the evidence for such an associated adaptive behaviour difficulty in Korsakoff amnesic subjects dependent upon cerebral pathology in the anterior portions of the brain.

Invalid use of the term syndrome

It is implicit in what has been said that if the term syndrome is used in an extremely broad sense then it fails to have meaning. One such usage was 'chronic brain syndrome'. Geschwind (1978) sums up the feeling of many: 'My objection to the term is that it carries an implication, however many qualifications are put on it, that there is such a thing as a single organic brain syndrome, something for which there is no evidence. The brain is the most complicated organ in the body, and thus one can expect many syndromes with different manifestations.'

The method of extreme cases

The syndrome comparison approach goes a long way to answering one of the principal objections to certain methods based solely on cutting scores derived from criterion groups. The assumption that a test validated on clearly defined brain-damaged groups will be useful for the day to day purposes of clinical diagnosis has been accepted uncritically. Yates (1966) pointed out that the fact that a test score (or range) has been validated on groups with clear cut cases may mean that its predictive validity may be quite low. If it can 'identify only those subjects whose brain damage is obvious, then the test serves no useful purpose, since it confirms what needs no confirmation' (Yates 1966). Study of the literature led Heilbrun (1962) to observe that a significant proportion of predictive hits seemed to come from those instances in which the neurological symptoms were fairly clear. It is also apparent that some neuropsychological test batteries gain much of their 'power of resolution' with regard to laterality of lesion from tests which are measures of sensory and motor processes, albeit more sensitive, refined and quantitative than those used in the normal clinical neurological examination.

Our present method is essentially what Kraepelin termed 'the method of extreme cases' (Zangwill 1978). Trainees are made familiar with a wide variety of syndromes both in their clinical presentation and the expression of difficulties in test performances. The training cases in the early stages are restricted to classical or extremely clear instances, i.e. the 'extreme case'. When these can be recognized with ease more complex cases are introduced to teach the range of variation that might be met with in clinical practice. We have found that this method facilitates the recognition of syndromes in their less dramatic or latent forms and makes it possible to detect characteristic patterns of neuropsychological deficit in their early stages of development. To date there have not been suitable studies of the efficacy of this method compared with more commonly used neuropsychological methods and there are obvious difficulties in doing so.

'A crucial study would be one in which the neurological group is made up entirely of subjects for whom neurologists disagree as to diagnosis or are unable to make a diagnostic statement at all at the time the psychological measure is obtained and for whom retrospective diagnosis is possible.' (Heilbrun 1962). Such predictive validity studies are few in number. One such study is that of Matthews et al (1966). These workers tested the predictive measures from the Halstead-Reitan Battery and the Wechsler scales on a group of subjects all of whom were initially suspected of neurological disease but in whom only half were subsequently confirmed as neurological, the other half being given a non-neurological diagnosis. The authors rather nicely refer to the latter group as 'pseudoneurologic'. Even in this more difficult diagnostic situation some of the measures discriminated at a high level. Further studies of predictive validity are obviously necessary.

One indirect measure of the clinical value of the syndrome method lies in the increasing demand for this type of clinical information where other types of psychological service have been, and continue to be, available. It may be, of course, that medical clinicians in particular find a common philosophy and terminology more attractive than purely psychometric reporting.

Double dissociation of function

This concept was put forward by Teuber (1955, 1959) and has been widely accepted and quoted by other workers. In discussing whether certain visual discrimination difficulties described after temporal lobe ablations in animals were specific to those particular areas, Teuber commented:

> To demonstrate specificity of the deficit for visual discrimination, we need to do more than show that discrimination in some other modality, e.g. somesthesis, is unimpaired. Such simple dissociation might indicate merely that visual discrimination is more vulnerable to temporal lesions than tactile discrimination. This would be a case of hierarchy of function rather than separate localization. What is needed for conclusive proof is 'double dissociation', i.e. evidence that tactile discrimination can be disturbed by some other lesion without loss on visual tasks and to a degree comparable in severity to the supposedly visual deficit after temporal lesions. (Teuber 1955)

A more general statement appeared a few years later in discussion of Teuber's findings in his extensive studies of human subjects with wounds to the brain:

> ...double dissociation requires that symptom A appear in lesions in one structure but not with those in another, and that symptom B appear with lesions of the other but not of the one. Whenever such dissociation is lacking, specificity in the effects of lesions has not been demonstrated. (Teuber 1959)

The concept or paradigm forms a useful tool in neuropsychology but despite acceptance of the notion in a general sense specific examples have accumulated slowly. The already considerable material on hemispheric dissociation of function continues to be expanded (e.g. Loring et al 1989) and the dissociation of visuoperceptual functions between the two sides of the brain posteriorly is becoming increasingly clarified (Newcombe et al 1987, 1989; Landis & Regard 1988), while the conceptual approach to the study of amnesia has proved a fertile field (e.g. Leng & Parkin 1988). Even difficulties such as perseveration, which at first sight might appear to be pervasive characteristics, turn out to be dissociable into different classes or subtypes (Kapur 1985). Numerous other examples of dissociation of part functions within a psychological domain have been well exploited in the long and elegant series of investigations headed by Warrington (Costello & Warrington 1987, McCarthy & Warrington 1987, 1988).

Kinsbourne has discussed the concept of dissociation in its research application to the study of *groups* of individuals with damage in different parts of the brain:

> If a patient group with damage centered at location A is superior to one damaged at B in respect to task P, but inferior in task Q, a double dissociation obtains between these groups. This permits the inference of at least one difference between the two groups specific to location of damage, for P may be a nonspecific task, relating, say, to general intelligence or some other variable in which the groups are imperfectly matched. But then it must be admitted that function Q must have been selectively impaired by a lesion at location A, since the inferiority in performing Q cannot be accounted for by failure of matching on the other task. The search for double dissociation is a valid means towards progress in neuropsychology. (Kinsbourne 1971)

This author warns that the converse situation, namely the failure to find dissociations, should not lead us to conclude that specific relationships do not exist between performance on specific tasks and particular anatomical sites or structures, since performance on a particular task may be affected by a number of factors. The recognition of the multiple determinants of the performance on many psychological tests should lead to the design of more 'discrete' tasks tied to single factors that might then be studied for their association with or dissociation from particular brain structures.

With the double dissociation paradigm Weiskrantz (1968) points out that 'the maximum information is conveyed when two treatments are alike in all but one critical aspect (e.g. for brain lesions—same mass, same damage to meninges, but different in locus) and that the two tasks similarly are alike in all but one critical aspect (e.g., same training procedure, same cue-response contingencies, but difference in sensory modality). This is simply to restate the essence of analytical control procedures, and the double dissociation paradigm is simply a way of combining two control procedures into a single pattern. But there are also great risks of reifying a dissociation between tests into a dissociation between functions and arguing that the affected function has been isolated by a single instance of dissociation.'

Clinical application—dissociation of homologous areas

The literature on mesial temporal lobe lesions and our own experience with unilateral anterior temporal lobectomy for complex partial seizures provides one of the clearest examples of arguing in the opposite direction, viz. from test findings to regional diagnosis. Lesions affecting the mesial aspects of the dominant temporal lobe produce a verbal memory deficit while nonverbal memory appears to be unaffected. The converse is true of corresponding lesions of the non-dominant side. The degree of deficit seems related to the extent of the lesion in the mesial temporal structures. With certain qualifications, lesions in other cerebral lobes do not affect memory. If we take tests which truly express the two types of disruption shown in the literature we might express it as follows, the negative sign representing less than expected performance:

Memory Tasks	LT	RT	Non-T
Verbal	−	+	+
Nonverbal	+	−	+

Thus an individual patient who performs poorly on a variety of verbal memory tasks while performing well on nonverbal memory tasks appears to share something in common with the group of 'dominant temporal lesion patients'. This presumption would be strengthened if there were information available about the differential performance of, say, temporal lobe patients on a different class of higher function. In our clinical experience Vignolo's (1969) finding of a different type of higher auditory analytic deficit related to the left (semantic-associative) and right (perceptual-discriminative) temporal lobes has been borne out:

Auditory tests	LT	RT	Non-T
Semantic−associative	−	+	+
Perceptual−discriminative	+	−	+

In a particular patient with the following set of performances we might feel more confident of diagnosing a left temporal lesion than on the basis of a single dissociation alone:

Verbal memory test	Poor
Semantic−associative auditory test	Poor
Nonverbal memory test	Normal
Perceptual−discriminative auditory test	Normal

This pattern might be termed a *congruent dissociation*. The dissociation in the instances cited is for homologous areas on either side of the brain so that we might use the term 'homologous dissociation'.

Care needs to be exercised in this situation in moving from test performance to function. Usually a single pair of tests is not enough because of the variations in the demands made by even seemingly similar tests.

One way of avoiding this pitfall is to look at the performance of the patient on several tests in the area, i.e. to apply a principle of syndrome analysis suggested by Luria and others. 'The initial hypothesis in this line of work is the assumption that in the presence of a given local lesion which directly causes the loss of some factor, all functional systems which include this factor suffer, while, at the same time, all functional systems which do not include the disturbed factor are preserved' (Luria 1973). From the psychologist's point of view one might look at the various poor test performances to see what Mack (1979) has called 'the shared variance'. This in turn requires that we know more than is usually the case about the factorial composition of the tests we use, and that we do not merely assume that the factor or process named by the test's authors is the only or even the principal cause of failure in every case. It is apparent that until we possess tests which are less multifactorial in their composition we will have to look carefully at the various possibilities for failure in each individual case.

Dissociation data also may influence inferences drawn from individual performances. Typical of the many dissociations shown by callostomy subjects is the finding by Loring et al (1989) of a specialization of response output of such a patient to verbal and visuo-spatial stimuli, even where free field stimuli were employed, i.e. the subject showed a differentially better performance with the right hand to verbal-spatial material and a superior performance to visuo-spatial material with the left hand. While the 'split brain' is an extreme example of a disconnection syndrome (Walsh 1987) many disconnection effects are produced by localized lesions but are not discovered or understood because of incomplete examination methods such as failing to examine the performance of each hand in appropriate cases.

Non-homologous dissociation

When attempts are made to relate complex and poorly delineated psychological functions to brain structures, regions other than homologues may become involved. The term spatial abilities will serve as an example. Teuber (1964) hypothesized that two sets of spatial abilities might be distinguished, (1) spatial orientation to external objects; and (2) spatial discrimination involving the subject's own body. These two subclasses of function he felt were mediated by the parietal and frontal regions respectively. Furthermore, there was a bias in the direction of the right parietal region being involved with tasks of extrapersonal space while the left frontal region was maximally involved with tests of personal or egocentric space. Though there is insufficient evidence on which to evaluate the hypothesis at present there are enough observations of this type to make the exercise worthwhile. The paradigm might be expressed:

Test	LF	RF	LP	RP	LT	RT
Personal Space	−	+	+	+	+	−
Extrapersonal space	+	+	+	−	+	+

Such a finding might be termed a non-homologous dissociation of function. In essence it is a restatement of the fact that tests should not be equated on a superficial basis, otherwise incorrect inferences may be drawn from test performances. In the above example failure on one spatial task has markedly different significance from failure on another.

The situation is even more complex when it is realized that some tests of spatial orientation/ability may require both types of ability for their solution.

Demonstration of dissociation of function by the Teuber paradigm forms a central part of the conceptual framework which is the basis for the method described in this work.

Dangers of the syndrome method

One of the risks in a syndrome methodology arises from the failure to recognize the principle of multiple determination of test failures, i.e. a particular test may be failed for a number of reasons. This is often coupled with equating poor performance with the 'most likely' cause in terms of group data. A common example might arise from the valid observations that certain WAIS sub-tests are most sensitive to right hemisphere damage, particularly in the parietal lobe (McFie 1975, Lezak 1976). However to take differentially poor performance on these tests as evidence of parietal damage in an individual case goes too far, since this is only one possible cause of poor performance, albeit the most common. Other causes of poor performance must be excluded if the conclusion is to be valid. This, of course, means that the neuropsychologist must know the sundry reasons for failure and have access to the means for testing them. This type of over simplified equation has given rise to such improbable inferences that alcohol impairs the right hemisphere to a greater degree than the left (see Ch. 2).

A second danger lies in the practice of accepting an explanation which fits most, but not all, of the clinician's observations or test data. The frequency of this error will be reduced, but not eliminated, with clinical experience and study of the literature. Significant features left unexplained often mean that the clinician was unaware of an alternative explanation which would cover *all* the facts. At the present time the relative dearth of well argued case analyses in the literature means that trainees must rely heavily on local instruction to improve this aspect of case work. The situation is not helped by illustrative cases in the literature which, while possibly committing this error, do not present sufficient data to check the probability of what may appear to the reader to be more satisfactory hypotheses. No doubt the present text will err in this regard on some occasions.

Clinical practice and theoretical development

Evidence derived from clinical material is of obvious importance in the development and refinement of theoretical models of neuropsychological functioning. However, there is currently much vigorous debate about the validity of drawing inferences from data derived from groups. There are strong proponents of the position that only data from 'unique' or single case studies permit valid inference about normal cognitive mechanisms from altered performance in those with disordered neurology (Caramazza & Badecker 1989), while others see a continuing use for both syndromic and single case analyses in neuropsychological research (McKenna & Warrington 1986, Zurif et al 1989).

INCORPORATING NEUROPSYCHOLOGICAL KNOWLEDGE

Perhaps the most important emphasis in an individualized approach to neuropsychological assessment should be on the continual incorporation of knowledge emerging from clinical and research studies. This enables the emerging 'psycho-anatomical' model to be used in an increasingly efficient manner in the understanding of individual cases. While the first steps are difficult, our training sessions have shown that those with the requisite background knowledge in neuropsychology, including basic neuroanatomy, rapidly become proficient in its use. Examples of application occur throughout the text but the following case will serve as the first illustration.

The psycho-anatomical model

Case: LD

A 53-year-old primary school teacher was referred by a neuro-ophthalmologist. Relevant extracts from the letter of referral outline the problem:

> LD was referred to me eight months ago. Her optometrist had found a field defect in February this year but she was unaware of difficulty with vision. She recalled two 'brown outs' during the 18 months but was not even certain when they occurred. She has had hypertension treated intermittently during the last two years ... Examination revealed a right upper quadrantic homonymous field defect which is congruous ... The field defect signifies a lesion in the left occipital lobe below the calcarine fissure. The CT scan of last March failed to show the lesion but curiously the more recent one in November 1st demonstrated an infarct on the medial aspect of the lower half of the occipital lobe. The blood pressure has been investigated and controlled.
>
> Throughout this illness Mrs D. has been troubled by depression and is currently taking amitriptyline. You will remember our discussion of patients with occipital lobe disease. I would be grateful if you would examine Mrs D. with neuropsychological studies. I have previously tried, both with the help of ... neuropsychologist and ... psychiatrist, to define the difficulties of patients with occipital lobe infarction. These patients appear more upset and depressed by their infarct than patients with lesions elsewhere in the cerebral cortex. One patient in fact was diagnosed as having hysterical loss of vision (and indeed she had suffered an infarct) and another patient, also with an obvious infarct, was so disturbed that the psychiatrist felt he could not have diagnosed her as having organic disease ...

The letter ended by citing several other cases where the patient had become depressed after occipital lobe infarction.

Our thinking in this case began with consideration of the pathological anatomy of such lesions rather than simply with the location of the lesion in the cerebrum. The occipital lesions described are in the territory of the posterior cerebral arteries. It seemed possible that structures other than those producing the visual field defect might have been affected by the pathological process that produced the infarction. One such major structure was the hippocampal formation and we were aware from earlier studies of others (e.g. Benson et al 1974) as well as from our own experience (Donnan et al 1978) that an amnesic syndrome of some severity can be produced when there is serious compromise or occlusion of the posterior vascular circulation. Subsequent work has strongly supported this relationship (Walsh 1987).

Many of our patients had been described as being confused and/or depressed and their amnesic difficulties had often one gone undetected. We were aware that bilateral lesions are necessary to produce a general amnesic syndrome. However, autopsy studies showed in some instances that apparently unilateral lesions were accompanied by lesser, silent, but nonetheless significant lesions in the other hemisphere, i.e. there was a bilateral but asymmetrical lesion. Thus we hypothesized that some of the distress shown by patients with occipital lobe infarction could be the result of lasting amnesic difficulties which were overshadowed by the attention given to the visual field defects.

A subsidiary hypothesis has received confirmation that, in purely unilateral cases, patients with left occipital lesions and verbal memory difficulties are more distressed than those with right occipital lesions accompanied by nonverbal memory problems. Of course, factors other than amnesic difficulties may be at work, but here is at least a point of departure for studying the effects of these lesions.

Neuropsychological examination

LD presented as a bright, alert woman without obvious sign of depressive mood:

Wechsler Memory Scale, Form I

Information	6	Digits Total	13 (7,6)
Orientation	5	Visual Reproduction	9
Mental Control	7	Associate Learning	9.5 (3,1;4,1;6,1)
Memory Passages	11		
MQ 112			

At first sight this would not seem to represent any gross degree of memory disorder. However, when LD failed to learn more than one of the four difficult pairs on the Associate Learning subtest she was asked to make a further effort to remember them. The three failed pairs were repeated with a preceding instruction for her to contrive a connection between them. She repeated them after the examiner and was allowed to rehearse them for a short time. After about fifteen minutes she was unable to recall any of the three. Of interest is the fact that the only pair she (a school teacher) had managed to retain was *school–grocery.* Delayed recall of one of the prose passages after twenty minutes produced only five points of the 22 given.

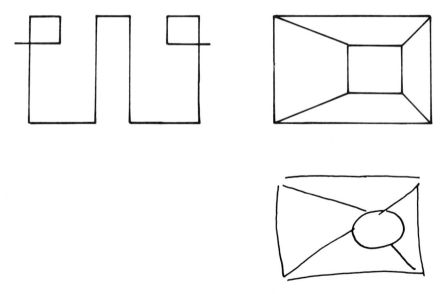

Fig. 1.5   Case LD. Card C, Visual Reproduction, WMS with patient's attempt.

At this stage LD was aware that she was having great difficulty with learning new material and what she did learn now on a day to day basis was rapidly forgotten. She had not discussed it with the other doctors she had seen.

An equivocal performance on the Visual Reproduction subtest left open the question as to whether the memory deficit was verbal-specific or general. On Card C she drew only one of the two figures, commenting that she was unsure as to whether it was a circle or square in the centre of the rectangle (see Fig. 1.5). Earlier in the testing it had been established that her visual field defect was not interfering with perception of detail or spatial relations.

Other tests were then given to check her visuo-spatial abilities and to see whether there was more widespread disruption of verbal functions.

Wechsler Adult Intelligence Scale

Information	12	Digit-Symbol	9
Comprehension	10	Block design	11
Similarities	12	Object Assembly	11
Digit Span	12		

These tests were all performed at about the expected level without any untoward qualitative features suggestive of localized cerebral pathology. Finally, the *Rey Figure* was given to check incidental memory with more complex material. On the copy she made one major distortion in the bottom left of the figure but corrected this spontaneously. She appeared unsure of her recall performed after a three minute delay and altered two components. The recall was much impoverished (Fig. 1.6).

The first examination concluded with the conviction that there was a memory difficulty, the nature of which needed further elucidation. Two possibilities were considered: (1) a general amnesic syndrome associated with bilateral pathology; or (2) a verbal specific memory difficulty associated with left posterior pathology. At this time the patient returned to her home in a distant town and was not seen until four months later.

Second examination

As some time had elapsed it was decided to repeat parts of the earlier testing as well as to extend the examination.

Wechsler Memory Scale, Form II

Information	6	Digits Total	10 (6,4)
Orientation	5	Visual Reproduction	14
Mental Control	8	Associate Learning	10 (5,0;6,0;6,1)
Memory Passages	9		
MQ 114			

Once again there was a pronounced difficulty with paired associate learning but this time there was no difficulty whatever on Visual Reproduction. Memory for prose was thought to be relatively poor considering her educational background.

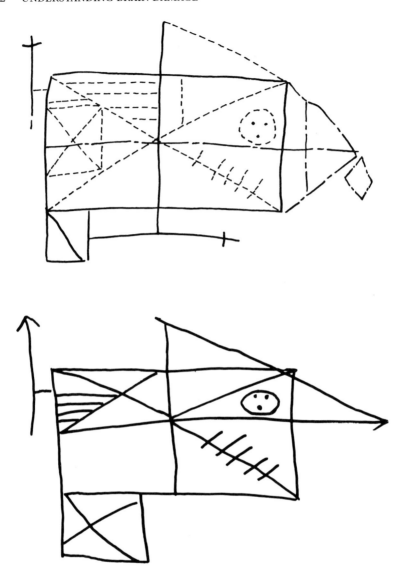

Fig. 1.6 Case LD. Rey Figure. Copy and Recall.

LD's copy of the *Rey Figure* was neater and better organized but her recall at four minutes was just as impoverished as it had been four months before. When asked, she said she was unsure whether she had seen the figure on the previous occasion. At this stage the examiner asked her about her memory in day-to-day situations. Mrs D. said that it had been pointed out that she repeated things to her friends, forgetting that she had already told them. She had found that she must write down things of importance or she was likely to forget. For the past few months she had kept a diary for the first time as an aide-mémoire. She had been managing her work as a teacher though her poor memory interfered at times. Fortunately she had been in the same teaching position for some years and so possessed a store of well established information from which to conduct her classes. She felt that she was withdrawing from social contact because of her memory problem.

On the *Rey Auditory Verbal Learning Test* she performed at a level clearly below that of her other verbal performances and showed a marked interference effect, being able to recall only four of the 15 items after interpolation of the second list. Her recognition memory was better and it was interesting to note that some of the words she recognized had not been recalled on any of the five learning trials.

List A	List B	List A	List A
Trial 1 2 3 4 5	Recall	Recall	Recognition
6 6 9 9 10	5	4	10

The patient's description of her subjective difficulties agreed with these findings. She had difficulty retaining information if this took place, for example, in a situation where she spoke to a number of people in turn. This fact tended to make her tense since she was aware that she tended to lose the information quickly with any outside distraction or interference. Despite this she felt that the problem did not adversely affect her work to any serious degree.

Repetition of parallel forms of the WAIS subtests showed no change over the period. Functions associated with the left hemisphere, such as reading, writing and colour naming, all appeared intact.

Thus, LD's main residual problem appeared to be a difficulty in memorizing new verbal material. Together with this she demonstrated poor recall for complex so-called 'nonverbal' material (Rey Figure) in the face of very good recall (a maximum score) for simpler visual designs (WMS Visual Reproduction). The recall deficit on the Rey Figure may have been due to the fact that its complexity actually requires some verbal encoding for recall. Such a hypothesis was put forward by Signoret & Lhermitte (1976) who observed similar performances in several patients with infarcts in the territory of the left posterior cerebral artery. The weight of evidence would seem to support the presence of a verbal specific memory defect which appears to be stable and is severe enough to be a constant strain on the patient, though she is able to cope fairly well in a very familiar work situation and home environment.

This patient, like others with unrecognized higher functional deficits, was helped in her adjustment by explanation of the relationship of her memory difficulty to its organic basis in her 'minor stroke'. It is noteworthy that she discarded the antidepressant medication she had been given and in the ensuing years managed well. It was explained that there was no reason to fear that the condition was a progressive on, and further help was provided by the reassuring lack of deterioration in serial examinations.

This case illustrates that the psycho-anatomical method can be productive in the individual case by using neuropsychological information to set up new hypotheses in situations where frequency comparison methods would be inapplicable because of absence of comparison on 'normative' data. Cognitive examination of the neurological patient is not synonymous with neuropsychological evaluation.

REFERENCES

Barbizet J 1970 Human memory and its pathology. Freeman, San Francisco

Beckner M 1959 The biological way of thought. University Press, New York

Benson D F 1979 Aphasia, alexia and agraphia. Churchill Livingstone, Edinburgh

Benson D F, Marsden C D, Meadows J C 1974 The amnesic syndrome of posterior cerebral artery occlusion. Acta Neurologica Scandinavica 50: 133–145

Benton A L 1961 The fiction of the 'Gerstmann syndrome'. Journal of Neurology, Neurosurgery and Psychiatry 24: 176–181

Ben-Yishay Y, Diller L, Mandelberg I, Gordon W, Gerstman L J 1971 Similarities and differences in Block Design performance between older normal and brain-injured persons: a task analysis. Journal of Abnormal Psychology 78: 17–25

Bruell J H, Albee G W 1962 Higher intellectual functions in a patient with hemispherectomy for tumors. Journal of Consulting Psychology 26: 90–98

Caramazza A, Badecker W 1989 Patient classification in neuropsychological research. Brain and Cognition 10:256–295

Chaplin J P 1968 Dictionary of psychology. Dell, New York, p 499

Christensen A L 1975 Luria's neuropsychological investigation. Munksgaard, Copenhagen

Costello A D, Warrington E K 1987 The dissociation of visuospatial neglect and neglect dyslexia. Journal of Neurology, Neurosurgery and Psychiatry 50: 1110–1116

Cronbach L J 1949 Essentials of psychological testing. Harper and Row, New York, p 233

Donnan G A, Walsh K W, Bladin P F 1978 Memory disorder in vertebrobasilar disease. Journal of Clinical and Experimental Neurology 15: 215–220

English H B, English A C 1958 Comprehensive dictionary of psychological and psychoanalytical terms. Longmans Green, New York, p 542

Eysenck H J, Arnold W, Meili R 1972 Encyclopedia of psychology. Search Press, London, p 311

Freeman F S 1962 Theory and practice of psychological testing, 3rd edn. Holt Rinehart and Winston, New York, p 14

Geschwind N 1978 Organic problems in the aged: brain syndromes and alcoholism. Journal of Geriatric Psychiatry 11: 161–166

Golden C J 1979 Clinical interpretation of objective psychological tests. Grune and Stratton, New York, p 209

Graham F K, Kendall B S 1960 Memory for Designs Test: Revised general manual. Perceptual and Motor Skills 11: 147–188

Grant A D, Berg E A 1948 A behavioral analysis of degree of reinforcement and ease of shifting to new responses in a Weigl-type card sorting. Journal of Experimental Psychology 38: 404–411

Hebb D O 1949 The organization of behavior. Wiley, New York

Heilbrun A B 1962 Issues in assessment of organic brain damage. Psychological Reports 10: 511–515

Heimburger R F, Demeyer W, Reitan R M 1964 Implications of Gerstmann's syndrome. Journal of Neurology, Neurosurgery and Psychiatry 27: 52–57

Kane R L, Goldstein G, Parsons O A 1989 A response to Mapou. Journal of Clinical and Experimental Neuropsychology 11: 589–595

Kaplan E 1983 Process and achievement revisited. In : Wapner S, Kaplan B (eds) Toward a holistic developmental psychology. Erlbaum. Hillsdale, New Jersey, p 143–156

Kaplan E 1988 A process approach to neuropsychological assessment. In : Boll T, Bryant B K (eds) Clinical neuropsychology: Research, measurement, and practice. American Psychological Association, Washington

Kapur N 1985 Double dissociation between perseveration in memory and problem solving tasks. Cortex 21: 461–467

Kertesz A 1979 Aphasia and associated disorders. Grune and Stratton, New York, p 78

Kinsbourne M 1971 Cognitive deficit: experimental analysis. In: McGaugh J L (ed) Psychobiology. Academic Press, New York, p 290–291 and 295

Kinsbourne M 1972 Contrasting patterns of memory span decrement in ageing and aphasia. Journal of Neurology, Neurosurgery and Psychiatry 35: 192–195

Korman M, Blumberg S 1963 Comparative efficiency of some tests of cerebral damage. Journal of Consulting Psychology 27: 303–309

Landis T, Regard M 1988 Hemianopia and agnosia. Klinische Monatsblatter für Augenheilkunde 192: 525–528

Leng R, Parkin A J 1988 Double dissociation of frontal dysfunction in organic amnesia. British Journal of Clinical Psychology 27: 359–362

Lewinsohn P M 1971 Assessment of clinical (diagnostic) skill: Illustration of a quantitative approach. Professional Psychology 2: 303–304

Lezak M D 1976 Neuropsychological Assessment. Oxford University Press, New York

Lezak M D 1980 An individualized approach to neuropsychological assessment (Unpublished manuscript)

Lezak M D 1988 I.Q : R.I.P. Presidential address, International Neuropsychological Society, New Orleans

Lhermitte F, Signoret J L 1972 Analyse neuropsychologique et différenciation des syndromes amnèsiques. Revue Neurologique 126: 161–178

Loring D W, Meador K J, Lee G P 1989 Differential–handed response to verbal and visual spatial stimuli : evidence of specialized hemispheric processing following callosotomy. Neuropsychologia 27: 811–827

Luria A R 1973 The working brain. Allen Lane Penguin Press, London, p 13–14

Luria A R, Majovski L V 1977 Basic approaches used in American and Soviet clinical neuropsychology. American Psychologist 32: 959–968

McCarthy R A, Warrington E K 1987 The double dissociation of short-term memory for lists and sentences. Evidence from aphasia. Brain 110: 1545–1563

McCarthy R A, Warrington E K 1988 Evidence for modality-specific meaning systems in the brain. Nature 334: 428–430

McFie J 1960 Psychological testing in clinical neurology. Journal of Nervous and Mental Disease 131: 383–393

McFie J 1969 The diagnostic significance of disorders of higher nervous activity. In : Vinken P J, Bruyn G W (eds) Handbook of clinical neurology. North-Holland, Amsterdam, vol 4, ch 1

McFie J 1975 Assessment of organic intellectual impairment. Academic Press, New York

Mack J 1979 Personal communication

McKenna P, Warrington E A 1986 The analytical approach to neuropsychological assessment. In : Grant I, Adams K M (eds), Neuropsychological assessment of neuropsychiatric disorders. Oxford University Press, New York, p 31–47

Mapou R L 1988 Testing to detect brain damage: An alternative to what may no longer be useful. Journal of Clinical and Experimental Neuropsychology 10: 271–278

Matarazzo J D 1972 Wechsler's measurement and appraisal of adult intelligence, 5th edn. Williams and Wilkins, Baltimore

Matthews C G, Shaw D J, Kløve H 1966 Psychological test performances in neurological and 'pseudo-neurologic' subjects. Cortex 2: 244–253

Mattis S, Kovner R, Goldmeier E 1978 Different patterns of amnestic syndromes. Brain and Language 6: 179–191

Meehl P E 1954 Clinical versus statistical prediction. University of Minnesota Press, Minneapolis

Meehl P E 1960 The cognitive activity of the clinician. American Psychologist 15: 19–27

Meehl P E 1961 Logic for the clinician. Contemporary Psychology 6: 389–391

Meehl P E 1972 Psychodiagnosis: selected papers. Norton, New York

Milberg W P, Herben N, Kaplan E 1986 The Boston process approach to neuropsychological assessment. In : Grant I, Adams K M (eds) Neuropsychological assessment of neuropsychiatric disorders. Oxford University Press, New York, p 65–86

Nadel A B 1938 A qualitative analysis of behavior following cerebral lesions: Diagnosed as primarily affecting the frontal lobes. Archives of Psychology No 224

Nelson H E 1976 A modified card sorting test sensitive to frontal lobe defects. Cortex 12: 313–324

Nelson H E 1982 The National Adult Reading Test manual. NFER-Nelson, Windsor, England

Nelson H E, O'Connell A 1978 Dementia: The estimation of premorbid intelligence levels using the new adult reading test. Cortex 14: 234–244

Newcombe F, Ratcliff G, Damasio H 1987 Dissociable visual and spatial impairments following right posterior cerebral lesions: clinical, neuropsychological and anatomical evidence. Neuropsychologia 25: 149 161

Newcombe F, de Haan E H, Ross J, Young A W 1989 Face processing, laterality and contrast sensitivity. Neuropsychologia 27: 523–538

Piercy M F 1959 Testing for intellectual impairment—some comments on tests and testers. Journal of Mental Science 105: 489–495

Poeck K, Orgass B 1966 Gerstmann's syndrome and aphasia. Cortex 2: 421–437

Reitan R M 1964 Psychological deficits resulting from cerebral lesions in man. In : Warren J M, Akert K (eds) The frontal granular cortex and behaviour. McGraw-Hill, New York

Reitan R M 1986 Theoretical and methodological bases of the Halstead-Reitan Test Battery. In : Grant I & Adams K M (eds) Neuropsychological assessment of neuropsychiatric disorders. Oxford University Press, New York p 3–30

Rosen H 1971 A comparison of two scoring systems for the Memory-for-Designs Test. Journal of Clinical Psychology 27: 79–81

Russell E W 1982 Theory and developments of pattern analysis methods related to the Halstead-Reitan Battery. In : Logue P E, Shear J M (eds) Clinical neuropsychology: a multidisciplinary approach. Thomas Springfield, Illinois

Russell E W, Neuringer C, Goldstein G 1970 Assessment of brain damage: A neuropsychological key approach. Wiley, New York

Shapiro M B 1951 Experimental studies of a perceptual anomaly. 1: Initial experiments. Journal of Mental Science 97: 90–100

Shapiro M B 1973 Intensive assessment of the single case. In Mettler P E (ed) The psychological assessment of mental and physical handicaps, Tavistock Publications, London, ch 21, p 652

Signoret J L, Lhermitte F 1976 The amnesic syndrome and the encoding process. In: Rosenzweig M R, Bennett E L (eds) Neural mechanisms of learning and memory . MIT Press, Cambridge, Massachusetts

Smith A 1973 Symbol Digit Modalities Test. Western Psychological Services, Los Angeles

Smith A 1975 Neuropsychological testing in neurological disorders. In: Friedland W F (ed) Advances in neurology, vol 7 Raven Press, New York

Sokal R R, Sneath P H 1963 Principles of numerical taxonomy. Freeman, San Francisco, p 13–14

Teuber H L 1955 Physiological psychology. Annual Review of Psychology 6: 267–296

Teuber H L 1959 Some alterations in behaviour after cerebral lesions in man. In: Bass A D (ed) Evolution of nervous control from primitive organisms to man. American Association for the Advancement of Science, Washington, p 187

Teuber H L 1964 The riddle of frontal lobe function in man. In: Warren J M, Akert K (eds) The frontal granular cortex and behavior. McGraw–Hill, New York, Ch 20

Vignolo L A 1969 Auditory agnosia: a review and report of recent evidence. In: Benton A L (ed) Contributions to clinical neuropsychology. Aldine, Chicago

Visser R S H 1980 Manual of the complex figure test. Swets and Zeitlinger, Lisse

Walsh K W 1987 Neuropsychology: a clinical approach, 2nd edn. Churchill Livingstone, Edinburgh

Weiskrantz L 1968 Some traps and pontifications. In: Weiskrantz L (ed) Analysis of behaviourial change. Harper and Row, New York

Yates A 1954 The validity of some psychological tests of brain damage. Psychological Bulletin 51: 359–380

Yates A 1966 Psychological deficit. Annual Review of Psychology 17: 111–144

Zangwill O 1978 Personal communication

Zurif E B, Gardner H, Brownell H H 1989 The case against group studies. Brain and Cognition 10: 237–255

2. Alcohol related brain damage

For convenience the effects of chronic alcohol abuse have been divided into two major divisions: the Korsakoff amnesic syndrome, and other non-amnesic psychological deficits. The reason for this division is that while both sets of changes frequently occur in the same individual, they can be seen dissociated and current evidence points to the strong possibility of two quite different aetiologies.

THE WERNICKE-KORSAKOFF SYNDROME

History

In 1881 Wernicke first described three cases of the syndrome which bears his name. The salient features were ataxia, ocular symptoms and mental confusion. Two of the cases were alcoholic. It was later established that the condition was related to poor nutrition, the specific deficiency being that of thiamine or vitamin B_1. This accounts for its frequent appearance in undernourished alcoholics although it also appears in other circumstances which produce thiamine avitaminosis.

In a series of reports from 1887 to 1891 Korsakoff reported the association of various mental disorders with polyneuritis. Sometimes the patient retained clear consciousness but was agitated while in others the agitation was part of a confusional state. In most of the patients an amnesic disorder was a prominent feature. Soon after these initial observations Korsakoff, along with others, noted that the amnesic syndrome could be seen without polyneuritis.

The most common aetiological factor, but by no means the only one, was heavy consumption of alcohol. Since that time there have been many attempts to clarify the description of the mental condition most often termed Korsakoff's psychosis. In recent years most studies have been directed to the most lasting and characteristic feature, namely the amnesia (see Barbizet 1970, Whitty & Zangwill 1977, Butters & Cermak 1980 for reviews).

Although a close association between Wernicke's disease and Korsakoff's psychosis was recognized by a number of writers at the turn of the century, the intimate clinical relationship was established by Bonhoeffer (1904) though pathological confirmation was not established firmly for about three more decades (see Victor et al 1971). Following resolution of the acute episode of Wernicke's encephalopathy patients were found to be suffering from the Korsakoff amnesic syndrome. Moreover, the pathological lesions appear to be identical in the two conditions. Because of the nature of the populations studied it is not always possible to ascertain whether Korsakoff patients have suffered from one or more episodes of Wernicke's disorder though this is usually the case. Most workers would agree with Victor (1976) that Korsakoff's psychosis is the psychic manifestation of Wernicke's disease.

Although it may turn out that all cases of acute encephalopathy develop the amnesic syndrome, it is still possible that the Korsakoff state may be reached without a florid encephalopathic episode. Multiple lesions in individual cases often appear to be of different ages suggesting that some subjects have had a number of separate episodes which may have cumulated to produce a fully developed Wernicke-Korsakoff syndrome. This would account for the wide range of combinations of amnesic and other cognitive deficits encountered in clinical practice.

The prevalence of the Wernicke-Korsakoff syndrome varies not only with the prevalence of alcoholism but also with the use of thiamine supplements such as used in flour. The absence of such supplements accounts in part for the relatively high prevalence in countries such as Australia (Harper et al 1989).

Neuropathology

The pathology of the Korsakoff and related amnesic syndromes has been reviewed by Brierley (1977) and Horel (1978) together with the classical description of the Wernicke-Korsakoff lesions by Victor et al (1971) and Victor (1976). In the Wernicke-Korsakoff group the mamillary bodies are affected in virtually every case (Harper 1979). In some cases with apparent macroscopic sparing, histological examination reveals the characteristic neuropathological changes. Other lesions are constantly found in the thalamus, hypothalamus, brain stem and cerebellum. Many of the cases also show associated cerebral atrophy often most prominent in the frontal regions (see below).

Victor (1976) considers the medial portion of the dorsomedial nucleus to be the region most strongly implicated in the production of the Korsakoff amnesic syndrome, though this is disputed by others, many of whom favour the mamillary bodies as the crucial structures. Certainly all the cases with amnesia in the Victor et al monograph had dorsomedial nucleus lesions while some with marked lesions of the mamillary bodies had had no history of amnesia. While individual cases show many areas affected in common there is a wide variety of pathology from case to case and some of the differences may be related to the quality and severity of amnesic and other deficits. Also, many patients who show typical post-mortem changes associated with the Wernicke-Korsakoff disorder are not diagnosed during life (as many as 80% of 131 cases in Harper's Australian study); at least, no record could be found to indicate the classical triad of ophthalmoplegia, gait disorder, and abnormal mental state (Harper 1983, Harper et al 1986). While some of the signs may have been missed this probably does not account for all the discrepancy, and Harper believes that many of the cases may be the end result of repeated subclinical episodes of thiamine deficiency.

Clinical features

The precise delineation of the Korsakoff amnesic syndrome is still somewhat unclear. Among the principal reasons, three deserve special mention:

1. The composition of groups which have been studied has varied with regard to the stage of development of the disorder and the degree to which the patients have been affected;

2. The variety of psychological tests and methods which has been used;

3. The collection of deficits seen in the typical Korsakoff patients may be the result of more than one pathological process (see below).

Nevertheless, the following description would find common agreement:

1. There is a profound difficulty or total inability in acquiring new material. This deficit encompasses both verbal and nonverbal material and is also independent of the sense modality through which the material is presented. For this reason the term *general* amnesic syndrome is used to distinguish it from the material-specific amnesias seen with unilateral lesions of the temporal lobes. Clinical tests demonstrate that material which appears to have been apprehended cannot be recalled after the passage of an unusually brief period which, in severe cases, may be down to minutes. As nothing new is learned there develops an increasing period of anterograde amnesia.

2. There is less complete agreement about the presence of retrograde amnesia but all agree that the Korsakoff patient has a profound difficulty of spontaneous recall of prior events. In endeavouring to extract a personal chronology from the patient several things are noticeable:

a. much more information can be elicited by direct questioning than by spontaneous recall

b. the amount of information decreases as questions move closer in time to the present

c. some of the information has no 'time tags' i.e., its temporal relations to other happenings appear to have been lost. The 'achronogenesis' has been stressed by several writers (see Barbizet 1970) and its presence should suggest very strongly an alcoholic aetiology.

Apart from these difficulties the patient will in the advanced stages tend to wander off the subject. Janet (1928) referred to the core of this difficulty as the 'problem of narration.'

Many clinical writers have described a temporal gradient in the sparing of memories, with those of childhood and early adult life being less affected than those of later periods. A test of the temporal gradient hypothesis by Sanders & Warrington (1971) found that the duration of the retrograde defect was very long indeed. However, more recent studies with larger samples and improved methodology have tended to give strong support to a temporal gradient theory (Seltzer & Benson 1974, Marslen-Wilson & Teuber 1975, Albert et al 1979). It may be that the severity of the condition plays a major role. Korsakoff himself noted that while remote sparing was often seen, in other cases 'even the memory of remote events may be disturbed' (Victor & Yakovlev 1955). Victor (1976) agreed that 'memories of the distant past are impaired in practically all cases of Korsakoff's psychosis and seriously impaired in most of them'.

3. An essential feature is the preservation of immediate memory, the audioverbal and visual spans being around 7.

4. Many aspects of learned behaviour are preserved. Clinical examination reveals no difficulties with speech, language, gesture and well-practised skills. There are no problems with the basic activities of daily living. However, outside a familiar environment, Korsakoff patients will get into difficulties especially if they need to incorporate new information for their behaviour to become adapted to a novel situation.

5. Confabulation had earlier been considered as necessary for the diagnosis of Korsakoff's psychosis but it is by no means a constant feature. It appears to be seen mainly in the acute state together with some confusion. Confabulation has been defined by Berlyne (1972) as 'a falsification of memory occurring in clear consciousness in association with an organically derived dementia'. It appears to be as common in dementia as it is in Korsakoff's disease and is also seen in other neurological disorders and a distinction has been made between different forms of confabulation (Kopelman 1987). There is some evidence that at least one form of confabulation may be related to a marked deficit in frontal lobe function (Stuss et al 1978, Kapur & Coughlan 1980). A study by Mercer et al (1977) using objective tests found that confabulation 'proved to be strongly related to the inability to withhold responses, to monitor one's own responses, and to provide verbal self-corrections'. Such a description would fit well with what is known of acute frontal lobe dysfunction. This is closely akin to the observation of experienced clinicians that confabulation is directly related to the absence of insight (Zangwill 1978). Certainly, confabulation is not a marked feature of the chronic state.

6. The patient often exhibits a lack of initiative and spontaneity together with a blunting of affect.

In addition there are associated cognitive deficits, often of a subtle nature, which are discussed below in relation to chronic alcoholism (without obvious amnesia).

Psychometric features

The Wechsler Memory Scale is often sufficient to establish a presumptive diagnosis. The amnesic syndrome is reflected in the following way:

1. Poor performance on the three subtests involving new learning, viz. Prose Passages, Visual Reproduction, and Paired Associate Learning. In the last named task the patient will usually be able to learn (or refresh) the 'easy' association pairs but will be completely unable to master the 'difficult pairs' which constitute new learning.

2. Digits Forward will be preserved to the level of six or more.

3. Orientation will be poor in the true Korsakoff patient but may be normal in the incipient or borderline case.

4. Mental Control will vary from case to case though preservation of these stereotyped mental operations is more generally the case.

A simple bedside test for new learning difficulties is supraspan learning. Having established the patient's digit span in the usual manner, a series of digits is chosen one or two above the span and the same series is repeated until the patient is able to repeat the series correctly. A suitable version with norms for several age groups and levels of education has recently come to hand (Hamsher et al 1980) and is well worth incorporating into the armamentarium.

Forms of axial amnesia

The type of amnesic syndrome seen in the Wernicke-Korsakoff disorder has been shown to be present in other conditions such as tumours of the third ventricle, herpetic encephalitis and posterior vascular occlusion. In fact, this type of amnesia appears to be produced whenever there is bilateral destruction of certain structures on the mesial or internal aspect of the cerebral hemispheres close to the central axis of the brain. For this reason the Korsakoff type of general amnesia has been called axial or mesial amnesia (Barbizet 1970). Structures thought to be important in its production are the hippocampus, mamillary bodies, part of the thalamus, and possibly other structures. Reviews are provided by Whitty & Zangwill (1977) and Horel (1978).

The finding of an axial amnesia in an adult individual who drinks alcohol on a regular basis strongly suggests a Korsakoff disorder. However, with the discovery that axial amnesia might have numerous causes, it became of clinical importance to determine whether there were differences in the amnesic syndrome according to aetiology. One such subdivision appears to separate alcoholic amnesia, with lesions in the mamillo-thalamic region, from the amnesia following herpetic encephalitis and other conditions where the lesions are maximal in the medial temporal areas (Lhermitte & Signoret 1972). Since that time it has become apparent that not only are there important differences in the amnesic syndrome according to lesion location but there are probably simultaneous deficits in two or more independent psychological processes in the Korsakoff variety (Mattis et al 1978, Kovner et al 1981, Squire 1981).

The principal findings from the Lhermitte & Signoret study are reproduced below (Table 2.1).

Details of the Lhermitte & Signoret tests are given in the Appendix. They are easily administered and have proved clinically useful in our experience in the differentiation of amnesic syndromes. The conceptual difficulties seen with the alcoholic form of the syndrome may well be due to associated pathology in the frontal system. This is discussed elsewhere.

Two features have immediate relevance in the management and rehabilitation of these two clinical sub-syndromes: (1) cued recall may be of limited benefit in aiding the alcoholic patient but is of no value to the medial temporal patient who has been described as having a syndrome of 'pure forgetting'; (2) conversely, the medial temporal patient is aided by having the material to be remembered incorporated into a system or matrix of conceptual relationships whereas even the intelligent alcoholic has great difficulty with conceptual ordering.

CHRONIC ALCOHOLISM WITHOUT AMNESIA

The second major set of changes is that seen in those alcoholics who, because of adequate nutrition, have not developed the amnesic syndrome.

Table 2.1   Differentiation of the amnesic syndrome according to locus of lesion

Clinical features	Mamillo-thalamic (Alcoholic)	Medial temporal (Post-encephalitis)
Delayed recall	May deny information was given	Says material has been forgotten
Confabulation	Variable	Absent
Chronology (long-term memory)	Disorganized	Satisfactory
Awareness of disorder	Lack of awareness or denial	No lack of awareness or denial
Test features (after Lhermitte & Signoret, 1972)		
A. Learning of spatial arrangement		
Trials to criterion	Very many more than controls	Very many more than controls
Errors	Numerous	Numerous
Spontaneous recall	Nil	Nil
Cued recall	Good	Nil
B. Learning of Logical arrangement	Failure	Normal
C. Learning of sequentially presented material		
Sequence of words	Failure	Normal
Sequences of coloured counters	Failure	Normal

Note: In addition, the two groups of patients showed qualitatively different types of errors during their learning trials on Test A.

Neuropathology of chronic alcoholism

Apart from the well documented localized Wernicke-Korsakoff lesions, chronic alcoholic excess leads to more widespread cerebral changes in a high proportion of cases. The cause of the changes is still unknown but they are believed by many to be due to toxic metabolic products rather than to a deficiency disorder resulting from poor nutrition. They have been reported quite early in the drinking history of the 'well nourished alcoholic'. A study by Lynch (1960) of eleven subjects with adequate nutritional status showed typical alcohol related brain changes at autopsy.

Although there had been earlier reports of such changes, the first extensive and systematic description was by Courville (1955). This author reported atrophy over much of the cortex but most marked in the upper part of the dorsolateral surface of the frontal lobes. This was often accompanied by subcortical loss which was reflected in ventricular dilatation. Subsequent workers have confirmed the findings, and radiological methods have been used in attempts to correlate indications of such pathology with the presence and degree of alcoholism. A small number of studies has also attempted to correlate radiological changes with psychological deficit.

Earlier studies of alcohol related brain changes employed pneumoencephalography. Among numerous studies, those by French workers in the 1950s left little doubt that there was a strong association between cerebral atrophy and chronic alcoholism (Lereboullet et al 1954, Pierson & Kirscher 1954, Pluvinage 1954, Peron & Gayno 1956, Postel & Cossa 1956). Another early study showed the presence of atrophy maximal in the parietal or frontoparietal regions in younger alcoholics (mean age only 32 years) in whom atrophy might not have been suspected (Tumarkin et al 1955). Such a finding has been confirmed subsequently (Skillicorn 1955, Haug 1968, Willanger et al 1968, Willanger 1970, Brewer & Perrett 1971, Iivanainen 1975). There were some indications from these studies that the cerebral changes could be associated with clinico-psychometric evidence of mental impairment. Over 90% of Brewer and Perrett's group showed evidence of atrophy and there was a positive correlation with psychological test measures of intellectual impairment. The high incidence of atrophy was somewhat surprising in view of their description of their patients as 'well dressed, well shaven and looking much like any other citizen'.

More recently, computerized axial tomography has added further weight to the relationship between alcoholic excess and brain atrophy (Fox et al 1976, Epstein et al 1977, Cala et al, 1978, Cala & Mastaglia 1980, Carlen et al 1978). Epstein et al concluded that alcoholic cerebral atrophy may be more frequent than previously believed, especially among younger individuals. Cala et al reconfirmed the diffuse bilateral nature of the atrophic changes in 73% of their cases. The maximal involvement was in the frontal regions in keeping with earlier studies. Their patients were free from amnesia but showed cognitive deficits similar to many psychological studies of chronic alcoholics, in the form of differentially poor performance on the WAIS subtests of Digit-Symbol Substitution, Block Design and Object Assembly. There was a significant correlation between these measures and cortical atrophy but not with the other subtests or the summarizing IQ measures.

The greater prominence of change in the frontal regions has been amply confirmed (Shimamura et al 1988) and post-mortem sampling shows significant, quantitative loss of cortical neurons in the superior frontal cortex, though not in the adjacent motor cortex (Harper et al 1987). The large neurones which have been shown to be affected differentially in Alzheimer's disease and in normal ageing have also been shown to be more affected in the chronic alcoholic brain (Harper & Kril 1989).

At least one study (Carlen et al 1978) has demonstrated with repeated CT scans that partial reversibility of 'atrophy' may occur with maintained abstinence and that this partial reversal is paralleled by some degree of functional improvement. However, the cognitive evaluation procedures were rather crude. It was also postulated at that time that improvement in the brain shrinkage might be related to improved cerebral hydration following abstinence but this does not seem to be the case (Harper et al 1988a). Moreover, the shrinkage seen on CT scan 'is singularly unimpressive when the brain is seen at autopsy' (Harper & Kril 1986).

The strong impression remains that cerebral atrophy is more common among heavy drinkers than their peers and that this atrophy is differentially distributed with the heaviest emphasis in the anterior regions. As Parsons (1977) points out, the contention that neuropsychological changes are related to cerebral atrophy 'remains at the stage of a good working hypothesis ... but the magnitude of the correlations leaves much of the variance unexplained'.

Psychological deficit in chronic alcoholism

General intellectual function

Reports in numerous reviews are unanimous in failing to find support for a generalized intellectual deterioration in chronic alcoholics even after many years of drinking. Much support for this point of view has come from the use of standardized intelligence tests in particular the summarizing IQ measures of the Wechsler Scales (Wechsler 1941, Murphy 1953, Kaldegg 1956, Peters 1956, Bauer & Johnson 1957, Wechsler 1958, Fitzhugh et al 1960, Plumeau et al 1960, Fitzhugh et al 1965, Malerstein & Belden 1968, Goldstein et al 1970, Goldstein & Shelly 1971, Smith et al 1973). This finding has been supported by studies employing other test measures (Jones 1971, Smith et al 1971, Tarter & Jones 1971, Smith & Layden 1972, Tarter 1973, Parsons 1974). Several studies have even found that their subjects have performed in the superior ranges of intellectual functioning.

Despite this apparently overwhelming evidence, care must be taken in interpreting a preserved IQ score as preservation of an effective intellect. The relative insensitivity of the summary scores of the WAIS, for example, to the presence of even large invasive lesions has been demonstrated (e.g. Case BC, Ch. 1). This insensitivity to intellectual deterioration may be even more marked where the changes, as in alcoholism, take place slowly over time or where the patient has been of a previously high level of intelligence. As mentioned elsewhere, part of this insensitivity lies in the failure to utilize qualitative as well as quantitative data from the standardized tests. It is significant that many of the 'negative' studies using the Wechsler Scales have shown a depression of the Performance measures in relation to the Verbal measures, and several subtests, notably Digit-Symbol Substitution, Block Design and Object Assembly, contribute much of the variance. This Verbal-Performance discrepancy has even been used to support the hypothesis that chronic alcoholism may affect the right hemisphere more than the left (see below—'The right hemisphere hypothesis').

Adaptive behaviour

There is a body of research data suggesting that tests measuring the more adaptive aspects of behaviour are those likely to show consistent loss after years of heavy drinking (Fitzhugh et al 1960, 1965; Vivian et al 1973). It seems that the more highly tests load on factors such as flexibility in problem solving, abstraction and other 'higher order' processes, the more likely they are to be affected in chronic alcoholism. Some studies also point to a continuing decline of certain abilities with duration of alcoholism (Lovibond & Holloway 1968, Tarter & Parsons 1971, Tarter 1973).

Perhaps the best documented cognitive change has been seen with tests of abstraction though the deficits do seem to be test dependent rather than a reflection of a general loss of abstract ability. The finding of a poor performance by alcoholic patients on the Halstead Category Test first reported by Fitzhugh et al (1960) has been replicated on numerous occasions (Fitzhugh et al 1965; Goldstein & Shelly 1971; Jones & Parsons 1971, 1972; Long & McLachlan 1974; Parker & Noble 1977, 1980; Schau & O'Leary 1977; Løberg 1980). Only one study employing a modified version of the Halstead Category Test has proved negative (Goldstein & Chotlos 1965). The Wisconsin Card Sorting Test has proved similarly sensitive to the effects of chronic alcoholism (Tarter 1971; Tarter & Parsons 1971; Tarter 1973, Parker & Noble 1977, 1980; Klisz & Parsons 1979).

The findings of conceptual problem-solving difficulties has received further support from studies employing other tests (e.g. Lhermitte & Signoret 1972, Pishkin et al 1972, Molloy, 1976). Despite this strong line of evidence there are enough studies with negative findings on similar tests to question the generality of a uniform conceptual deficit in all alcoholics (Jonsson et al 1962, Claesson & Carlson 1970, Jones & Parsons 1972, Johnson et al 1973). It is possible that a qualitative examination of responses to the various tests might reveal the common characteristics associated with success or failure.

Several studies have shown poor performance by chronic alcoholics on the Trail Making Test (Fitzhugh et al 1965, Goldstein & Shelly 1971, Løberg 1980). KIeinknecht & Goldstein (1972) consider this test to be a combined measure of psychomotor speed and problem solving but an important element is the ability to shift flexibly between two sets of well known mental operations and it would not be difficult to establish whether this was of major importance in producing a performance deficit in this group of patients. We are constantly being reminded that the determinants of performance on even seemingly simple tests is, indeed, quite complex.

Moreover, as argued below, because of the variation in pathology found in individual cases, it is highly unlikely that chronic alcoholics form a uniform group with a narrow range of psychological deficits. Nevertheless, there appears to be a good deal of agreement that in a high proportion of chronic alcoholics 'the ability to solve problems, to perform complex psychomotor tasks and to manipulate abstract concepts appears to be particularly affected'. (Ron 1977).

Memory and Learning

Until quite recently it had been generally believed that there was little to suggest that memory and learning functions were significantly affected in the detoxified alcoholic who did not show evidence of the Korsakoff syndrome. Most reviewers felt that, while many alcoholics had neuropsychological deficits, these could not be attributed to impaired memory functioning (Parsons & Prigitano 1977). At least two reviews have reported that chronic alcoholics do not perform poorly on the Wechsler Memory Scale (Kleinknecht & Goldstein 1972, Goodwin & Hill 1975). Further negative evidence may be cited for paired-associate learning (Jonsson et al 1962, Claesson & Carlsson 1970, Berglund & Sonesson 1976), Kendall's Memory for Designs (May et al 1970, Berglund & Sonesson 1976, Donovan et al 1976) and the memory measure on the Tactual Performance Test (Fitzhugh et al 1960, 1965).

Nevertheless, the consistently poor performance of alcoholics on the Benton Visual

Retention Test (Claesson & Carlsson 1970, Brewer & Perrett 1971, Page & Linden 1974, Berglund & Sonesson 1976) and serial verbal learning (Allen et al 1971, Weingartner & Faillace 1971, Weingartner et al 1971) means that the presence of some form of memory deficit cannot be lightly dismissed. As with other cognitive deficits in alcoholism, the test-dependent nature of the findings might form a starting point for an examination of their nature.

The 'continuity hypothesis.' In 1980 Ryan and Butters revived interest in the 'continuity hypothesis' first put forward by Ryback in 1971, namely that there might be a continuity between the memory deficits in cocktail-party drinking, alcoholic amnesia and the Wernicke-Korsakoff disorder (Ryan & Butters 1980a). Employing a sophisticated set of measures which increases information-processing demands, these authors have been able to demonstrate 'subtle, but real, learning and memory deficits in alcoholics who report no obvious problems with memory'. The deficits were more marked in alcoholics with subjective complaints of memory problems and, of course, were very marked in a Korsakoff group.

These two latter groups also performed poorly on the three subtests of the Wechsler Memory Scale which require new learning (Logical Memory, Visual Reproduction and Associate Learning). Ryan and Butters support their argument for continuity by pointing to evidence that, for other cognitive deficits, chronic alcoholics perform at a level intermediate between Korsakoff and non-alcoholic control subjects (Oscar-Berman 1973, Butters et al 1977, Glosser et al 1977, Kapur & Butters 1977).

On the anatomical side Ryan and Butters cite only one study (Feuerlein & Heyse 1970) in supposedly intact alcoholics where periventricular atrophy was inferred from echoencephalography. This is, of course, one of the regions consistently implicated in the amnesic syndrome.

The latent or borderline amnesic patient.   One of the practical values arising out of such studies is that it might be possible to detect the degree of risk of memory impairment using these more refined measures. The group of alcoholics with subjective complaints of memory difficulty are termed 'borderline Korsakoff' by Ryan and Butters. This group differs from the true Korsakoff in the degree of preservation of insight, orientation and attempts at compensation. They are capable of slowly acquiring new information and 'this residual memory capacity is sufficient to allow the borderline subject to live on his own' (op. cit. p 196). The findings demonstrate an apparent clinical continuity, but are not sufficient evidence (even if they receive further confirmation) that the memory difficulty in the Korsakoff and non-Korsakoff groups has the same aetiology. At present a two-factor theory appears equally tenable.

Social drinking and cognition

The claim of Parker & Noble (1977) that even social drinking may cause cognitive impairment has received apparent support from studies such as Cala et al (1983). These workers have claimed to show an association between brain shrinkage and fall-off with very low levels of alcohol consumption. Unfortunately, they do not produce data which can be examined, and direct replications of the Parker and Noble study have failed to reveal satisfactory evidence of any general cognitive impairment with social drinking though each study has reported association between one or more measures of consumption and various cognitive test measures (MacVane et al 1982, Parsons & Fabian 1982, Hannon et al 1983). In a later replication study Hannon et al (1987) again found several inverse relationships between cognitive performance and drinking but could not confirm any specific correlations. In both studies they found relationships which would not be predicted by a hypothesis of a harmful effect of social drinking. Furthermore, repeated testing following two weeks of abstention in half the group showed no resulting difference.

Similarly, Carey & Maisto (1987) found no differential improvement after three weeks' abstention in half their group of female social drinkers compared with those who continued to drink, nor was cognitive performance related to drinking pattern in the preceding six months for the whole group.

Bowden (1987) has pointed to the methodological shortcomings of studies reputedly showing cognitive loss from social drinking and found that all the data presented in support of the hypothesis could be explained parsimoniously by an association between innate ability, demographic variables and drinking behaviour. His group (Bowden et al 1988) also directly tested the toxic effect theory (or 'hangover hypothesis') that there is a residual effect on the brain after blood alcohol levels have returned to zero, and found no support for this notion.

Since cognitive changes in chronic alcoholics are well established it follows that those at the upper end of social drinking, variously defined, are probably at risk. Waugh et al (1989) divided their healthy male volunteer drinkers into three groups according to daily consumption: (1) 40g or less; (2) 41-80 g; and (3) 81-130. Only those in group (3) performed poorly and the deficits, while not as severe, were of the same pattern as those of chronic alcoholics. We have used the detection of such a pattern of incipient cognitive change in those at risk as an integral part of the counselling process.

Finally, while pathological evidence is scarce, Harper et al (1988a) found moderate lowering of volume in the brains of moderate drinkers although these did not reach significance.

Evolution of cognitive change

The development of cognitive change is shown schematically in Figure 2.1 and might be hypothesized as follows:

1. Heavy consumption of alcohol results in an increasing danger of cognitive deficit, particularly of the more adaptive functions. There is evidence that such deficit may be detectable even in the so-called social drinker (Parker & Noble 1977, 1980; Jones & Jones 1980). The frequent finding of neuropathological changes in the anterior parts of the brain would tend to support this contention since these regions are differentially involved in adaptive behaviour.

2. With increased drinking, higher levels of information processing become increasingly involved. In our experience, heavy drinkers without a clinically apparent

amnesic difficulty perform poorly on learning or memory tasks which require the subject to organize the material for the process of committing it to memory. Thus we find that patients perform poorly on longer verbal serial learning tasks and complex maze learning (Hunt 1979). Qualitative features strongly suggest that this is a 'frontal' amnesia. This allows a parsimonious explanation of all the cognitive changes, namely that they are caused by some pathological process which affects wide regions of the brain but particularly affects the anterior regions. This point of view is cogently expressed by Ryan (1980):

> It is suggested ... [by Flavell 1971] ... that remembering is a skill, very much like problem-solving, for both demand planful, intentional, goal-directed, future oriented behaviour. According to this view, memorizing new information requires the learner to generate various encoding and retrieval strategies and to test for effectiveness over the course of learning so that inadequate strategies can be located and improved or discarded. With practice, a person may become so skilled at remembering that, under certain circumstances, this process occurs automatically. Given the oft-reported difficulty alcoholics have in problem-solving, it may be more accurate to view alcoholics' encoding and retrieval deficits as by-products of a more general problem-solving deficit. They perform poorly on memory tasks for the same reason they perform poorly on concept-formation tasks: they use inappropriate strategies.

ALCOHOL RELATED BRAIN IMPAIRMENT

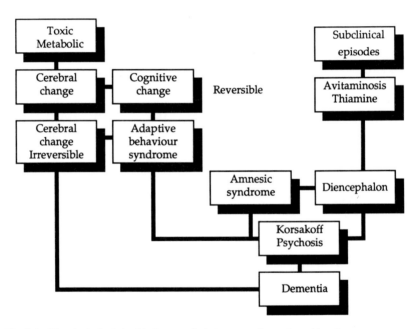

Fig. 2.1 Hypothesized relationship between alcohol consumption and cognitive change.

3. Following the advent of the mentioned cognitive changes some alcoholics continue to drink heavily, develop a poor state of nutrition and suffer the *added* central lesions due to thiamine avitaminosis, consequently developing the Korsakoff amnesic syndrome. Thus every patient with an alcoholic amnesic syndrome should, of necessity, demonstrate on testing the characteristic cognitive difficulties of the frontal variety as well as the amnesia. Such associated difficulties are constantly seen in the

Korsakoff amnesic patient though they are not seen in other amnesic disorders (Janowsky et al 1989). Similarly, the well nourished alcoholic should show clear evidence of loss of these other deficits without the Korsakoff amnesic disorder. Typical cases appear at the end of the chapter.

4. The final end-point of prolonged heavy drinking will be an alcoholic dementia possibly as an extension of whatever process produces the non-amnesic cognitive changes. For obvious reasons alcoholic dementia is often seen coupled with an extreme form of the amnesic syndrome. Cutting considers this accelerated psychological deterioration to be the same in nature but more severe in degree to the 'subclinical psychological deterioration' of 1. and 2. above. 'However, its gradual development, its relative independence of nutritional factors, a longer drinking history, the age and sex composition, and most of all the intellectual decline which is evident, justify its status as separate from Korsakoff's syndrome. Some degree of recovery is the rule rather than the exception.' (Cutting 1978). In summary, the term Korsakoff psychosis refers to a total clinical picture made up of the Korsakoff or general amnesic syndrome plus the non-amnesic cognitive changes of different aetiology plus personality changes.

Reviews of psychological deficits have been given by Kleinknecht & Goldstein (1972), Goodwin & Hill (1975), Grant & Mohns (1975), Tarter (1975, 1976), Parsons (1977), Ron (1977) and Bolter & Hannon (1980). The most extensive recent review is by Bowden (1987). The neuropsychological findings have often been used to infer the nature, extent and location of cerebral damage and have given rise to at least three types of explanation. The first hypothesis, namely that alcohol causes a general intellectual degradation, cannot be sustained in the light of the evidence already outlined. The other hypotheses warrant further consideration. The first of these is the right hemisphere hypothesis.

The right hemisphere hypothesis

Stated simply this hypothesis would read: 'alcoholism disturbs cognitive functions subserved by the right hemisphere more than those subserved by the left'. The fact that this hypothesis could be taken seriously reflects a blind acceptance by some of a simple equation between test score and localization or lateralization of functional deficit.

One major piece of evidence cited in support is the frequent finding on the Wechsler scales of a poorer PIQ than VIQ score in chronic alcoholics. This is then taken to mean greater right than left hemisphere dysfunction since the proponents of this hypothesis appear to take any differential lowering as evidence of lateralization. That such an assumption is unwarranted is shown by lack of clear supporting evidence and has been discussed elsewhere (Walsh 1987). The following scheme is suggested for considering Wechsler scores in relation to laterality of lesion:

1. Brain lesions tend to depress the brain's efficiency irrespective of their location or laterality, i.e. have a nonspecific effect (Satz 1966).
2. Brain lesions also have specific effects according to their laterality. Left-sided

lesions do often depress verbal performances and right-sided lesions do depress visuospatial and visuoconstructive tasks whose performance depends on functions usually allotted to the right hemisphere.

3. Timed tests will be more sensitive to general depression of brain efficiency than well established stereotypes of the kind found on the most commonly used verbal tests. In the Wechsler scales the timed tests are almost exclusively on the Performance scale.

These assumptions would lead to certain expectations, e.g., in left-sided lesions of moderate size (effect) the nonspecific factor may be equal to or greater than the specific (verbal) effect. In all right-sided lesions the specific and nonspecific effects will be additive in depressing scores on the Performance scale. As left-sided lesions expand, the specific (verbal) effect will become greater than the nonspecific with resulting depression of the Verbal score in relation to the Performance score.

Thus: (1) where VIQ and PIQ are equal there may still be a lateralized lesion; (2) a small difference with PIQ less than VIQ may be seen with either a left- or right-sided lesion; (3) a PIQ markedly lower than VIQ suggests a right-sided lesion; (4) a VIQ less than PIQ is strongly suggestive of a left-sided lesion. This logic has borne up well in a large number of cases in our clinic. The general rule needs to be used against a background of other factors, e.g. the fact that the frequency of PIQ greater than VIQ tends to increase towards the lower end of the continuum.

A similarly simple equation of test score to laterality has been made for specific tests such as visuo-constructive tasks like Block Design. This has been discussed in relation to alcohol by Bolter & Hannon (1980) and in the broader context of inference making by Lezak (1976). It is sufficient to repeat here that the score obtained on many tests loosely ascribed to one or other hemisphere or brain system often has a complex determination by factors, only some of which are related to laterality . It is also unwise to compare tests which are relatively stable in the face of cerebral impairment with those which, because of the need for dealing with novel material and new problem-solving have a 'lower threshold of disruption' (Bolter & Hannon 1980). This comment has been made in a number of places, e.g. Chandler & Parsons (1977). An adequate test of the right hemisphere hypothesis would only come by making a comparison between equally sensitive tests differing only in their proven reference to one side of the brain.

The anterior or frontal hypothesis

This hypothesis is by far the most attractive. It asserts that much of the psychological impairment seen in the chronic alcoholic is attributable to brain damage in the anterior regions of the brain. We will use the term 'frontal hypothesis' to accentuate the fact that many of the features can be explained parsimoniously in terms of damage to the frontal lobes. This form of explanation can be examined in the light of both neuropathological and behavioural evidence. The former has already been outlined. The behavioural evidence comes from two areas: (1) cognitive deficit; and (2) personality changes. Of these, the study of cognitive deficits has received by far the most attention.

Cognitive deficit

In 1975 Tarter summarized the evidence in support of the hypothesis and this has been updated by Bolter and Hannon (1980). Neither review was able to confirm the hypothesis in its simple form though the hypothesis did appear 'to account for most of the psychological deficits and [was able to] conceptualize them into a systematic and coherent framework' (Tarter 1975, p361). Evidence cited includes: (1) poor abstract ability or conceptual shifting; (2) lack of flexibility in changing cognitive set; (3) deficient adaptive problem solving; (4) decreased planning capacity; (5) poverty of error utilization; (6) deficient spatial scanning; and (7) disrupted motor regulation. The similarity to the intellectual components of the 'frontal lobe syndrome' can be seen in comparison with any review of frontal lobe function (Walsh 1987). Many of these deficits, especially in their subtle form, may escape detection where only quantitative data from standardized tests are used.

Despite this accumulation of evidence, apparent exceptions have militated against the use of the hypothesis in clinical situations. Some of the reluctance revolves around the absence of single pathognomonic tests. Bolter and Hannon comment that such theories 'should be investigated using tests known to be highly sensitive to brain damage in selective brain regions. Since relatively few such tests exist at the present time, however, researchers should be very cautious about implying that the results on a given test indicate damage in a given area of the brain.' (1980, p 176). Much of the argument against the anticipated efficacy of single tests in the localization of cerebral damage was outlined in Chapter 1. It is worth repeating that the same objection does not apply to the syndrome approach. If an alcoholic subject shows a deficiency on a range of tests, poor performance on which has been shown by 'frontal' patients, it becomes increasingly likely that the deficits are associated with frontal damage. After all, it is possible to diagnose localized frontal pathology reliably with neuropsychological examination even though some elements (test performances) may not be present in the individual case.

A related problem is that not all 'frontal phenomena' have been found in alcoholics (Tarter 1971, 1973). Again, we should not find this surprising since not all patients with proven frontal pathology have all the symptoms and signs that have been abstracted from the literature and claimed as an important part of the frontal lobe syndrome. There is evidence that there may be sub-syndromes related to different areas of the frontal lobes (dorsolateral, basal and medial—see Ch. 5). If this is so, then it may well be that with greater accent on dorsolateral atrophy shown in neuropathological studies, corresponding differences of intellectual regulation may be more commonly associated with alcohol related brain damage than, say, difficulties of self motivation or the flexible control of excitation/inhibition which are more characteristic of damage to the medial and basal areas respectively.

Finally, it would be surprising if any simple hypothesis would account satisfactorily for all the data considering the known variation in pathology, e.g. while the frontal regions appear to be those most frequently and severely affected, this is often accompanied by more widespread damage. In other cases the frontal regions may be less affected than the parietal or temporal areas with a corresponding change in symptomatology. The importance of both the pathological and behavioural evidence is that it should alert the clinician to seek evidence for functional deficits which can be subtle yet pervasive and which may present a serious impediment to management and rehabilitation.

Personality change

Finally, changes in personality have. often been described in chronic alcoholism but there is little systematic evidence in support of any neurological basis for these changes. Suffice it to say that while such findings do not confirm a predominantly anterior (fronto-limbic) hypothesis, they are certainly not contrary to it.

Implications of psychological deficit

The importance of the loss of adaptive abilities was stated very clearly three decades ago by Fitzhugh et al: 'One aspect of continuing sobriety and post-treatment adjustment is perhaps associated with generating constructive alternative solutions to problems or using personal resources in an adaptive fashion. Frequently the discharged alcoholic fails to arrive at alternative solutions even though standard psychometric techniques indicate generally adequate intellectual levels.' (1960, p 402) Such an important implication has been reinforced in recent publications: 'The alcoholic maintains those kind of abilities that would contribute to the appearance of intactness in many of the situations of everyday living, but he also has more difficulties in situations in which high level adaptive functioning is required. Situations of this type often involve such capacities as planning and foresight and the ability to make the appropriate decision on the basis of available evidence.' (Goldstein 1976, p 129). (See also Smith et al 1973, Schau & O'Leary 1977).

It is this 'appearance of intactness' that the neuropsychologist should be able to penetrate for the better management of the person and the greater understanding by his advisors, many of whom are told by psychologists on the basis of standardized test measures that there is no evidence of intellectual loss. The lowering of adaptive abilities often remains concealed until the alcoholic loses his job and needs to seek another or attempts to undertake retraining. Gordon et al (1988) point to the need to utilize knowledge of the alcoholic's neuropsychological deficits as well as psychological factors in assessing the person's ability to benefit from treatment procedures. The present author has found that, like head injured patients, the success of therapy often depends crucially to the degree to which adaptive functions are preserved or compromised.

Premature ageing

The similarity between the nature of the cognitive deficits with alcoholism and those seen with normal ageing has led some to postulate that chronic alcohol abuse may exert its noxious influence by accelerating the biological processes of normal ageing. One of the first studies to suggest this hypothesis was that of Fitzhugh et al (1965).

Support for the hypothesis has come from Kish & Cheney (1969) who found that alcoholics in their thirties performed like non-alcoholic controls at least ten years older. A recent test of this hypothesis by Blusewicz et al (1977) using a broad battery of sensory, perceptual and higher cognitive tests showed a similarity in the differentially poor performance of both young alcoholic and normal elderly subjects on the higher cognitive tasks. This confirmed an earlier finding by others (Goldstein & Shelly 1971, Jones & Parsons 1971). More recently Ryan & Butters (1980b), using experimental tests of memory and learning, showed that the scores of alcoholics were identical with those of older non-alcoholics.

However, there should be caution in taking the similarity of test scores to indicate a common aetiology. The opinion stated frequently in this volume is echoed by Ryan and Butters: 'Different individuals may obtain the same score on a particular test for very different reasons. As a consequence, information about the neuropsychological processes which underlie a subject's performance can only be provided by a detailed qualitative analysis of his responses.' (op. cit.)

Reversibility, recovery and prognosis

There is a growing list of studies demonstrating improvement in cognitive measures after several weeks of abstention from alcohol (Jonsson et al 1962, Carlsson et al 1973, Long & McLachlan 1974, Page & Linden 1974, Clarke & Houghton 1975, Page & Schaub 1977, Hester et al 1980, Schau et al 1980). This list is far from exhaustive but there is general agreement that there may be considerable improvement particularly in the first few weeks of treatment. However, this improvement may be far from complete especially since subtle but incapacitating deficits may still be present in many patients. There do not appear to be any systematic studies of alcoholics who have remained abstinent over considerable periods of time. Cases such as that of WD (see below) suggest that complete recovery may be a rare event.

There is some evidence that there may be a progressive decline in certain abilities with increasing duration of alcoholism (Lovibond & Holloway 1968, Jones & Parsons 1971, Tarter & Parsons 1971, Tarter 1973) and recovery may be less complete in the more chronic (Tarter & Jones 1971). A greater degree of cognitive impairment may suggest a poor prognosis (Berglund et al 1977) or predict relapse (Gregson & Taylor 1977).

CASE EXAMPLES

The following cases illustrate part of the range of difficulties to be seen in individual patients.

Korsakoff psychosis

Case : QT

This 55-year-old former court reporter was referred with a history of anxiety and depression, as well as alcoholism which had resulted in hepatic cirrhosis. He had been retired on a pension five years previously because of ill health. He had had some part-time employment since but was aware of having a good deal of difficulty with his memory.

Just prior to retirement, he had undergone standard intellectual assessment at his regional veterans' hospital. It was noted that his WAIS VIQ was 134 and that his PIQ was 110. The psychologist had concluded that there were 'slight signs of intellectual decline' but no details were available apart from the summary scores, nor was there any evidence that any standard memory examination had been done.

The referral requested an estimate of the extent of his assumed brain impairment with specific reference to his future management. In view of his history of alcoholism the examination began with an appraisal of memory.

Wechsler Memory Scale, Form I

Information	4	Digits Total	14 (8,6)
Orientation	3	Visual Reproduction	2
Mental Control	9	Associate Learning	6.5 (2,0;4,0;5,1)
Memory Passages	3.5		
MQ 86			

The psychometric features of the amnesic syndrome are shown very clearly. The excellent performances on routine mental operations (Mental Control) and immediate memory (Digits) contrast sharply with very poor performances on new learning of both verbal (Memory Passages and new Paired Associates) and the nonverbal task (Visual Reproduction). The Memory Quotient itself, though of less importance, clearly shows a profound lowering when contrasted with the estimate of premorbid cognitive ability based on the high level of his former occupation and the WAIS Verbal IQ of 134 found five years before. The findings were a firm substantiation of the patient's subjective complaints of memory difficulty. In keeping with the presence of insight he did not confabulate. The degree of memory impairment was further tested with the *Rey AVLT*:

List A						List B	List A	List A
Trials	1	2	3	4	5	Recall	Recall	Recognition
Correct	6	8	7	8	9	3	5	13

This test served to confirm the presence and severity of his memory deficit. His ability to acquire new verbal information was exceedingly poor for a man of his background. On each trial most of the correctly recalled words came from the end of the list (recency effect) and he continued to produce one response word from outside the list. This was the same word which he had produced earlier as an incorrect response in paired-associate teaming. There was interference from the interpolated list. However, in keeping with findings in the literature as well as clinical experience, his recognition memory was vastly superior to his spontaneous recall.

To examine memory for more complex visual material the *Rey Figure* was used. His first attempt was both poorly organized and poorly executed (Fig 2.2).

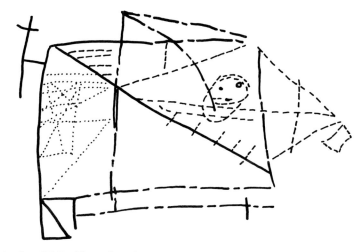

Fig. 2.2   Case QT. Rey Figure. Copy 1.

He was asked to copy the figure again taking more care. This produced some improvement (Fig. 2.3) and largely negated the possibility that a visuo-constructive deficit lay at the basis of his poor copying performance.

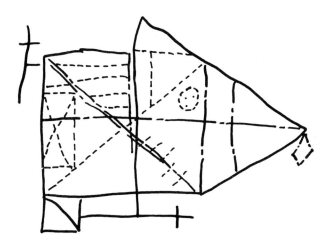

Fig 2.3   Case QT. Rey Figure. Copy 2.

Despite this added experience with the second attempt, the recall at three minutes produced virtually nothing (Fig 2.4). It had become apparent that the patient had an amnesic syndrome of marked severity.

In line with the findings of intellectual deficits in the chronic alcoholic, QT was given a series of tests related to adaptive abilities, including some which may be

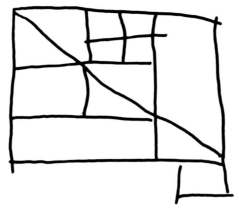

Fig. 2.4 Case QT. Rey Figure. Recall.

considered sensitive to frontal lobe dysfunction. On several of these he produced unexpectedly good results:

Colour-Form Sorting Test. No difficulty whatsoever.

Verbal Fluency. F-18; A-17; S-23. No apparent difficulty.

Trial Making Test. A. 38 seconds. B. 51 seconds. Marginally slow but unremarkable.

However, he encountered more difficulty with maze learning:

Porteus Maze Test. Despite an overall mental age score of 13.5 years, he failed the first trial on Years VIII, IX, X and XII. This would be well below his premorbid intelligence level as estimated five years previously.

Austin Maze Test. He applied himself diligently and continued to concentrate although he made little or no progress until the test was finally abandoned:

Trials	1	2	3	4	5	6	7	8	9	10
Errors	64	25	51	27	27	24	16	19	22	21

Trials	11	12	13	14	15	16	discontinued			
Errors	51	25	22	14	20	50				

While his severe memory deficit no doubt accounted for much of his poor performance, he also showed some of the qualitative features that we have noted in chronic alcoholic patients without clinical or psychometric evidence of a memory deficit (Hunt 1979), in patients with closed head injuries where the impact quite literally falls on the frontal lobes, and in patients with confirmed frontal lobe lesions.

He continued to make prohibited diagonal moves, turned back along previously successful parts of the maze, and moved more than one step at a time. This rule breaking was not due to his failure to remember the instructions as he often commented that he realized he should not do these things thus showing the classical 'dissociation between knowing and doing'. He also realized the parts of the maze with which he was having difficulty but was unable to utilize this fact to bring about some degree of learning. It seemed likely that his complex learning was made virtually impossible by a compounding of his memory difficulty with the 'problem of error utilization' (see Walsh 1987).

At this level of difficulty he showed no evidence whatsoever of new learning. The opinion was given that the prognosis for effective collaboration with rehabilitation was exceedingly poor despite the preservation of a degree of insight into the presence of his memory defect.

There was little evidence at the time to indicate whether this patient would remain in his present state or progress to an ultimate state of alcoholic dementia. The probability of this latter eventuality was rendered more likely when the patient admitted that he was still drinking at weekends despite all efforts of his doctors to persuade him to abstain.

This case also illustrates the common finding that not all aspects of 'frontal' disorders of intellectual regulation or conceptual difficulty will be seen in an individual case. This is also true of cases (such as cerebral tumours) with unequivocal frontal lesions. The frontal lobe syndrome is an abstraction derived from groups of patients and care should be taken not to rule out frontal lobe dysfunction on the basis of absence of one or more commonly reported signs.

Case: TH

TH, a factory worker, was admitted to hospital at the age of 57 with a six month history of lethargy and weakness. The referring physician commented 'We think her symptoms and signs are largely due to alcohol. Her drinking has increased over the past 17 months since her separation from her husband and the death of her son-in-law. She also has hypercalcaemia for which she is being investigated. A CT scan shows frontal lobe atrophy but no discrete lesions'. No reference was made to any loss of higher intellectual functions.

One of the hospital psychologists carried out an abbreviated memory and intellectual examination after the patient had been in hospital for two weeks.

WMS, Form I

Information	3	Digits Total	10 (6,4)
Orientation	1	Visual Reproduction	2
Mental Control	1	Associate Learning	4.5 (3,0;3,0;3,0)
Logical Memory	2 (3,1)		
MQ 67			

TH was sure of her age, birthdate, the present political leader, and the current year, but was unable to give even an approximation to the month and day. She presented well in everyday conversation which, if kept to simple, familiar topics gave no indication of the severity of her amnesic syndrome.

The examining psychologist felt that her scores on selected WAIS subtests were probably not significantly below what might have been expected from her education, occupation and social background, and the quality of her verbal responses. The possible exception was a slow performance on Digit-Symbol substitution.

WAIS (age scaled scores)

Information	9	Digit-Symbol	7
Comprehension	7	Block Design	10
Similarities	8	Object Assembly	9
Digit Span	10		

On the Colour-Form Sorting Test TH carried out form sorting with correct verbalization: 'set of squares, set of round rings, set of triangles. Asked to sort the pieces another way she produced the following:

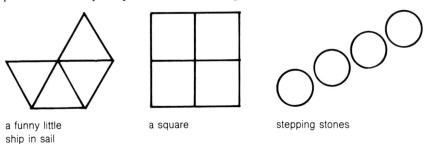

a funny little   a square   stepping stones
ship in sail

She was unable to arrive at the colour sorting and had difficulty in grasping this second possibility even when it was demonstrated to her. Although no further exploration of 'frontal' functions was carried out, the characteristics of her performance on this task would be in keeping with the known evidence of frontal atrophy in this case.

On interview this patient was completely unable to give a consistent chronology of the principal events in her life though she could recall some of them as isolated items especially on direct questioning. No details of anything she recounted from recent months made any coherent sense.

It seems surprising that this woman was said to have been coping in her day-to-day life though she admitted to numerous instances of forgetting, e.g. coming home without having purchased items for which she had set out. It was also noted that, in common with other patients with preserved insight, she did not confabulate.

When the physicians received the diagnosis of 'Korsakoff amnesic syndrome' they were surprised since she presented so well on direct questioning. The diagnosis was readily accepted after a demonstration at the bedside where, despite being able to repeat seven digits with relative ease, she failed supraspan learning (eight digits) despite an almost endless repetition of the same series. Further strong confirmation of her amnesia came from the nurses' description of her ward behaviour.

This is a typical example of the degree to which a person may be able to continue in a familiar environment despite an advanced amnesic syndrome.

Borderline Korsakoff psychosis

Case: QS

QS was referred by a neurologist with the following information: 'This former boxer, aged 56 years, who overuses alcohol considerably, has been becoming more and more depressed and amnestic lately and is determined to do something about it. He has an idée fixe about certain subjects which amounts at times to a paranoia—at least a flavour of same—and all in all it is thought by both myself and the general practitioner that he is slowly dementing'.

A neuropsychological examination with special regard to memory was requested to see whether the clinical impression was borne out on examination.

Neuropsychological examination

The history of his subjective complaints, excessive alcohol intake, and possible effects from repeated trauma arising from his period as a professional boxer, suggested a broad intellectual examination beginning with an examination of memory. The possibility of presenile dementia was kept in mind, together with other less likely causes for his memory disorder.

WMS, Form I

Information	5	Digits Total	12 (7,5)
Orientation	5	Visual Reproduction	6
Mental Control	6	Associate Learning	6.5 (3,0;5,0;5,0)
Memory Passages	6.5		

MQ 93

Although the Memory Quotient could be considered in the normal range, especially for a man of his occupational and educational background, the differential pattern was consistent with a general amnesic syndrome of the type seen in the 'borderline Korsakoff' patient (Ryan & Butters 1980a). QS was correctly oriented, had good immediate memory and, though a trifle slow, carried out routine mental operations without mistakes. In contrast, all forms of new learning were poor and he had insight into his memory shortcomings. Further evidence of amnesic difficulty came with the Rey Figure (Figs. 2.5 and 2.6). His copy was complete and carried out in an orderly sequence with spontaneously corrected errors. (Copy score 35, 90th centile). In contrast there was marked impoverishment in the reproduction from memory, which reached only the 10th centile.

Having established the presence of an amnesic syndrome the examination was then extended to see whether the neurologist's suspicion of 'dementia' could be supported.

It was noted that immediate memory span was preserved, an unusual finding in any measurable degree of dementia. Several other possibilities suggested themselves, viz. general intellectual impairment associated with his career as a boxer, presenile dementia, or cognitive deterioration associated with chronic alcoholism. Our experience suggested that if any of these were the cause of the severe memory disorder they should be accompanied by an obvious and general fall-off in adaptive functions. On tests of this hypothesis he performed as follows:

Colour-Form Sorting Test. QS had no difficulty verbalizing the two concepts and shifting readily from one to the other.

Porteus Maze Test. A mental age score of 14.5 years with none of the features seen

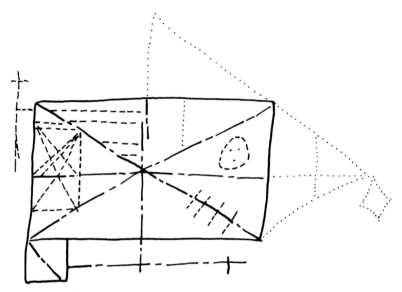

Fig. 2.5   Case QS. Rey Figure. Copy.

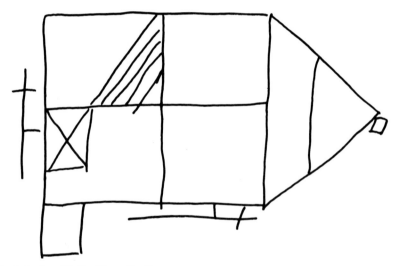

Fig. 2.6   Case QS. Rey Figure. Recall.

with clearly defined frontal (or widespread) pathology.

Verbal Fluency. The patient's mean score of 13.7 was above that anticipated. He did, however, disregard the instructions by giving many capitalized words. These were not included in the scoring.

Trail Making Test. Although this test is not specifically related to frontal lobe functions, since it is affected by lesions in many locations, it does provide an opportunity to observe on Part B the difficulty which frontal subjects have in flexibly shifting sets and resisting the tendency to run on an 'inert stereotype' (Luria 1973).

Our patient was a little slow on Part A (43 seconds) and much more so on Part B (115 seconds) but did not make any errors.

In the testing time available two verbal and two performance subtests of the WAIS were given:

Information	10	Digit-Symbol	6
Similarities	9	Block Design	4

Testing was terminated when QS was having difficulty solving the intermediate level items of the Block Design subtest. There were indications that he was unable to handle the material when it became complex. No constructional deviations were seen.

Although the examination was less than ideal the opinion was given that there was strong confirmation of the presence of an axial-type amnesia together with indications of decline in other intellectual processes which were also markedly slowed. The overall pattern was thought to be more probably due to alcohol than to any other cause, though trauma from boxing may have contributed. The opinion was also given that further impairment from alcohol would produce an obvious alcoholic dementia.

Postscript: The report of the CT scan became available after this examination: 'The appearances are those of moderate cortical and cerebellar atrophy, particularly affecting the frontal lobes'.

A Korsakoff variant

Case: AY

This 55-year-old female clerk was seen at a rehabilitation hospital to which she had been admitted with a three week history of difficulty in walking and paraesthesia of the lower limbs. On admission she was quite unable to walk unaided. Her gait was markedly ataxic and it soon became apparent that she also had a disorder of recent memory. A diagnosis of peripheral neuropathy and central nervous system damage due to alcoholism was made. Supplementary vitamin therapy was commenced. The psychologist was asked to comment on the presence and severity of any alcohol related cognitive impairment.

AY was unable to provide a coherent account of her educational, occupational and social history though many discrete items could be elicited on specific questioning. She thought that she had left school at about the age of 17 years and remained at home for some time before gaining employment as a clerk. She was unable to recall why she had not gone straight to work upon completing school. She was vague about the details of her marriage but she thought that she was in her early twenties when she married a builder. The marriage was childless and she and her husband separated after sixteen years but have remained good friends. Her most recent work had been serving meals to the patients in a large private hospital, which she enjoyed. She could not, however, remember when or why she stopped work there. She lived alone in a flat and admitted to drinking two or three bottles of beer every day after work, and occasionally spirits as well.

First examination

AY was slightly nervous, had an agreeable manner, and co-operated fully with testing. She persevered in the face of considerable difficulties. The marked similarity between the standard intellectual and memory tests on two occasions a month apart can be seen from the following summary. The pro rata values entered by the psychologist in the reports one month apart have been retained solely for comparison over time.

WMS	Form I	Form II
Information	3	2
Orientation	4	4
Mental Control	6	6
Memory Passages	2.5	4
Digits Total	13 (7,6)	12 (7.5)
Visual Reproduction	11	13
Associate Learning	9.5 (5,0;6,0;6,1)	7.5 (5,0;5,0;5,0)
MQ	96	96

	WAIS	NHAIS (one month later)
Information	11	11
Comprehension	13	9
Similarities	12	13
Digit Span	12	11
Digit-Symbol	4	5
Block Design	7	5
Object Assembly	6	8
Prorated VIQ	116	110
Prorated PIQ	89	91

The first examination revealed a profound difficulty with recent memory for new verbal material in the presence of well preserved old verbal information and intact immediate memory. However, the pattern differed from that of a general amnesic syndrome in the relatively good performance on Visual Reproduction. There was no evidence of confabulation.

In order to check the possible preservation of nonverbal memory the Rey Figure was given. There were several minor inaccuracies in the copy (score 32, 50th centile) which was also very poorly planned (Fig. 2.7).

Only a modicum of information (score 7, below the 10th percentile) was recalled after three minutes (Fig. 2.8). It had been noted in her attempts on the WMS Visual Reproduction that the patient had been unsure of her recall and would have reproduced very little had she not been encouraged to put down what she thought the designs looked like no matter how uncertain she felt. This encouragement did not help with the Rey Figure.

Performances on the selected subtests of the WAIS showed the usual differential features seen in chronic alcoholic and Korsakoff patients in favour of 'cystallized' tests. A subsequent reappraisal of the Block Design subtest seemed to suggest a problem solving difficulty with an inability to deal with the 'embedded' designs (see Ch. 1).

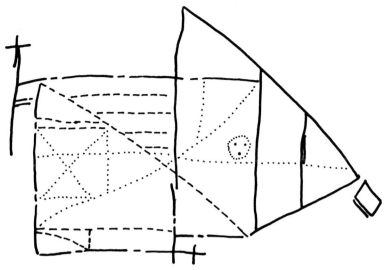

Fig. 2.7   Case AY. Rey Figure. Copy.

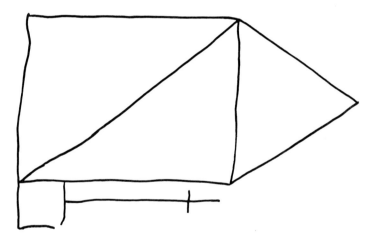

Fig. 2.8   Case AY. Rey Figure. Recall.

Second examination

After four weeks of energetic vitamin supplement therapy the patient was re-examined. It was discouraging to note that there had been absolutely no change in the standardized memory and intellectual tests. Another nonverbal memory task, the Benton Visual Retention Test, at this examination yielded a score of 3 correct with 13 errors (expected 7 correct and 3 errors, or better) which further supported the presence of a general, i.e. nonspecific memory disorder. Other tests were consistent with an alcoholic aetiology. This case is presented because we have seen this pattern of performance in a number of patients, all of whom have had clearly evident alcoholic damage with no other neurological manifestations. Psychometrically the features are:

1. exceedingly poor memory for verbal material
2. preserved immediate memory for digits, both forwards and backwards
3. apparently preserved nonverbal memory as tested by the Visual Reproduction of the WMS but poor performance on other nonverbal memory tests (Benton VRT, Rey Figure).

The reasons for the apparent sparing of one nonverbal memory test (while perhaps due to the short time between presentation and recall) invite study. In the meantime we prefer to think of it as a variant of the Korsakoff Syndrome and it was reported as such in this case. The severity of the amnesia and the failure of this and other associated intellectual impairment to improve in the slightest degree was thought to indicate a poor prognosis and a sheltered environment was suggested for continuing medical care with neuropsychological review after one year.

All cases of this kind we have seen in the decade since AY's presentation have shown a uniformly poor prognosis.

Borderline Korsakoff syndrome

Case: VQ

This 47-year-old man who worked as a leather cutter in a shoe factory was referred from a general medical unit of our hospital where he was being treated for cardiac failure. He was said to be an alcoholic with a poor dietary history and the physicians wished to know whether there was evidence of organic brain impairment.

He stated that he had commenced drinking at the age of 14 and freely admitted that he had drunk an average of 24 to 30 glasses of beer a day for the past 20 years. He was firm in his denial of being an alcoholic though he said he had known people who were. Such people, he said, 'can't help themselves. They fall over all the time and get into trouble with the police'. He did however admit to having been arrested for drunkenness some dozen times and volunteered the fact that he often missed meals because he was drinking. He had suffered three attacks of rheumatic fever at the ages of 12, 17 and 19 years. He cooperated readily with testing which began with the *Wechsler Memory Scale*, Form I:

Information	6	Digits Total	12(8,4)
Orientation	4	Visual Reproduction	5
Mental Control	6	Associate Learning	10.5 (2,1;4,2;5,2)
Memory Passages	8		
MQ 93			

There was no evidence of confabulation. While the overall score did not appear depressed below that anticipated from his educational, social and occupational background he did appear to have some difficulty with retaining new material (Memory Passages, Visual Reproduction, difficult Paired Associates). In contrast, his immediate memory (Digits Forward) was very good and he was correctly oriented in time and place. The memory examination was then extended:

RAVLT

List A						*List B*	*List A*	*List A*
Trial	1	2	3	4	5	Recall	Recall	Recognition
Correct	6	10	9	10	9	3	7	15

An examination of the pattern of recall showed that this varied from trial to trial suggesting that VQ was unable to develop an effective strategy to aid recall. When this is taken with the plateau effect in the learning curve and the excellence of recognition memory the performance is typical of many alcoholics we have seen in the stage before a disorder of memory becomes clinically apparent. There was also an interference effect apparent in the recall of List B. A separate check of homogeneous interference using two triads of words as described by Christensen (1975) yielded the same result. The memory and learning difficulty has all the characteristics of 'frontal amnesia' where the principal problem appears to lie in disruption of the intellectual processes of organizing the material for the purpose of committing it to memory. Such an interpretation is supported by VQ's performance on the Rey Figure (Figs. 2.9, 2.10). The copy was somewhat careless and carried out in a piecemeal fashion without an apparent plan. (Score 32, 50th centile).

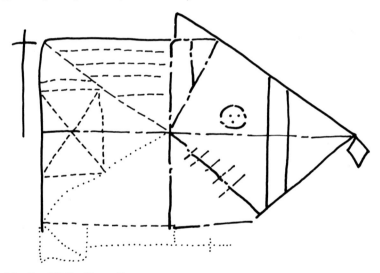

Fig. 2.9 Case VQ. Rey Figure. Copy.

There was considerable impoverishment in the recall at three minutes (Score 13.5, 10th centile).

A short form of the *WAIS* was used to sample other areas of cognitive functionings:

Information	11	Digit-Symbol	16
Similarities	11	Block Design	7
Digit Span	11	Object Assembly	6

The pattern of verbal subtests suggested a native intellectual endowment at least in the bright normal range, which reinforced the idea that his performance on the

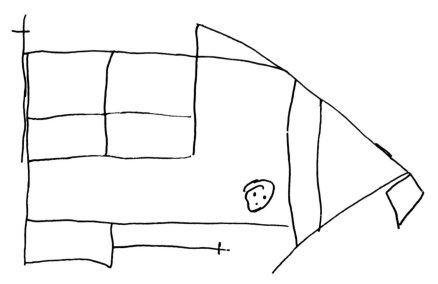

Fig. 2.10 Case VQ. Rey Figure. Recall.

Wechsler Memory Scale was below par. The relatively poor showing on the selected Performance Scale subtests was suggestive of alcohol related brain damage but insufficient qualitative information was provided by the psychologist to warrant further comment. It is noteworthy that VQ failed both trials of Item 2 on Block Design and was unable to solve others when extra time was allowed. Like frontally damaged patients VQ solved the problems quickly when a grid was placed over the designs thus providing a partial programme for their solution.

Trail Making Test. Part A–65 seconds. Part B–165 seconds. Apart from being generally slow on both parts, VQ had difficulty in alternating the two sequences of Part B, where on three occasions he could not resist the impulse to follow the alphabetical stereotype (e.g. G-H instead of G-8, J-K instead of J-11) although he clearly knew what to do and indicated this by the time of his first error. This difficulty with inhibiting competing response tendencies is also seen frequently in frontal lobe impairment and thus is not an unexpected finding in the performance of many chronic alcoholics on this test.

The difficulties encountered by this patient might be classified as a borderline Korsakoff syndrome.

A non-alcoholic memory disorder in a heavy drinker

Case: YN

A 38-year-old man whose jobs had included labouring and truck driving was referred for neuropsychological assessment from a half-way house for alcoholics because of his complaints of poor memory. He had been a heavy drinker for about twenty years but had been sober for ten weeks prior to testing. He complained of periods of confusion and 'mini-blackouts' after which he was unable to recall what he had said or thought.

This confusion was also apparent during his ten weeks of sobriety. He stated that his memory difficulty interfered with his day-to-day living and, for example, he would read a section of a book without remembering the details and would not remember if he had read the book previously.

YN had sustained a head injury in a road traffic accident 20 years previously at the age of 18 when he had fallen from his motorcycle. The patient himself believed that it was from this date that he had experienced difficulty in remembering. The details of the accident, including the nature and severity of the patient's injuries, and associated loss of consciousness, were unknown after this long interval.

First examination

Examination began with the *Wechsler Memory Scale*, Form I:

Information	5	Digits Total	11 (5,6)
Orientation	5	Visual Reproduction	14
Mental Control	6	Associate Learning	8 (4,0;6,0;6,0)
Memory Passages	5		
MQ 93			

Two things are immediately apparent. Firstly, YN was having marked difficulty with acquiring new information. Secondly, this memory difficulty was quite specific to verbal material. He produced a perfect score on Visual Reproduction. Despite the strong alcoholic history such an amnestic disorder cannot be considered under the rubric of the Korsakoff amnesic syndrome, which is general, not material-specific. Verbal specific memory difficulties are normally associated with lateralized lesions, being most clear-cut with damage to the deep or medial portions of the left (dominant) temporal lobe (Walsh 1987).

It was decided to compare the three Performance Scale subtests most frequently associated with chronic alcoholism with a short form of the Verbal Scale of the WAIS. There was a relatively poor performance on Digit-Symbol Substitution but scores on the other Performance tests were not significantly different from the verbal scores. There were no qualitative features in any of his performances to suggest other focal or general cerebral impairment. At least part of the depression of the Digit-Symbol score may also have been due to his memory difficulty.

WAIS

Information	13	Digit-Symbol	7
Similarities	12	Block Design	11
Digit Span	10	Object Assembly	10

The findings were thought to support the patient's attribution of his memory difficulty to the head injury sustained many years before. His Memory Quotient of 93 was well below that expected on the basis of his better intelligence test subscores. The difference appeared solely related to the verbal-specific memory difficulty. The dissociation between YN's ability to learn verbal and nonverbal material was strongly reinforced by his near perfect score (34 out of 36) in the recall of the Rey Figure whereas he required three attempts before he could recall correctly two triads of simple words. Further evidence that YN's memory disorder was material specific rather than general was that he retained the sensorimotor illusion of Charpontiev in a normal way suggesting that his incidental memory in this nonverbal sphere was normal. Amnesic patients with bilateral involvement of the memory structures of the temporal lobes immediately lose the illusion following interfering activity (Luria 1973).

The organizers of the half-way house were informed that there appeared to be a specific memory disorder apparently of long standing, related not to his alcoholism, but to an earlier injury. It was possible that, superimposed on this, there may have been episodic worsening of memory performance related to his alcoholic blackouts. The relation of alcoholic blackouts to memory disorders needs further elucidation (Tarter 1976). The need to cease drinking altogether was stressed to the patient to ensure that his already depressed verbal memory was not compounded by an even more severe bilateral amnesic syndrome.

YN was next seen some two and a half years later. He appeared healthy and well nourished and was neat and tidy. He said that he had continued to be abstinent since his previous visit and had been in his present job for over a year. He was alert and well oriented and eager to do well on the tests. It was decided to re-examine his memory and also to check other adaptive abilities in case subtle changes were present, especially as the first examination had been somewhat restricted in scope.

Second examination

WMS, Form II

Information	6	Digits Total	10 (6,4)
Orientation	5	Visual Reproduction	12
Mental Control	8	Associate Learning	7 (3,0;4,1;3,1)
Memory Passages	3		
MQ 90			

Once again he displayed a differentially poor verbal memory, the pattern being almost identical with that on the first examination.

The *Rey AVLT* strongly confirmed the verbal memory difficulty:

List A						List B	List A	List A
Trial	1	2	3	4	5	Recall	Recall	Recognition
Correct	5	6	7	7	8	3	6	9

The verbal-specific nature of the patient's problem was highlighted by his good performance on nonverbal memory tasks:

Lhermitte and Signoret tests

Spatial memory task. All items were correctly recalled on only the second trial. His spontaneous recall at five minutes was without error.

Logical memory task. All items were correctly recalled on the first trial. YN was able to verbalize the principles on which the matrix was set out on the test board.

Austin Maze Test. The level of performance was free of qualitative errors and at or above the level expected from his educational and occupational background. There was not the slightest indication of any adaptive behaviour syndrome that would have been anticipated on the basis of an alcohol aetiology.

Trials	1	2	3	4	5	6	7	8	9	10	11
Errors	11	6	6	4	4	2	1	1	1	1	0

Porteus Maze Test. YN made only one error in the total series of problems.
Colour-Form Sorting Test. In keeping with his immediate grasp of the Lhermitte logical memory task, YN was able to execute and verbalize both categories.

In summary, this patient continues to have a quite marked verbal–specific memory defect which has remained stable over a considerable period. There was no evidence of any associated neuropsychological deficits indicative of alcohol related brain damage.

YN's second visit provided an interesting addendum. Very little information on his occupational background had been available from the early file. Apparently this was communicated to the patient, who arrived for assessment having compiled a social, educational, and occupational history which included no less than 25 residential addresses and the names of 34 individuals or firms for whom YN had worked over more than two decades. Most of the jobs involved simple labouring work. The compilation was made largely by the patient himself and though it was not possible to check, there were certain internal consistencies which suggested that the chronology was correct. Thus, even before the examination began, it was apparent that YN was able to retain detailed information over very long periods and the 'achronogenesis' which so often characterizes alcoholic memory defects was not in evidence.

A non-amnesic intellectual disorder

Case: WD

This former university graduate and college lecturer was first seen at the age of 46. He suffered from a chronic anxiety state and gave a history of heavy drinking for the previous eight years. He had commenced drinking at the age of 20 and had been compulsorily retired from his post some time before his referral to us because the continuation of his psychiatric condition and alcoholism had rendered him unable to cope. His marriage had broken down and his psychiatrist was pessimistic about his prognosis. At that time he showed clear signs of alcoholic liver damage and peripheral neuritis. He was worried by blank periods in his memory, and inability to think clearly and to recall names and dates.

Despite these difficulties he continued treatment for his alcoholism and (apart from one brief relapse) had remained abstinent, living mostly in semi-sheltered environments and continuing contact with his medical advisors throughout. Shortly after becoming abstinent he recommenced his legal studies and successfully completed the academic requirements for a law degree. It is noteworthy that he was able to cope with little more than half an academic workload each year although he was not engaged on other work and, on a number of occasions, he passed his subjects only with supplementary examinations or after repeating the subject. Throughout these years he complained of difficulty in concentration and memory, aggravated by periods of anxiety and depression.

Five years later he was again referred for assessment. His doctor was concerned about his ability to work effectively in his proposed new profession and wondered whether neuropsychological assessment might help with planning his future employment. He reported that during the current year WD had entered a full-time professional preparation course of supervised assignments and had found a full day's work and concentration very difficult. The quality of his assignments was so far below the expected standard that doubts were expressed about his ability to carry out unsupervised professional work.

Scaled Scores	First examination (age 46) WAIS	Second examination (age 51) NHAIS
Information	17	-
Comprehension	18	-
Similarities	17	-
Digit Span	10	13
Verbal IQ	134	-
Digit–Symbol	14	11
Block Design	7	6
Picture Arrangement	9	9
Object Assembly	5	6
Performance IQ	104	99
WMS MQ	122	143

The first testing results were made available from another centre. They show some features frequently seen with chronic alcohol abuse, a WAIS PIQ considerably below the VIQ—the result of extremely poor performance on the Block Design and Object Assembly tasks together with a relatively poor showing on Picture Arrangement. On the constructional tasks he failed consistently when the items became complex but showed no constructional deviations or other qualitative features of the type seen with localized lesions in the posterior portions of the right hemisphere. The difficulties on the performance subtests were so marked as to raise the possibility in the psychologist's mind at that time of a right hemisphere lesion, but his opinion was that these difficulties arose from problem-solving deficiencies possibly associated with alcoholic damage to the frontal lobes. It was suggested that the patient be referred again for further psychological exploration of his difficulties but this was not done.

At the second testing five years later there was a remarkable similarity on comparable subtests of intelligence. There had been an improvement in the Wechsler Memory Scale where the patient reached the MQ ceiling of 143. The Rey AVLT was commenced but discontinued when the patient achieved a perfect score of 15 on the second trial with every item placed in the correct order. It seemed unlikely that any measurable degree of amnesic syndrome could be present with such results. It should be remembered at this stage that the patient was complaining of difficulty with 'memory' and one explanation of this might be the presence of a 'frontal' amnesia.

With intelligent subjects who have preserved many of their well-tried strategies of learning this difficulty may not emerge unless the material is both novel and complex. The presence of a stable and long-standing cognitive deficit was clearly possible in the light of the unimproved scores on several of the performance subtests of the NHAIS. At this juncture it was decided to utilize more complex memory and learning tasks:

Rey Figure (Figs. 2.11, 2.12). There was a marked fall in score from an almost perfect copy (score 35) to a recall score around the 50th centile (score 22.5). It would have been tempting to classify this as an example of frontal amnesia. However, the sequential order of the copy followed a logical sequence unlike those described elsewhere. All that could be concluded was that the patient had difficulty recalling novel complex spatial material.

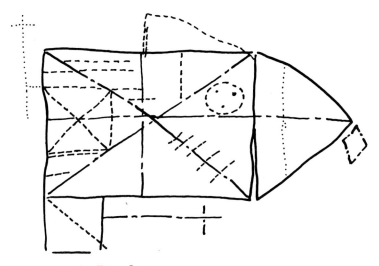

Fig. 2.11   Case WD. Rey Figure. Copy.

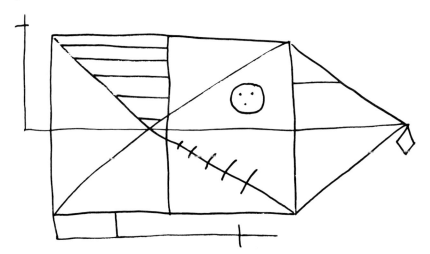

Fig. 2.12   Case WD. Rey Figure. Recall.

Austin Maze. WD experienced considerable difficulty in learning the Milner pathway. He was quite clearly surprised at his inability to eradicate errors that he was well able to verbalize. In line with other cases his error-free performance on the 20th trial should not be taken as evidence that he had 'learned' the pathway.

Trial	1	2	3	4	5	6	7	8	9	10
Errors	16	11	7	7	9	3	1	7	3	3

Trial	11	12	13	14	15	16	17	18	19	20
Errors	7	7	1	1	2	2	2	6	1	0

His inability to utilize the information from his errors to produce an error-free performance stood in sharp contrast to the excellence of his performance on the Rey AVLT and an estimate of his premorbid ability based on the verbal subtests of the WAIS. We would have expected an errorless performance in no more than six to eight trials on these figures.

The difficulty seemed to be one of error utilization. We have seen such a deficit most clearly in patients with proven frontal lobe lesions, where it forms one of the most reliable indicators of frontal pathology. The sensitivity of the maze test in bringing out this difficulty has been confirmed in many cases in our clinic since the distinction between error recognition and error utilization was made by Konow and Pribram in 1970. It is important to note that a deficit of error utilization has also been described in alcoholics (Tarter 1973) and we have confirmed this finding in a group of alcoholics without clinical or psychometric evidence of a memory disorder (Hunt 1979).

It is important to know that most patients with this difficulty continue to make single or multiple errors on many trials even after reaching a criterion of one errorless trial. This failure to eradicate errors may have disastrous consequences outside the testing situation.

On the basis of the findings we hypothesized that WD might be suffering from alcohol related cerebral damage with consequent lowering of adaptive abilities associated with the frontal and possibly other areas of the cortex. A CT scan shortly after the second testing revealed cerebral atrophy of mild to moderate degree maximal in the frontal regions. If this patient was having trouble with his professional assignments due to diminution of the organizing and adaptive abilities which depend upon the integrity of the frontal lobes, his history of difficulty in the last year where he had had to organize assignments for himself becomes a little clearer. He may have achieved his passes in academic subjects in the preceding years because his instructors had been standing over him acting as a surrogate set of frontal lobes. Thus it was felt worthwhile to extend this examination at a later session to ascertain the extent of disruption of WD's adaptive abilities but, once again, the patient became unavailable for testing.

Certainly this case illustrates the fact that deficits of complex intellectual behaviour may be present after a considerable period of abstention from alcohol. The fact that the deficits may be subtle does not mean that they are minor. It remains to be seen whether this patient and others like him are able to cope with occupations and professions which demand the constant application of adaptive abilities and not the mere repetition of inert stereotypes (Luria 1973) either acquired before the ravages of alcoholism or handed on to them by others. All our clinical experience would suggest the contrary. In a number of them a purely psychiatric basis for their inability to cope had been postulated before these subtle but disabling disorders were revealed by neuropsychological examination. Like the present patient most of them had been thought to be intellectually intact on the basis of 'normal' to 'above average' summary scores on the Wechsler scales and their impressive social presentation.

Thus, subtle but incapacitating cognitive deficit may continue to exist in patients, even after years of abstention, without any *obvious* clinical or psychometric features of impairment.

REFERENCES

Albert M S, Butters N, Levin J 1979 Temporal gradients in the retrograde amnesia of patients with alcoholic Korsakoff's disease. Archives of Neurology 36: 211–216

Allen R, Faillace L, Reynolds D 1971 Recovery of memory functioning in alcoholics following prolonged alcoholic intoxication. Journal of Nervous and Mental Disease 153: 417–423

Barbizet J 1970 Human memory and its pathology. Freeman, San Francisco

Bauer R, Johnson D 1957 The question of deterioration in alcoholism. Journal of Consulting Psychology 21: 296

Benton A L, Hamsher K deS, Varney N R, Spreen O (eds) 1983 Contributions to neuropsychological assessment. Oxford University Press, New York

Berglund M, Leijonquist H, Horlen M 1977 Prognostic significance and reversibility of cerebral dysfunction in alcoholics. Journal of Studies of Alcohol 38: 1761–1770

Berglund M, Sonesson B 1976 Personality impairment in alcoholism: its relation to regional cerebral blood flow and psychometric performance. Quarterly Journal of Studies on Alcohol 37: 298–310

Berlyne N 1972 Confabulation. British Journal of Psychiatry 120: 31–39

Blusewicz M J, Dustman R E, Schenkenberg T, Beck E C 1977 Neuropsychological correlates of chronic alcoholism and aging. Journal of Nervous and Mental Disease 165: 348–355

Bolter J F,Hannon R 1980 Cerebral damage associated with alcoholism: a re-examination. The Psychological Record 30: 165–179

Bonhoeffer K 1904 Der Korsakowsche Symptomen–complex in seinen Beziehungen zu den verschiedenen. Krankheitsformen Allgemeine Zeitschrift für Psychiatrie 6: 744–752

Bowden S C 1987 Brain impairment in social drinkers? No cause for concern. Alcoholism 11 : 407–410

Bowden S C, Walton N H, Walsh K W 1988 The hangover hypothesis and the influence of moderate social drinking on mental ability. Alcoholism 12: 25– 29

Brewer C, Perrett L 1971 Brain damage due to alcohol consumption: an air-encephalographic psychometric and electroencephalographic study. British Journal of Addiction 66: 170–182

Brierley J B 1977 Neuropathology of amnesic states. In: Whitty C W M, Zangwill O L (eds) Amnesia, 2nd edn. Butterworths, London

Butters N, Cermak L S 1980 Alcoholic Korsakoff 's syndrome. Academic Press, New York

Butters N, Cermak L S, Montgomery K, Adinolfi A 1977 Some comparisons of the memory and visuoperceptive deficits of chronic alcoholics and patients with Korsakoff's disease. Alcoholism 1: 73–80

Cala L A, Jones B, Burns P, Davis R F, Stenhouse N, Mastaglia F L 1983 Results of computerized tomography, psychometric testing and dietary studies in social drinkers with emphasis on reversibility after abstinence. Medical Journal of Australia 2: 264–269

Cala L A, Jones B, Mastaglia F L, Wiley B 1978 Brain atrophy and intellectual impairment in heavy drinkers: a clinical psychometric and computerized tomography study. Australian and New Zealand Journal of Medicine 8: 147–153

Cala L A, Mastaglia F L 1980 Computerized axial tomography in the detection of brain damage. Medical Journal of Australia 2:193–198

Carey K B, Maisto S A 1987 Effect of a change in drinking pattern on the cognitive function of female social drinkers. Journal of Studies on Alcohol 48: 236–242

Harper C, Kril J 1986 Pathological changes in alcoholic brain shrinkage. Medical Journal of Australia 144: 3–4

Harper C, Miles G, Finlay–Jones R 1986 Clinical signs in the Wernicke–Korsakoff complex: a retrospective analysis of 131 cases diagnosed at necropsy. Journal of Neurology, Neurosurgery and Psychiatry 49; 341–345

Harper C, Kril J, Daly J 1987 Are we drinking our neurones away? British Medical Journal (Clinical Research) 294: 534–536

Harper C, Kril J, Daly J 1988a Does a moderate alcohol intake damage the brain? Journal of Neurology, Neurosurgery and Psychiatry 51: 909–913

Harper C, Kril J, Daly J M 1988b Brain shrinkage in alcoholics is not caused by changes in hydration: a pathological study. Journal of Neurology, Neurosurgery and Psychiatry 51 : 124–127

Harper C, Kril J 1989 Patterns of neuronal loss in the cerebral cortex in chronic alcoholic patients. Journal of the Neurological Sciences 92: 81–89

Harper C, Gold J, Rodriguez M, Perdices M 1989 The prevalence of the Wernicke–Korsakoff syndrome in Sydney, Australia: a prospective necroscopy study. Journal of Neurology, Neurosurgery and Psychiatry 52: 282–285

Haug J 1968 Pneumoencephalographic evidence of brain damage in chronic alcoholics. Acta Psychiatrica Scandanavica 203: 135–143

Hester R K, Smith J W, Jackson T R 1980 Recovery of cognitive skills in alcoholics. Journal of Studies on Alcohol 41: 363–367

Horel J A 1978 The neuroanatomy of amnesia. A critique of the hippocampal memory hypothesis. Brain 107: 403–445

Hunt M 1979 A preliminary neuropsychological investigation of frontal lobe disorders found in alcoholism. Unpublished Masters thesis, University of Melbourne

Iivanainen M 1975 Pneumoencephalographic and clinical characteristics of diffuse cerebral atrophy. Acta Neurologica Scandanavica 51: 310–327

Janet P 1928 L'évolution de la mémoire et la notion du temps. Chahine, Paris

Janowsky J S, Shimamura A P, Kritchevsky M, Squire L R 1989a Cognitive impairment following frontal lobe damage and its relevance to human amnesia. Behavioral Neuroscience 103: 548–560

Janowsky J S, Shimamura A P, Squire L R 1989b Source memory impairment in patients with frontal lobe lesions. Neuropsychologia 27: 1043–1056

Johnson G, Parsons O, Holloway F, Bruhn P 1973 Intradimensional reversal shift performance in brain-damaged and chronic alcoholic patients. Journal of Consulting and Clinical Psychology 40: 253–258

Jones B, 1971 Verbal and spatial intelligence in short- and long-term alcoholics. The Journal of Nervous and Mental Disease 153: 292–298.

Jones B M, Parsons O A 1971 Impaired abstracting ability in chronic alcoholics. Archives of General Psychiatry 24: 71–75

Jones B M, Parsons O A 1972 Specific vs generalized deficits of abstracting ability in chronic alcoholics. Archives of General Psychiatry 26: 380–384

Jones M K, Jones B M 1980 The relationship of age and drinking habits to the effects of alcohol on memory in women. Journal of Studies on Alcohol 41: 179–186

Jonsson C O, Cronholm B, Izikowitz S 1962 Intellectual changes in alcoholics. Quarterly Journal of Studies on Alcohol 23: 221–242

Kaldegg A 1956 Psychological observations in a group of alcoholic patients. Quarterly Journal of Studies on Alcohol 17: 608–628

Kapur N, Butters N 1977 An analysis of the visuoperceptual deficits in alcoholic Korsakoffs and long-term alcoholics. Quarterly Journal of Studies on Alcohol 38: 2025–2035

Kapur N, Coughlan A K 1980 Confabulation and frontal lobe dysfunction. Journal of Neurology, Neurosurgery and Psychiatry 43:461–463

Kish G, Cheney T 1969 Impaired abilities in alcoholism measured by the General Aptitude Test Battery. Quarterly Journal of Studies on Alcohol 30: 384–388

Kleinknecht R A, Goldstein S G 1972 Neuropsychological deficits associated with alcohol. A review and discussion. Quarterly Journal of Studies on Alcohol 33: 999–1019

Klisz D K, Parsons O A 1979 Cognitive functioning in alcoholics: the role of subject attrition. Journal of Abnormal Psychology 88: 268–276

Konow A, Pribram K H 1970 Error recognition and utilization produced by injury to the frontal cortex in man. Neuropsychologia 8: 489–491

Kopelman M D 1987 Two types of confabulation. Journal of Neurology, Neurosurgery and Psychiatry 50 : 1482–1487

Kovner R, Mattis S, Goldmeier E, Davis L 1981 Korsakoff amnesic syndrome: the result of simultaneous deficits in several independent processes? Brain and Language 12: 23–32

Lereboullet J, Pluvinage R, Vidart L 1954 Les limites de la désintoxication alcoolique. Bulletins et mémoires de la société médicale des hôpitaux de Paris 70: 527–528

Lezak M D 1976 Neuropsychological Assessment. Oxford University Press, New York

Lhermitte F, Signoret J L 1972 Analyse neuropsychologique et différenciation des syndromes amnésiques. Revue Neurologique 126: 161–178

Løberg T 1980 Alcohol misuse and neuropsychological deficits in man. Journal of Studies on Alcohol 41: 119–128

Long J, McLachlan J 1974 Abstract reasoning and perceptual-motor efficiency in alcoholics: impairment and reversibility. Quarterly Journal of Studies on Alcohol 35: 1220–1229

Lovibond S, Holloway I 1968 Differential sorting behaviour of schizophrenics and organics. Journal of Clinical Psychology 24: 307–311

Luria A R 1973 The working brain. Allen Lane Penguin Press, London

Lynch M J G 1960 Brain lesions in chronic alcoholics. Archives of Pathology 69: 342–353

MacVane J, Butters N, Montgomery K, Farber J 1982 Cognitive functioning in men social drinkers. Journal of Studies on Alcohol 43: 81–95

Malerstein A, Belden E 1968 WAIS,SILS and PPVT in Korsakoff's syndrome. Archives of General Psychiatry 19: 743–750

Marslen-Wilson W D, Teuber H L 1975 Memory for remote events in anterograde amnesia: recognition of public figures from news photographs. Neuropsychologia 13: 353–364

Mattis S, Kovner R, Goldmeier E 1978 Different patterns of amnestic syndromes. Brain and Language 6: 179–191

May A, Urquhart A, Watts R 1970 Memory for designs test: a follow-up study. Perceptual and Motor Skills 30: 753–754

Mayes A R, Meudell P R, Mann D, Pickering A 1988 Location of lesions in Korsakoff's syndrome: neuropsychological and neuropathological data on two patients. Cortex 24: 367–388

Mercer B, Wapner W, Gardner H, Benson D F 1977 A study of confabulation. Archives of Neurology 34: 429–433

Molloy M P 1976 A neuropsychological investigation of the memory disorder found in chronic alcoholism. Unpublished Masters thesis, University of Melbourne

Murphy M 1953 Social class differences in intellectual characteristics of alcoholics. Quarterly Journal of Studies on Alcohol 14:192–196

O'Carroll R E, Gilleard C J 1986 Estimation of premorbid intelligence in dementia. British Journal of Clinical Psychology 25: 157–158

Oscar-Berman M 1973 Hypothesis testing and focussing behavior during concept formation by amnesic Korsakoff patients. Neuropsychologia 11: 191–198

Page R D, Linden J D 1974 'Reversible' organic brain syndrome in alcoholics: a psychometric evaluation. Quarterly Journal of Studies on Alcohol 35: 98–107

Page R D, Schaub L H 1977 Intellectual functioning in alcoholics during six months abstinence. Journal of Studies on Alcohol 38: 1240–1246

Parker E S, Noble E P 1977 Alcohol consumption and cognitive functioning in social drinkers. Journal of Studies on Alcohol 38: 1224–1232

Parker E S, Noble E P 1980 Alcohol and aging process in social drinkers. Journal of Studies on Alcohol 41: 170–178

Parsons O A 1974 Brain damage in alcoholics: altered state of consciousness. Alcohol Technical Reports 2: 93–105

Parsons O A 1977 Neuropsychological deficits in alcoholics: facts and fancies. Alcoholism 1: 51–56

Parsons O A, Prigitano P 1977 Memory functioning in alcoholics. In: Birnbaum I M, Parker E S (eds) Alcohol and human memory. Lawrence Erlbaum Associates, New Jersey

Parsons O A, Fabian M S 1982 Comments on 'cognitive functioning in men social drinkers: a replication study'. Journal of Studies on Alcohol 43:178–182

Peron N, Gayno M 1956 Atrophie cérébrale des éthyliques. Revue Neurologique 94: 621–624

Peters G 1956 Emotional and intellectual concomitants of advanced chronic alcoholism. Journal of Consulting Psychology 20: 390

Pierson C A Kirscher J P 1954 La pneumoencéphalographie chez l'alcoolique. Revue Neurologique 90: 673–676

Pishkin V, Fishkin S, Stahl M 1972 Concept learning in chronic alcoholics: psychophysiological and set functions. Journal of Clinical Psychology 28: 328–334

Plumeau F Machover S Puzzo F 1960 Wechsler-Bellevue performances of remitted and unremitted alcoholics and their normal controls. Journal of Consulting Psychology. 24: 240–242

Pluvinage R 1954 Les atrophies cérébrales des alcooliques. Bulletins et mémoires de la Société Médicale des Hôpitaux de Paris 70: 524

Postel J, Cossa P 1956 L'atrophie cérébrale des alcooliques chroniques: étude encéphalographique. Revue Neurologique 94: 604–606

Ron M A 1977 Brain damage in chronic alcoholism: a neuropathological, neuroradiological and psychological review. Psychological Medicine 7: 103–112

Ryan C 1980 Learning and memory deficits in alcoholics. Journal of Studies on Alcohol 41: 437–447

Ryan C, Butters N 1980a Further evidence for a continuum-of-impairment encompassing male alcoholic Korsakoff patients and chronic alcoholic men. Alcoholism: Clinical and Experimental Research 4: 190–198

Ryan C Butters N 1980b Learning and memory impairment in young and old alcoholics: evidence for the premature aging hypothesis. Alcoholism: Clinical and Experimental Research 4: 288–293

Ryback R 1971 Continuum and specificity of the effects of alcohol on memory: a review. Quarterly Journal of Studies on Alcohol 32: 995–1016

Sanders H I, Warrington E K 1971 Memory for remote events in amnesic patients. Brain 94: 661–668

Satz P 1966 Specific and non-specific effects of brain lesions in man. Journal of Abnormal Psychology 71: 65–70

Schau E J, O'Leary M R 1977 Adaptive abilities of hospitalized alcoholics and matched controls. Journal of Studies on Alcohol 38: 403–409

Schau E J, O'Leary M R, Chaney E F 1980 Reversibility of cognitive deficit in alcoholics. Journal of Studies on Alcohol 41: 733–744

Seltzer B, Benson D F 1974 The temporal pattern of retrograde amnesia in Korsakoff's disease. Neurology 24: 527–530

Shimamura A P, Jernigan T L, Squire L R 1988 Korsakoff's syndrome: radiological correlates. Journal of Neuroscience 8: 4400–4410

Skillicorn S 1955 Presenile cerebellar ataxia in chronic alcoholics. Neurology 5: 527–534

Smith J, Burt D, Chapman R 1973 Intelligence and brain damage in alcoholics: a study of patients in middle and upper social class. Quarterly Journal of Studies on Alcohol 34: 414–422

Smith J, Johnson L, Burdick J 1971 Sleep, psychological and clinical changes during alcohol withdrawal in NAD-treated alcoholics. Quarterly Journal of Studies on Alcohol 32: 982–994

Smith J, Layden T 1972 Changes in psychological performance and blood chemistry in alcoholics during and after hospital treatment. Quarterly Journal of Studies on Alcohol 33: 379–394

Squire L R 1981 Two forms of human amnesia: an analysis of forgetting. Journal of Neuroscience 1: 635–640

Stuss D T, Alexander M P, Lieberman A, Levine H 1978 An extraordinary form of confabulation. Neurology 28: 1166–1172

Tarter R E 1971 A neuropsychological examination of cognition and perceptual capacities in chronic alcoholics. Doctoral dissertation, University of Oklahoma

Tarter R E 1973 An analysis of cognitive deficits in chronic alcoholics. Journal of Nervous and Mental Disease 157: 138–147

Tarter R E 1975 Psychological deficit in chronic alcoholics: A review. The International Journal of the Addictions 10: 327–368

Tarter R E 1976 Neuropsychological investigations of alcoholism. In: Goldstein G, Neuringer C (eds) Empirical studies of alcoholism. Ballinger, Cambridge, Massachusetts

Tarter R E, Jones B 1971 Motor impairment in chronic alcoholics. Journal of Nervous Diseases 32: 632–633

Tarter R E, Parsons O A 1971 Conceptual shifting in chronic alcoholics. Journal of Abnormal Psychology 77: 71–75

Tumarkin B Wilson J, Snyder G 1955 Cerebral atrophy due to alcoholism in young adults. U S Armed Forces Medical Journal 6: 57–74

Victor M 1976 The Wernicke-Korsakoff syndrome. In : Vinken P J, Bruyn G W (eds) Handbook of clinical neurology. North-Holland, Amsterdam, vol 28, ch 9

Victor M, Adams R D, Collins G F 1971 The Wernicke-Korsakoff syndrome. Davis, Philadelphia

Victor M, Yakovlev P I 1955 S S Korsakoff's psychic disorder in conjunction with peripheral neuritis: a translation of Korsakoff's original article with brief comments on the author and his contribution to clinical medicine. Neurology 5: 394–406

Vivian T, Goldstein G, Shelly C 1973 Reaction time and motor speed in chronic alcoholics. Perceptual and Motor Skills 30: 136–138

Walsh K W 1987 Neuropsychology: a clinical approach, 2nd edn. Churchill Livingstone, Edinburgh

Waugh M, Jackson M, Fox G A, Hawke S H, Tuck R R 1989 Effect of social drinking on neuro-psychological performance. British Journal of Addiction 84: 659–667

Wechsler D 1941 The effect of alcohol on mental activity. Quarterly Journal of Studies on Alcohol 2: 479–485

Wechsler D 1958 The measurement and appraisal of adult intelligence. Williams and Wilkins, Baltimore

Weingartner H, Faillace L 1971 Alcohol state dependent learning in man. Journal of Nervous and Mental Disease 153: 395–406

Weingartner H, Faillace L, Markley H 1971 Verbal information retention in alcoholics. Quarterly Journal of Studies on Alcohol 32: 293–303

Whitty C W M, Zangwill O L 1977 Amnesia: clinical, psychological and medicolegal aspects, 2nd edn. Butterworths, London

Willanger R 1970 Intellectual impairment in diffuse cerebral lesions. Munksgaard, Copenhagen

Willanger R, Thygesen P, Nielsen R, Peterson O 1968 Intellectual impairment and cerebral atrophy: a psychological, neurological and radiological investigation. Danish Medical Bulletin 15: 65–94

Zangwill O L 1943 Clinical tests of memory impairment. Proceedings of the Royal Society of Medicine 36: 576–580

Zangwill O 1978 Personal communication

3. Intellectual decline

DIAGNOSIS OF DEMENTIA

Despite numerous attempts to qualify it or dispense with it entirely the term dementia seems here to stay. It remains a general descriptive term denoting not one but many brain disorders of known or unknown aetiology which have in common the fact that they produce widespread dissolution of human mental capabilities and social functions. The slowly progressive deterioration of intellect, emotion and will occurs in the presence of unimpaired consciousness.

It is not surprising that under this broad rubric there exists a wide variety of clinical presentations due not only to the varied aetiology and subsequent pathology but also to the individual differences between subjects (e.g. Pearce & Miller 1973, Slaby & Wyatt 1974, Smith & Kinsbourne 1977, Wells 1977, Katzman et al 1978). Post (1975) also points out that the term is applied differently by neurologists and psychiatrists. Neurologists may use it simply as a synonym for impairment of higher mental function not necessarily either widespread or irreversible. On the other hand, psychiatrists usually mean to convey a disorder which has a widespread effect on higher functions and is both progressive and (usually) irreversible. In this regard it is important to emphasize that although the most common form of dementia, Alzheimer's disease and several other common dementias still have no effective treatment, over 10% of the disorders causing dementia are reversible or arrestable. In a further 25% of cases correct diagnosis may suggest specific therapy for the underlying disorder. Harrison & Marsden compared the results of studies in three different hospitals and found the same pattern of findings emerging in cases of dementia—approximately a quarter were treatable conditions, a quarter had definable but basically untreatable causes and about one half were cerebral atrophy of unknown origin (Marsden & Harrison 1972, Freemon 1976, Harrison & Marsden 1977).

The dementias have also been divided into primary types due to parenchymatous cerebral degeneration, and secondary types associated with known conditions. The secondary dementias may be subdivided into those associated with systemic or neurological disease. In the primary type the dementia is the only evidence of disease while in the secondary type features of neurological or other systemic disorder may present before cognitive signs. As the following table illustrates, at least some causes of dementia can now be identified.

Table 3.1 Diagnosis in 417 patients fully evaluated for dementia (from Wells 1979b)

Diagnosis	% of total
Dementia of unknown cause	47.7
Alcoholic dementia	10.0
Multi-infarct dementia	9.4
Normal pressure hydrocephalus	6.0
Intracranial masses	4.8
Huntington's chorea	2.9
Drug toxicity	2.4
Post-traumatic	6.7
Other identified diseases	6.7
Pseudodementia	6.7
Uncertain	1.7

As Strub & Black (1981) remarked: 'The outlook for the demented patient is still not overly hopeful in general; but, compared to the futile view of the past, the diagnostic and treatment possibilities available today offer hope to many patients' (p 169-170). The résumé which follows concentrates particularly on those conditions in which the neuropsychologist may be called upon for an assessment.

Alzheimer's disease

Clinical features

The term Alzheimer's disease was coined by Kraepelin following the original descriptions of Alzheimer in the early part of this century. It is a primary degenerative disease of unknown aetiology.

Although this disorder was first described in a patient of middle age, there is little to distinguish it clinically from the most common type of dementia in the elderly, formerly termed 'senile dementia', and both conditions exhibit the same pathological changes (Newton 1948). There is a clear sex difference, females being affected about twice as often as males. Detailed clinical descriptions appear in most textbooks of psychiatry and neurobehavioural science (e.g. Strub & Black 1981). A brief summary cannot do justice to the complexity of the clinical picture but Roth (1981), in updating his classical description of 1955, stresses the importance of the natural history and says that three of the following four features must be present for the diagnosis to be made: '(1) a gradual and continually progressive failure in work performance and some of the common activities of everyday living; (2) impairment in memory ...; (3) deterioration in general intellectual ability with impairment of grasp, capacity for reasoning, inference, and conceptual and abstract thought; and (4) disorganization of personality and its characteristic features with deterioration in self care, blunting of emotional sensibility, and impairment of social adjustment...' At the outset noncognitive changes may be more obvious than the loss of higher intellectual function especially if the person has a well established repertoire of programmes of action to suit a variety of situations in his or her work or social situations. In these cases an apparently sudden decompensation may occur due to unexpected situational stress such as the death of a spouse, loss of occupation for external reasons, or sudden illness.

Emphasis is rightly placed on the progressive nature of the disorder and Roth (1981) suggests the term 'organic mental impairment' for clearly nonprogressive types of cases such as those described by Roth et al (1979). There is little known about such cases and the author has found it useful to employ at least two examinations several months apart before conveying the diagnosis (which implies prognosis) to the patient, relatives or even those professionals who might unwittingly convey it. In the nonprogressive or slowly progressing case, the demonstration of the absence of obvious deterioration is very reassuring for the patient.

Personal history. A carefully taken history is probably the most important single factor in diagnosis. This is particularly aided by perceptive relatives and friends though these are not always to hand. It should be the first part of any neuropsychological assessment and, in doubtful cases, the use of social workers to check the home or work setting often proves invaluable. Lapses of behaviour out of keeping with the patient's usual conduct are of particular significance and may appear before any apparent cognitive loss. At this stage, performance on psychological tests of intelligence has been said to be unhelpful because of the many instances where such testing has been negative. This has usually occurred where insensitive measures have been employed.

On the contrary, it is quite common to find in such latent cases marked changes in the ability to acquire and retain new material, and to cope with problem solving for which the patient does not already have a well developed strategy or programme for solution. In particular, intelligent patients and those with a broad life experience may escape notice while they remain in a familiar situation because of their established skills which are relatively resistant to cerebral impairment. However, the patient's problem-solving difficulties become 'particularly evident when the patient attempts to solve complex novel problems in which he cannot rely upon well established routinized skills and strategies' (Strub & Black 1981, p 124). It is because of this difference in loading on well stored information and skills versus new learning and problem solving that the WAIS Performance score is usually well below the Verbal (Bolton et al 1966, Roth et al 1979). In any case, if a sensitive, appropriate examination is negative, the cause of the change in behaviour probably lies elsewhere.

In many cases cognitive changes are the first feature noticed by the patient and the relatives. Many of these cases are self-referred and show clear signs of incipient decline. They are often mildly depressed, perhaps in response to the sensing of their own intellectual degradation, and may be confused. Distinguishing features are present in the cognitive examination (see below). Memory disturbance is by far the most common complaint and must be distinguished from the numerous conditions which may give rise to amnesic syndromes. Alzheimer's disease should not be diagnosed in the absence of accompanying signs of other intellectual deficits.

Pathological changes

The most obvious feature morphologically is the presence of pronounced brain atrophy with increased width of sulci and dilatation of ventricles. The pathological changes are not confined to one part of the brain. However, in most cases the cortex of the frontal and temporal lobes is much more affected than the parieto-occipital regions though narrowly localized atrophy is rare. The atrophy might be said to be widespread but not uniform. The limbic grey matter of the temporal lobes (amygdaloid nucleus and hippocampus) is usually markedly affected.

Tomlinson et al (1968) have noted the presence of cerebral softenings due to small infarctions in some patients with characteristic Alzheimer pathology. For this reason the distinction between Alzheimer dementia and multi-infarct dementia may not be clear cut.

Alzheimer's first patient, a woman aged 51 years, showed widespread changes in the neurones of the cerebral cortex. The changes have been studied intensively since that time and take the form of thickening and tortuosity of fibrils, or neurofibrillary tangles, within the cytoplasm of the nerve cell, and neurofibrillary degeneration. This is now recognized as an intermediate process in the death of these cells which begins with degeneration of the cell extensions which permit transmission between cells, and further degeneration within the cells which result in the appearance of the second major characteristic feature, the senile plaque of Marinesco. Other histopathological features are also described.

Kemper (1978) was one of a number of authors who have drawn attention to the heavy concentration of neuropathology in the hippocampal region. This observation has received much support in quantitative studies (e.g. Dayan 1970b, Hooper & Vogel 1976, Ball 1977). Kemper commented : 'The relationship of a lesion in this location to the memory deficit appears well documented and it seems likely that the changes noted in these brains are in some way related to this prominent and early feature of senile dementia.' (op. cit. p 112) It now appears that plaque formation may spread outward from the region of the hippocampus and amygdala.

All the pathological features of Alzheimer's disease are also to be found in the brains of elderly non-demented individuals (Dayan 1970a). This study shows an increased prevalence with age, in subjects over 60, of pathological changes similar to those of Alzheimer's disease. However, the changes appear to be less intense and the neurofibrillary changes are largely restricted to the hippocampi in the normal aged. This similarity has raised the question as to whether Alzheimer's disease is an acceleration of the ageing process. The matter is unresolved but it is important to remember that similar neuropathological changes might be brought about by different factors. More detailed descriptions of the pathology may be found in Adams et al (1984).

As well as the suggested hippocampal pathology and amnesia one might also hypothesize that destruction of the anterior cortical regions is directly related to the loss of adaptive behaviour which is such a characteristic feature of this disease. This is why the present author suggests that an examination placing emphasis on adaptive aspects of intellectual behaviour together with searching memory examination will be most productive in latent or incipient cases of dementia. Psychological examinations, on the other hand, which are too heavily loaded with tests of long stored information and well practised skills, may miss the early cases especially if valuable information is lost by combining scores on several different tests into a summarizing score such as the IQ.

In recent years the fact that Alzheimer's disease is associated with changes in the cholinergic system stimulated research with the possibility of arresting or reversing the pathological process. Certainly, abnormal biochemistry in the form of abnormal acetylcholine synthesis and choline acetyltransferase activity is a constant feature. However, serotoninergic, noradrenergic and other chemical compounds related to neurotransmission have also been demonstrated so that the possibility of replacement therapy akin to the paradigm of Parkinson's disease seems less likely. One might expect that if the spread is essentially *anatomical* rather than biochemical, chemical therapy might be unproductive.

Finally, the EEG may be helpful in distinguishing Alzheimer's from other primary dementias in the presenile group. The characteristic feature in Alzheimer's disease is nonspecific slow wave activity in the theta and delta range.

Non-Alzheimer primary dementia

Even before Alzheimer described his work on primary dementia Pick had described a form of presenile dementia which was characterized by circumscribed frontotemporal atrophy and clinical features which in retrospect we recognize as being predominantly of anterior origin, e.g. loss of social grace, disinhibition or apathy, and frequently aphasia. Subsequently neuronal inclusions, now termed Pick bodies, were found which are pathognomonic of this uncommon disorder.

In the past five years the evidence from biopsy and autopsy studies has made it increasingly evident that there are a significant number of patients with presenile dementia with atrophy concentrated in the frontal and temporal regions, only some of whom display characteristic Pick bodies. In a prospective study of 158 cases of dementia Brun (1987) found predominant frontal or frontotemporal atrophy in 26 and, of these, only 4 could be classified as Pick's disease. The large remaining subgroup can be designated as dementia of the frontal type (DFT) and it remains to be seen whether it is related to Pick's disease. What is of interest is the closely similar picture which is described for this latter group in recent reports from different centres (Hagberg & Gustafson 1985, Neary et al 1986, 1987, 1988; Gustafson 1987, Johanson & Hagberg 1989).

The disorder has an insidious onset and the first signs are usually a set of changes which can be subsumed under the rubric of alteration in personality, and which has a characteristic 'frontal' flavour. There is loss of interest in usual activities including work, and a bland indifference, which is soon followed by loss of interest in personal appearance and hygiene, and emotional unconcern. A disregard for others with unaccustomed rudeness is sometimes what first alerts those around to the changes. When these are mentioned the patient shows both lack of concern and lack of insight. There may be periods of crude jocularity or unwarranted euphoria despite a lowering of spontaneity and initiative. Occasionally the patient appears depressed.

A feature which clearly distinguishes the group from Alzheimer's disease is the relative preservation of memory. Fluctuating forgetfulness may be a function of inattentiveness since formal testing reveals preserved ability to learn new material. In keeping with this Knopman et al (1989) found a relative preservation of memory in six cases of Pick's disease despite marked impairment of executive functions. For a considerable time, visuo-spatial abilities also remain largely normal. The most typical neurobehavioural change is progressively reduced speech and language with stereotypy. Frank aphasia does not appear in the early stages. There is a progression later in some cases to mutism. In their psychometric analysis Johanson & Hagberg (1989) found expressive speech changes to be the most characteristic finding. Associative verbal fluency tasks are particularly sensitive.

Although scores on standardized intellectual tests such as the WAIS remain unchanged for some considerable time, the patients may prove difficult to examine because of their indifferent or flippant attitude or because they tend to be perseverative. Those tests with a high loading on so-called executive functions which are so useful in all disorders with suspected frontal involvement also prove most useful here. No case of suspected dementia should be cleared on the basis of preservation of appropriate levels. Early detection of such cases allows planning for the patient's future and will become increasingly important, should curative or arresting therapies emerge.

In the elderly population self-neglect is a not uncommon problem and with the apparent preservation of intellect and memory it is probable that many elderly patients with frontal lobe wasting have not come under neurological or neuropsychological scrutiny (Orrel et al 1989). Emerging knowledge of brain wasting will undoubtedly uncover many more such cases.

Investigations

The diagnosis of the non-Alzheimer disorders has been improved by CT and MRI scanning and made even clearer by positron emission tomography (PET) (Szelies & Karenberg 1986, Kamo et al 1987, Heiss et al 1989, Salmon & Franck 1989). A study of regional cerebral blood flow by Risberg (1987) showed differential reduction of flow in the frontal regions in keeping with the clinical frontal picture in nine cases of non-Alzheimer dementia and four cases of Pick's disease, the most pronounced changes being in the latter. Using single proton emission computed tomography (SPECT), a more readily available and less expensive method, Weinstein et al (1989) have shown temporoparietal hypoperfusion in Alzheimer's disease and frontal hypoperfusion in Pick's disease. Such techniques lend themselves to correlative studies with clinical neurological and neuropsychological evaluations which should help in defining types of dementing disorders.

Finally, in contrast to the Alzheimer patients, the EEG tends to be normal in patients with dementia of the frontal type.

The remainder of primary dementia cases comprises a miscellany of less common entities.

Dementia and cerebrovascular disease

Until about a decade ago the diagnosis (or misdiagnosis) of cerebral arteriosclerosis as a cause of dementia was quite frequent. About that time studies began to demonstrate a lack of relationship between cerebral vessel atheroma and the parenchymatous changes described in a high proportion of cases of dementia coming to autopsy. A growing body of opinion supported the contention of Fisher (1968): 'In brief, cerebrovascular dementia is a matter of strokes large and small.' This was a matter of wrongly inferred aetiology and a difference in terminology. It does not invalidate the detailed clinical descriptions given, for example, by Slater & Roth (1969) of a group of cases they termed 'arteriosclerotic psychosis'. The new term 'multi-infarct dementia' became widespread after the publication of Hachinski et al (1974) though recognition of two separate forms of dementia, one of which had a vascular basis, had been recognized for several years. Hachinski et al pointed out that the infarcts tended to be small and multiple and were seen in association with hypertension. The cavities of the old infarcts appear as small holes or lacunes in different parts of the brain, particularly the diencephalon, brain stem and deep cerebral white matter. The presence of a number of lacunes had been known since the description of *'foyers lacunaires de déstintégration'* by Pierre Marie (1901) the final state being termed, *'l'état lacunaire'*. Marie pointed out that the lacunes were usually small, often no larger than a grain of millet.

The infarcts of multi-infarct dementia are now known to arise from the heart or from atheromatous plaques often situated in extracerebral vessels such as the carotid arteries and 'in only a small minority of cases are cerebral softenings caused by in situ thrombosis of cerebral vessels' (Lhermitte et al 1970). The association with hypertension and vascular pathology means that many cases of dementia might be prevented or arrested by appropriate medical or surgical treatment.

The clinical picture is characterized by 'abrupt episodes which lead to weakness, slowness, dysarthria, dysphagia, small-stepped gait, brisk reflexes and extensor plantar responses. All these signs are usually present by the time that mental deterioration occurs. Pathological laughing and crying are common' (Hachinski et al 1974). Such descriptions emphasize the importance of careful history taking and observation over a period longer than the usual clinical interview. Thirteen of the characteristic features described by Slater and Roth (1969) and others were drawn up into a crude scale by Hachinski et al (1975) to derive an 'ischemic score'. Their comparison of Alzheimer and multi-infarct patients showed a bimodal distribution with no overlap in scores. It is questionable whether an observant clinician gains any more useful information by quantifying signs and symptoms in this way, but the tabulation may serve as a useful checklist for the less experienced. Of more value is the careful and detailed qualification of each of the features given in Roth's review (Roth 1981), e.g. he points out with regard to 'fluctuation' (one of the 13 points) that this variation of behaviour may be found in sundry forms of dementia. What he stresses is 'the periodic return to relatively efficient intellectual functioning and good or normal emotional rapport that characterizes these cases during the first few years, when opportunities for treatment may still be open in some cases' (p 32-33).

An added difficulty in differentiating between primary degenerative dementia and multi-infarct dementia is the sizeable number of patients who show clear evidence of both types of pathology (Tomlinson et al 1968, Todorov et al 1975, Jellinger 1976, Tomlinson 1977).

CT scan and multi-infarct dementia

Though areas of low attenuation are more common in the scans of patients with multi-infarct dementia than in those with Alzheimer's disease they are uncommon in both groups (Du Boulay et al 1979). These authors inferred that 'in multi-infarct dementia many of the infarcts are invisible by CT. If we cannot expect to visualize the final effects of small infarcts, *we are not justified in accepting a normal scan as evidence of no damage after transient ischemic attack*'. [my italic]. Other workers agree that it is sometimes clinically difficult to differentiate between Alzheimer's and multi-infarct dementia even with the aid of neuroradiological techniques such as angiography and CT scan (Radue et al 1978, Jacoby & Levy 1980). This question is taken up again in Chapter 6 in connection with the neuropsychological examination in relation to vascular lesions. At the present time there is little psychological documentation of multi-infarct dementia apart from studies comparing levels of performance on standardized intelligence tests (e.g. Perez et al 1975) and Brust (1983) considers that vascular dementia is still being overdiagnosed.

Normal pressure hydrecephalus

In the 1960s several writers drew attention to cases of chronic hydrocephalus in which the cerebrospinal fluid pressure was apparently normal (McHugh 1964, Adams et al 1965, Ojemann et al 1969). Recently it has been shown that short bursts of raised pressure are probably the cause of the trouble. Shunting has been successful in some cases in resolving neurological and, sometimes, psychological function.

The principal early features noted were 'mild impairment of memory, slowness and paucity of thought and action, unsteadiness of gait and unwitting urinary incontinence' (Adams et al 1965, p 122). To this may be added certain signs suggestive of frontal lobe involvement, e.g. euphoria or apathy, and disinhibition.

This form of hydrocephalus occurs from middle age onwards and so must be distinguished from other conditions, notably endogenous depression and Alzheimer's disease.

In distinguishing early cases from Alzheimer's disease, Adams et al comment: 'In Alzheimer's disease the principal disability is loss of memory to which other defects in cognitive function (calculation, speech and thinking) are later added; only late in the illness will mental and physical slowness, disturbance of gait and lack of urinary control appear. The development of the deficit usually extends over a much longer time (years) than in our cases of 'normal pressure hydrocephalus', in which the impairment of function appeared over a period of only a few months' (op. cit. p 123). Progression of the disorder varies in rate but early shunting seems to carry the most favourable results. The criteria for shunting are by no means clear and have been reviewed by Strub & Black (1981).

The neuropsychologist may be called upon to confirm the memory difficulty and early signs of frontal lobe involvement in the early stages. Neuropsychological assessment is also of value in monitoring change before and after shunting. Where dementia is more prominent in the early stages than the gait disorder, prognosis seems less favourable. Even in cases where alertness is restored and the gait disorder and incontinence disappears, some residual intellectual impairment may still be in evidence.

Other forms of dementia

The great number of less common causes of dementia precludes discourse here. Readers are referred to works on dementia (Wells 1977) or organic brain syndromes (Strub & Black 1981). Neuropsychologists have become involved with research into a number of these, e.g. Huntington's disease, Parkinson's disease and multiple sclerosis, and referrals appear to be increasing for examination of patients with renal and other systemic disorders suspected of intellectual decline. Treatment itself is not without its drawbacks, as witnessed by the emergence of dialysis dementia which makes it mandatory to monitor patients' neuropsychological functions in such situations. Finally, industrial toxicology is bringing to light increasing evidence of environmental hazards to healthy brain functioning.

PSEUDODEMENTIA

The term 'pseudodementia' can be traced back several decades. It was most often discussed in relation to hysteria and to the Ganser syndrome in particular, though some writers inferred rather than documented its presence in other situations (Mapother & Lewis 1937). However, the term first came into prominence with the article by Kiloh (1961) which remains the most comprehensive treatment of the subject. He drew attention to situations in which 'the diagnosis of dementia is entertained but has to be abandoned because of the subsequent course of the illness', i.e. unexpected recovery. Pseudodementia thus referred to a situation in which the behavioural changes were mimicked, at times so closely as to mislead all but the most astute observers.

While recognizing the Ganser state (Goldin & MacDonald 1955) as perhaps the best known example of the condition, Kiloh was careful to point out that this was only one of a number of conditions which might mimic the picture of dementia. The Ganser state was a rather rare though dramatic subset from a broader and more common group of cases he termed 'hysterical pseudodementia'. Discussion of the relation of the Ganser syndrome to hysterical pseudodementia, together with case examples of the latter, is given in Chapter 4. In general this group should present little difficulty in differential diagnosis to experienced clinicians.

Even more common than the hysterical group is depressive pseudodementia which appears to make up the greater proportion of cases cited in the literature (e.g. Post 1975, Wells 1979b, Caine 1981). Kiloh (1961) and subsequent writers have stressed an even wider range of non-organic conditions which may mimic dementia (Smith et al 1976, Wells 1979a, Caine 1981). The frequency with which these conditions are observed will vary, being rare in general practice but more commonly observed by those 'whose practices include significant numbers of elderly patients or patients with neuropsychiatric problems' (Wells 1979a). Minor degrees of pseudodementia are very frequent (Kiloh 1981) and the mimicking of only certain restricted features of dementia such as the memory disorder may resemble cognitive deficits produced by localized neuropathology. This gives rise to a number of referrals of these suspect or atypical cases from neurologists and psychiatrists to their colleagues in neuropsychology and neuropsychiatry. Many such referrals raise the possibility of malingering in the differential diagnosis (see Ch.4).

With the revived interest in pseudodementia there has been a tendency to speak of it as a syndrome (Wells 1979a, Caine 1981). In his original article Kiloh was careful to point out that the 'name can of course have no place in any nosological system; it is purely descriptive and carries no diagnostic weight'. More recently he has reiterated this point, stressing that the 'illusion of dementia' may appear with any of a number of psychiatric syndromes and should not be granted the rank of a syndrome in its own right (Kiloh 1981). Certainly the descriptions given do not seem to warrant the reification of the term 'pseudodementia' into a neuropsychiatric syndrome in the strict sense of the term 'syndrome' discussed in Chapter 1. Used in this sense the word syndrome takes on the over-general meaning it held in the usages 'chronic brain syndrome' or 'organic brain syndrome' with the deficiencies of such a general usage pointed out by authors such as Seltzer & Sherwin (1978).

A novel conception of the basis of pseudodementia comes from Caine (1981) who argues that: 'Neuropsychological abnormalities are usually associated with structural CNS pathology. The presence of such deficits in the context of treatable, remitting psychiatric disorders suggests that these abnormalities may reflect specific impairments of brain functioning'. (op. cit. p 1363). Unfortunately the 'neuro-psychological abnormalities' are largely unspecified and to equate poor test performance on so-called neuropsychological tests is to disregard the many nonstructural reasons for poor performance discussed elsewhere (Chs. 1 and 4). On the other hand, if true neuropsychological abnormalities can be substantiated the term pseudodementia would be inappropriate.

Although reports vary greatly as to the misdiagnosis of dementia, studies over the past decade have shown that retrospective examination of cases originally classified as dementia, or in whom the diagnosis had been seriously considered, reveals a proportion of cases who demonstrate by their recovery or failure to deteriorate over time that the diagnosis was incorrect (Marsden & Harrison 1972, Nott & Fleminger 1975, Post 1975, Freemon 1976, Smith et al 1976, Roth et al 1979, Wells 1979a, Caine 1981). The difficulty of clinical differentiation is shown, for example, by the need for special ancillary investigations such as neuroradiological examinations in a high proportion of cases before a definitive diagnosis could be made (Smith et al 1976). The problem has been eased but not completely obviated by the advent of computerized tomography (see below).

Depression, dementia and pseudodementia

The relationship between depression and dementia is not a simple one and the fact that depression is the most common condition to masquerade as dementia, particularly in the elderly, requires some clarification. Brent (1979) has objected that Wells' attempt (Wells 1979a) to create a dichotomy of clinical features which differentiates between dementia and pseudodementia 'may obscure the true complexity of the clinical situation'. He warns that signs favouring one side of the dichotomy need to be examined with care and points to a common enough situation in which dementia may go unrecognized 'until an environmental change or interpersonal loss precipitates an acute decompensation'. Shraberg (1979) describes an elderly man with a subacute onset of what appeared to be dementia in a person with a prior history of affective illness. Mental status and psychological testing showed clear evidence of intellectual impairment and the patient was unable to cope. Following drug treatment (imipramine) there was improvement to the degree that he was able to return home, and he continued to manage. Psychological testing showed some improvement, between pre- and post-treatment examinations but significant losses of higher mental functions were still obvious. Brent (op. cit.) points out that this set of events might easily be characterized as 'acute onset' and thus bias the clinician in favour of a pseudodementia if he followed the oversimplified notion of a dichotomy between dementia and pseudodementia. In the case cited the process is interactive and highlights the fact that intellectual decline is only one of the factors involved in producing the social picture of dementia. Brent's dissertation continues with an examination of the role of psychosocial factors in creating and alleviating 'demented' behaviour.

In other situations depression appears to be an integral part of the dementing picture particularly in the early stages of Alzheimer's disease in the elderly. 'Often these disorders are self-fuelling, with the depression arising out of the patient's growing awareness of his cognitive losses. The resultant pseudodementia not only potentiates the primary deficit but leads to a further deterioration as self-esteem-promoting vocational and interpersonal functioning are compromised' (Brent 1979). Roth (1981) refers to these cases as dementia with 'depressive coloring'. He describes features which may help in distinguishing the depression associated with dementia, particularly multi-infarct dementia, from depressive pictures unaccompanied by organic changes.

There is general agreement that endogenous depression, especially when severe, is more likely to provide a diagnostic problem than neurotic depression (e.g. Kiloh 1981). The depressed patient's impaired concentration, lack of interest and psychomotor retardation give rise to such poor performance on tasks of memory, calculation and the like, that they raise the possibility of dementia. The patient often describes a difficulty with thinking which may reinforce the suspicion of dementia not only in examining professionals but also in the patient himself. Further reinforcement may be given by the depressed patient's social withdrawal and loss of self-care. McHugh & Folstein (1979) refer to this as the 'dementia syndrome of depression'.

Differentiation of the early stages of dementia from depression may be difficult in that the onset of dementia may be characterized only by some decline in general efficiency of performance, loss of initiative and apathy, and so may resemble affective conditions closely. Careful attention to the history, characteristics of the clinical picture and appropriate cognitive examination will clarify the diagnosis in most cases.

Numerous authors have emphasized the paramount importance of careful history taking as the most important factor contributing to correct diagnosis (Post 1975, Wells

1979, Kiloh 1981, Roth 1981). 'As a general rule, depression starts with loss of interest, confidence and drive, but objective failure at work or a memory disorder will become a problem only by the time depression has been well established .... In contrast symptoms that might be attributed to an affective illness usually occur in the course of cerebral failure after cognitive deterioration has been progressing for some time' (Post 1975, p 105-106). The onset of depression is often more readily dated within a short period of time while the temporal onset of failure with dementia is often difficult for family and friends to specify. In retrospect, friends of dementing patients will usually be able to back-date, the onset some considerable time. The rapid rate of progression is more characteristic of depression than dementia. Further details of the natural history of dementia are available in the descriptions of Roth (1955, 1981).

Psychological test performance and depression

Memory and learning. The frequency and severity of memory disorder in dementia has long suggested that tests of memory and learning might be useful in differentiating dementia from other disorders. Memory tests have been used in such a situation for some three decades. However, the fact that memory troubles are also commonly reported in other conditions suggests some caution. The following survey of a sample of studies may clarify some of the issues. Methodological shortcomings or failure to describe the samples in enough detail render the conclusions tentative.

In one of the first studies using the Wechsler Memory Scale, Walton (1958) found that those patients who were subsequently classed as brain damaged showed significantly more difficulty in new learning than those who were subsequently given the label 'functional', though the latter did show some difficulty. Cronholm & Ottosson (1961) confirmed a poor performance for depressives when compared with normals on both immediate recall and after a delay of three hours in the presence of normal immediate memory span. However, there was no significant difference for normal or depressive subjects on measures of retention or forgetting. This is a most important finding since *both* learning and retention are affected in dementia. Little attention has been given to this finding in the literature. Friedman (1964) compared 55 severe depressives with a well matched control group of 65 subjects and found no difference on either paired associate learning or the Memory for Designs Test (Graham & Kendall 1960).

It was during this period that attempts to discover single tests or indices of 'organicity' or 'brain damage' reached their height (or depth). This was often in the context of trying to find an effective screening device between functional and organic cases (see Ch. 1). A promising test of new learning for this purpose was the Modified New Word Learning Test (Walton & Black 1957). Bolton et al (1967) reviewed studies reporting the effectiveness of this test as a unitary screening device. While some showed promising results others yielded too high a percentage of misclassifications for the test to be used in this way. The errors were often in the direction of false positives e.g. in their own study Bolton et al found some 29% of elderly patients with affective disorders scored in 'the organic range'. It was obvious that such a procedure could not be used on its own. Similar unsatisfactory misclassification was reported for a similar task, the Synonym Learning Test (Kendrick et al 1965) while the misclassification rate rose very sharply if the population contained a large proportion of pseudodementia cases.

Studies such as that of Coughlan & Hollows (1984) have continued to demonstrate that impairment over a range of memory tasks is not significantly greater than with a group of matched controls. There is also some evidence that the memory problems of depressed patients may be distinguished from those of organic amnesics by the use of self-report techniques (Squire & Zouzounis 1988).

The findings of Whitehead (1973) pointed the way to differentiating between the memory and learning performance of depressive versus dementing patients. She compared two such groups on tests of immediate memory (digit span forward), long-term memory (vocabulary), and short-term memory, that included several tests of rote learning, logical memory and recognition. Depressive patients were tested both during their 'ill' phase and in remission. While there was no difference between the two groups for the immediate and long term tests 'ill' depressives scored at a higher level on all short-term memory tasks and depressive patients in remission showed gains on two tests of synonym learning and one of serial verbal learning. The tests of logical memory and recognition memory showed no such improvement with remission, indicating the stability of these two tests in the presence of depression. Steinberg & Jarvik (1976) likewise found that the greater the improvement in depression the greater was the improvement in short-term memory while long-term memory remained stable before and after treatment. Further confirmation is given by Caine (1981) who found that although depressed patients performed poorly, they demonstrated ability to learn new information. Also their delayed verbal recall tested after ten minutes was usually adequate and their recognition memory unimpaired. These results emphasize the fact that not all memory tests are sensitive to depression. Furthermore, the types of error differed between the two groups. While both groups made omission errors the dementing group made significantly more random errors and more false positives on a recognition task but significantly less transposition errors. The poorer performance of elderly patients with very clear evidence of memory disorder on recognition as well as free recall measures had been reported earlier by Inglis (1957,1959) though the diagnosis of dementia was not offered definitively in these patients.

Although some authors suggest the possibility of a common mechanism lowering the performance of both depressive and dementing patients, 'an alternative possibility is that the immediate causes of deficits are entirely different, since a great many factors are obviously involved in determining the actual score gained on a verbal learning task' (Whitehead 1973, p 283). This statement agrees with the argument made about the complex determination of most test scores in Chapter 1. Even the nature of the material may affect recall. In testing hospitalized depressed patients on the recall of prose material Breslow et al (1981) found that most of the deficit was due to poor recall of the positive themes in the story as opposed to the negative or neutral themes.

The evidence thus suggests that, if the patient is willing to co-operate, even a brief examination will demonstrate preserved new learning in depressed patients and this alone may be sufficient to direct the examination away from Alzheimer's disease. The author finds the Paired-Associate learning subtest from the Wechsler Memory Scale and supraspan digit learning the most sensitive screening measures. A good performance on these almost certainly excludes most forms of dementia.

Intelligence and other functions. In contrast to clinical impression, standard tests of intelligence appear to be little affected by depression. Butler & Perlin (1963), in an intensive study of 47 elderly men with mild depressive symptoms, found no effect on the eleven subtests of the WAIS or Raven's Progressive Matrices, but speed of reaction was affected. Similar findings are apparent in the data of Kendrick & Post (1967) for more depressed patients. Friedman's patients (Friedman 1964) were also severely depressed but an extensive testing which took a full day and yielded 82 test scores showed that only three scores were significantly lower than matched controls. Two of these involved speed of responding while the other was a test of binocular far acuity. Faibish & Kimbell (1977) specifically selected seven subtests of the WAIS which had earlier been suggested to be sensitive to depression (Rapaport et al 1945). Although employing conservative measures they found low correlations between test scores and ratings for depression. Added measures of psychomotor performance had a somewhat higher correlation but still did not reach significance.

Finally Donnelly et al (1982) examined a large group of patients in whom depression was severe enough to warrant hospitalization. The WAIS summarizing scores (VIQ, PIQ, FSIQ) were compared on admission and again on remission. Though these measures did improve between the two testings the magnitude of the rise was within the test-retest practice effect of this test suggesting once again the stability of these intellectual measures in the face of depression.

In summary it would seem that except in extreme cases of withdrawal and failure to co-operate, cognitive testing may be a useful adjunct in the differential diagnosis of depression and dementia. Intellectual measures are preserved in depressive cases even of moderate to marked severity while learning deficits, if they occur, are of less severity and are characterized by good recognition memory and retention of recently acquired material together with qualitatively different types of errors on rote learning.

Despite this general finding the recent report of Kral & Emery (1989) sounds a note of caution. In following elderly patients with so-called depressive pseudodementia they found that cognitive function improved after treatment and even after further relapses. Nevertheless, on long term follow-up, 90% of their 44 subjects developed dementia of the Alzheimer type. Perhaps it would be wise to continue to review elderly patients who experience periods of depression. Certainly we have found that demonstration of their intactness through the cognitive examination has been considerably reassuring for our patients.

It is worth stressing that depression and dementia may co-exist and there is consensus that all evidence of depression should be treated seriously even where there is clear evidence of organic deterioration (Post 1975, Kiloh 1981). A treatment trial may be of great value in doubtful cases especially where it is difficult to elicit a satisfactory history or decompensation is suspected as described earlier.

Psychological testing and pseudodementia

There is a widespread opinion that psychometric testing is of very limited value in distinguishing dementia from pseudodementia (Kiloh 1961, Post 1975, Smith et al 1976, Caine 1981, Roth 1981). The present author would agree with this if the term 'psychometric' is restricted to the use of level of performance only, on standardized measures of the Wechsler variety. Unfortunately the word 'psychometric' is used interchangeably by some with 'neuropsychological'. 'The patterns of intellectual impairment seen in patients with pseudodementia resembles, in many aspects, the kinds of cognitive abnormalities observed in patients with 'organic' disorders: clinicians who evaluate pseudodementia cannot use *neuropsychological testing* [my italic] as an infallible method for discriminating 'organic' from 'functional' disorders' (Caine 1981, p 1363). Two points might be made in reply to this. Firstly, neuro-psychological assessment has as one of its most valuable contributions the ability to demonstrate clearly how pseudoneurological conditions can usually be distinguished from them with a high degree of confidence by properly trained neuropsychologists. Secondly, neuropsychological assessment does not lay claim to be the sole basis on which to make a diagnosis of dementia. We would agree with Roth (1981) that clinical examination incorporating many lines of evidence is the correct way to proceed. Neuropsychological assessment provides part of the evidence upon which a diagnostic decision may be based. Sometimes this evidence is crucial.

Wells, on the other hand, found neuropsychological assessment useful in the diagnosis of pseudodementia: 'in none [of the nine cases] did the psychologists suggest that the clinical picture resulted from diffuse cerebral dysfunction such as is characteristic of dementia. All of these patients performed poorly on one or more of the tests usually used to measure organic dysfunction, but it was their inconsistent performance from test to test that argued most strongly against attributing their clinical dysfunction primarily to organic disease ...' (Wells 1979a). Though he admits other possible reasons for the results differing from those of other workers, Wells considers an equally plausible reason to be the more skilful interpretation by the psychologists involved.

Syndrome or artefact?

Some of the diagnostic difficulty between real dementia and pseudodementia has been produced by the failure to recognize that there are multiple causes for a clinical picture which may resemble dementia (Kiloh 1961). While admitting this, some writers have grouped the symptoms and signs together under the one heading or syndrome (Wells 1979a, Caine 1981). It might be preferable to attempt to separate the clinical features which belong to the subcategories. An examination of Well's table (1979a) listing the major clinical features differentiating pseudodementia from dementia shows statements which clearly refer to depressive pseudodementia, e.g. 'Patients usually communicate strong sense of distress'—a point in favour of pseudodementia. Kiloh (1981) points out that Roth & Myers (1975) listed this sense of distress as a characteristic feature of *depressed* pseudodementia and contrasted it with the empty and poorly communicated affect of the demented patient. Thus this symptom clearly refers to one particular class of pseudodementia. It is inappropriate to use it to represent part of a general syndrome. It clearly does not apply to the other major class of pseudodementias, viz hysterical pseudodementia. On the other hand, some of Wells' discriminating features do apply to this second group of hysterical pseudodementia and its congeners—'patient highlights failure', 'patient emphasizes disability'. Still other features might be applicable to either subgroup.

While stressing the non-unitary nature of the term pseudodementia, checklists may usefully turn the attention of clinicians to qualitative features which might allow an efficient screening of dementia from its imitators, thus allowing a more detailed appraisal of the nature and possible aetiology in individual cases.

CEREBRAL PATHOLOGY AND BEHAVIOURAL CHANGE

CT scan, atrophy and cognitive loss

Although there seems to be general agreement that a relationship exists between the presence of neuropathological changes and decline in higher mental functions, the nature, degree and determinants of this relationship are still unclear. A simple linear relationship between loss of brain integrity and behavioural incompetence was challenged several decades ago by studies comparing autopsy reports with observations of behaviour prior to death. These studies revealed exceptions in both directions, namely, individuals with wasted brains whose behaviour had not been characterized by apparent gross intellectual decline, and individuals with markedly deteriorated intellectual behaviour whose brains showed no evidence of wasting (e.g. Gallinek 1948, Gal 1959). This led some authors to postulate that behavioural breakdown was due to a combination of brain changes and the individual's capacity to compensate for such changes. This earlier literature contains numerous reports of various forms of treatment which improved the behaviour of individuals suffering from apparent dementia. These treatments included psychotherapy, drugs, electroconvulsive therapy and a variety of psychosocial manipulations. Though it is likely that these studies contained a number of patients who would now be classified as pseudodementia they probably also contained a number of patients of the types described by Shraberg (1979) who decompensated through a combination of neuropathological and psychosocial factors.

Computerized axial tomography

The advent of computerized tomography offered considerable advantages over pneumoencephalography in visualization of the state of the brain and rapidly replaced this latter procedure in most cases. From its inception, attempts were made to correlate the CT visual evidence of brain wasting with the clinical state, the latter sometimes including objective measures of cognitive function. Sundry measures of the CT image were used—mainly estimates of ventricular enlargement or cortical atrophy or a combination of the two. Early enthusiasm for the use of CT scanning in the diagnosis of dementia waned as experience accumulated and negative findings came to the fore. Roberts & Caird (1976) looked at 66 patients from 62 to 90 years who ranged from mentally normal to severely impaired. There was a broad relationship between increasing ventricular dilatation and increasing mental impairment. No such relationship was shown for cortical atrophy. Claveria et al (1977) found 'a rough correlation between signs of cortical atrophy and psychometric assessment [but] these are not statistically significant, owing to a wide scatter of values' (p 214). Some workers originally optimistic were less so as their studies became more definitive (Fox et al 1979, Kaszniak, Garron & Fox 1979, Kaszniak et al 1979) and their results confirmed a relatively weak correlation between degree of atrophy and degree of cognitive dysfunction. Fox et al (1979) reminded readers that the two terms cerebral atrophy and dementia are not synonymous 'cerebral atrophy is a radiologic or pathologic observation whereas dementia is a clinical diagnosis'. This opinion is shared by others (Levy 1975, Claveria et al 1977). Jacoby & Levy (1980) reported group differences but within the group of primary dementia there were only weak correlations between measures of cognitive impairment and ventricular measures but not of cortical atrophy.

The work of de Leon et al (1979, 1980) made it clear that the size of the correlation depended to some extent on the types of measure that were used, both radiological and psychological. They devised a method of 'blind' CT rating to produce a continuum of increased ventricular dilatation and increased sulcal prominence which were each correlated with 28 memory measures, seven psychomotor measures and two global measures of mental status and deterioration. As in other studies the ventricular measures proved superior to the cortical measures with 17 of the memory scores and five of the psychomotor being significant, compared with only seven of the memory scores and one psychomotor measure correlating with cortical atrophy. It seems that the presence and degree of relationship will vary with the measures adopted. Since appropriate details are not always provided it is difficult to compare studies. In an unpublished study of our own we found a nonsignificant correlation between purely quantitative psychometric data and CT appearance, but a significant correlation when the same data were rated for presence or absence of dementia by an experienced neuropsychologist who was provided with all the psychological test findings, both qualitative and quantitative, and who was 'blind' to the clinical state of the patient and the radiological findings.

Need for normative CT data

One of the other emerging requirements is the collection of normative data, since the degree of atrophy must be seen in relation to that found in the normal ageing population. Jacoby et al (1980), studying 50 elderly subjects considered to be both psychiatrically and neurologically normal, found a reciprocal relationship between a global rating of CT atrophy and a test of memory and orientation. However, the significance disappeared when controlled for age. In other areas where atrophy is produced in younger subjects, e.g. heavy drinkers, normative data is beginning to emerge (Roth 1977).

Even in the diagnosis of multi-infarct dementia, where one might expect computerized tomography would be most helpful, there must be reservations. Jacoby

& Levy (1980) found a significant excess of infarcts in dementia of the Alzheimer type when compared with normals even though patients with cerebrovascular disease had been excluded in selection.

Numerical versus visual methods. Recently a promising method of CT evaluation has been investigated. This makes 'direct use of the numerical output of the scanner instead of relying on visual reconstruction ... [this] exploits the computer component of the scanner rather than using this sophisticated equipment as a traditional X-Ray machine' (Naguib & Levy 1982). Several research papers have already appeared. Naeser et al (1980) examined the scans of patients with a provisional diagnosis of presenile dementia and found the CT density numbers showed different values for those with confirmed dementia compared with suspected cases in whom dementia had been ruled out. There was no overlap of the two distributions of numbers for their small groups. The density measures were independent of the presence or absence of prominent sulci. Bondareff et al (1981) similarly found regional differences in density between clinically demented patients and normal controls. The regional differences in density numbers followed the known distribution of Alzheimer's pathology, being most marked in the frontal and temporal regions. Once again this would emphasize the importance of incorporating into the neuropsychological examination tests which are sensitive to this type of regional pathology. The study of Naguib & Levy (1982) studied the follow-up of 40 subjects from the previous study of Jacoby and Levy (1980) after 28 months. Those surviving at this time had performed better on a number of tests, particularly measures of speech and constructional ability. Measures of atrophy and ventricular dilatation had no predictive value but density measures were significantly lower in the right parietal region in the non-survivors.

This research technique might find ready clinical application. Hence, with the refinement of both CT measures and the appropriate and sensitive neuropsychological assessment methods, we might return to the earlier state of optimism.

Cognitive testing

Neuropsychological assessment in cases of suspected dementia requires consideration of four major factors which might affect differential diagnosis: (1) the effects of normal ageing; (2) the effects of local or generalized neuropathology; (3) sensitivity of the cognitive measures to psychopathological factors; and (4) an estimate of the individual's premorbid level of ability. At times there may be an interaction of two or more of these.

Ageing

Methodological difficulties in gathering accurate, representative data in the elderly population has resulted in a relative dearth of clear information. This situation is being redressed, e.g. Savage (1973) and Kramer & Jarvik (1979) have reviewed most of the methods used to assess intellectual performance in older subjects with and without cerebral pathology. Some reviews limit themselves largely to particular sets of measures such as the Halstead-Reitan Battery (Klisz 1978) or to specific functions such as memory (Botwinick & Storandt 1974). Albert & Kaplan (1980) provide both qualitative as well as quantitative information on neuropsychological deficits in the elderly.

Of particular value is the substantial body of knowledge which indicates that slowing of perceptual, psychomotor and cognitive processes is characteristic of normal ageing. This knowledge must form part of the frame of reference for judging the significance of a particular performance especially as brain impairment also affects speed of response. The possibility of an interaction effect was demonstrated by Benton (1977) who showed that while brain damage slowed the reaction time of young subjects, it slowed older subjects much more. The interaction of a speed factor with other psychological processes is of crucial importance in determining the outcome on many tests. This area is reviewed extensively by Birren et al (1979). However, psychomotor slowing should not be construed simply as a pathophysiological process. It has been noted that reaction time in ageing individuals may be improved by appropriate adjustment of preparatory intervals. Likewise, altering the rate of presentation may improve the efficiency of learning in the elderly. Slowing in itself does not always mean the loss of ability to adapt behaviour to situation.

'The aura of ageing as a pathogenic process is difficult to dispel' (Baer 1972). Limited support for the hypothesis that normal ageing does not, of necessity, imply a general decline of intellectual functioning is provided by studies such as that by Benton, Eslinger and Damasio (1981). In generating normative data for nine tests in volunteers from 65 to 84 years they found little evidence for a general cognitive decline before the age of 80. Those over this age showed a higher overall failure on the tests but 70% of the over-80 group made no more than one failure on the nine tests.

One of the practical difficulties for workers in the field of ageing is that, while test manuals provide some information, much normative data of value is scattered throughout the literature. This needs to be corrected not only for comparison purposes in dementia but also because it is important to understand the cognitive abilities retained as well as lost. It is also apparent that most studies of performance in the elderly have confined themselves to establishing levels of performance. 'To ask at what level of cognitive functioning an older person is performing is only part of the evaluative task. It is more important to determine the mechanisms underlying less than optimal performance' (Kramer & Jarvik 1979, p259). This suggestion is, in fact, an extension to the normal aged of the notion of multiple causation of failure, particularly on complex tasks, which is the central theme of this text, i.e. the focus should be on *process* as well as level. The reliability of normative information in ageing will depend on appropriate methodology used in its gathering. The pitfalls are discussed by Baltes & Willis (1979) and Kramer & Jarvik (1979). Roth (1981) is one of many authors who have pointed to the fact that cross-sectional studies which have compared the performance of different age groups may have tended to give an exaggerated view of the amount of cognitive decline which may be attributed to normal senescence. It is obvious, too, that longitudinal studies may become increasingly loaded with the more fit, both mentally and physically. A large number of studies has shown a clear correlation between intellectual performance and survival (Jarvik & Falek 1963, Lieberman 1965, McDonald 1969, Palmore 1969, Blum et al 1970, Kay 1977).

Neuropathology

Effective differential diagnosis in dementia and pseudodementia necessitates familiarity with the whole gamut of neurological disorders that may produce cognitive impairment. Even geographically localized lesions, e.g. tumours, may have widespread effects via oedema, disconnection and diaschisis. Particular attention should be given to conditions such as neurovascular disorders (Ch. 6) which show an increase in frequency with age. Some workers have provided extensive clinical and research data in particular areas, e.g. Miller's work on the memory disorder in presenile dementia (Miller 1973, 1975, 1977, 1978). The present text assumes a general familiarity with such material as a requisite for development in clinical neuropsychology. Special attention should be paid to sensory disturbances which are particularly common with advancing age (Fields 1975).

Psychopathology

It is not uncommon for organic pathology and psychopathology to exist in the same patient. For this reason the simple dichotomy—functional versus organic—is often inappropriate and it behoves the examiner to be aware of the effects of such factors as anxiety, depression and preoccupation on the measures being used. Apart from cognizance of their presence it may be advisable to gain some estimate of their severity by means of personality assessment techniques. It is assumed throughout this text that neuropsychological assessment is taking place in a context where such information may be readily obtained. Most neuropsychologists, indeed, possess these skills themselves. Further reference to psychological factors is made in Chapter 4.

Premorbid ability

A reliable estimate of the individual's premorbid level of ability is essential for deficit measurement. This may take the form of using the best of a range of scores from a sample of the patient's performance on a variety of tasks such as the subtests of the Wechsler scales (Lezak 1976), or utilizing tasks which hold up well in the face of ageing or cerebral impairment. Of the latter, vocabulary has been widely accepted as such a stable measure. In 1975 Nelson & McKenna reported that the ability of patients to read aloud from the Schonell Graded Word Test was less affected by dementia than the commonly used Vocabulary subtest of the WAIS. In essence the mean reading scores for the dementing and control subjects were almost identical.

This led Nelson and her colleagues to derive a seemingly more robust test for the purpose of estimating former intellectual levels (Nelson and O'Connell 1978). The test is termed the New Adult Reading Test (NART). Words were selected which can be read correctly only 'if the subject knows of the word and recognizes its written form'. This was achieved by choosing 'irregular' words which differ from 'regular' words in that the former do not follow the usual transition from visual appreciation of the written form to its pronunciation. This obviates guessing to a large degree by excluding unfamiliar 'regular' words which might be read by literate subjects via application of common rules of pronunciation. Examples of 'irregular' words are 'subtle', 'gaoled', 'banal', 'labile' and 'prelate'. The test has a high ceiling and is thus suitable for a wide range of patients. Our clinical experience suggests it as a valuable adjunct to examination, particularly as it is brief and is well accepted by patients. O'Carroll & Gilleard (1986) have shown that the NART is independent of behavioural and cognitive measures of severity in demented patients—a further confirmation of its usefulness.

Rating scales

There have been numerous attempts to standardize and quantify the mental status examination. The earliest appears to be the Mental Test Score of Roth & Hopkins (1953). A variation of this scale was used in the well known study of Blessed et al (1968). A similar mental status questionnaire by Kahn et al (1960), used in screening a large number of persons over 65, also found a high correlation with the clinical presence and severity of organic brain impairment. Robinson (1979) provides a brief review of rating scales in dementia while more extensive treatment is provided by Raskin & Jarvik (1979).

Perhaps the most documented rating scale is the Mini Mental State test devised by Folstein et al (1975). It concentrates on cognitive functions only (orientation, registration, attention, calculation, recall and language) and includes eleven questions generating scores from zero to 30. It can be given in five to ten minutes, thereby not taxing the attention and co-operation of elderly subjects. The test has shown some promise as a screening procedure and it correlates well enough with CT evidence of both atrophy and focal lesions to commend its use in some situations (Tsai & Tsuang 1979). However, the finding of measurable overlap between the scores of some depressed patients and some with Alzheimer's disease, despite significant group mean differences, urges caution in its use (McHugh & Folstein 1979). Rating scales have also been devised to follow stages in the progression of dementing states (Hughes et al 1982).

CASE EXAMPLES

Case: YN

This 55-year-old farmer presented with the complaint of difficulty with reading which had progressively worsened over the preceding year. He was also concerned about the fall-off in his ability to remember things both recent and remote. He claimed that he had no difficulty carrying out his work as a farmer. He had taken up farming after the end of the Second World War and had been successful in his work.

He had completed eight years of primary education before serving as a private throughout the war.

At interview YN expressed concern about his recent difficulties, but described a word-finding difficulty rather than a general memory problem. He said that he had difficulty calling to mind the right words when asked specific questions. By contrast, he reported, and demonstrated in interview, intact ability to carry on less structured conversation about familiar topics in a fluent manner provided these were of a simple nature. His chronology of past events was, however, noted to be somewhat jumbled, and his narrative was rambling and a little disjointed. As the interview proceeded it became obvious that YN's intellectual problems were widespread.

With a view to excluding presenile dementia, neuropsychological assessment began with an examination of memory:

Wechsler Memory Scale, Form I

Information	1	Digits Total	8 (5, 3)
Orientation	3	Visual Reproduction	0
Mental Control	0	Associate Learning	abandoned
Memory Passages	2		

Almost at the outset it was clear that the patient had a severe, pervasive memory problem which was strikingly at variance with the air of apparent preservation in the early part of the interview, though not unexpected in the light of more and more problems which had emerged as the interview proceeded. He showed a profound inability to learn new information and the paired associate learning subtest had to be abandoned as he was only able to hold for a very brief interval just what it was he was supposed to be attempting. His immediate memory was somewhat low and after the WMS further questioning confirmed that his long-term memory was also affected, for example, he was unable to give even approximate dates for the Second World War despite its salience as an event within his personal history. An attempt was then made to sample other intellectual abilities.

Wechsler Adult Intelligence Scale (scaled scores)

Information	8	Picture Completion	3
Similarities	10	Block Design	0
Digit Span	6	Object Assembly	0

On the WAIS Information and Similarities subtests YN obtained scores that approximate to what might be expected from his educational, occupational and social history. However, these two scores on tests utilizing his store of old information were isolated peaks in an otherwise very poor performance on a wide range of tasks. Once confronted with even the simplest of new tasks, he demonstrated clearly his general fall-off in all areas of ability. He could not manage the simplest Block Design item even with demonstrations and was totally unable to piece together any of the Object Assembly figures. His writing and spelling were also seriously affected.

During this testing YN showed that he was aware that he was not able to do many things which he felt he could have done with ease previously. With this degree of insight he was understandably anxious and depressed about his deficits. For this

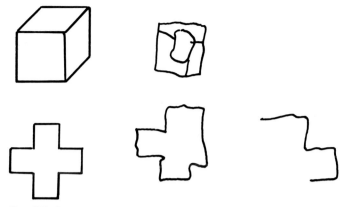

Fig. 3.1   Case YN. Attempts at copying simple drawings.

reason testing was not extended beyond what was necessary to make clear the wide-ranging nature of his difficulties. A diagnosis of presenile dementia was made. There was nothing in the history or subsequent medical examination which contradicted this diagnosis and a CT scan showed marked generalized cerebral atrophy.

The case is somewhat unusual in view of the patient's awareness of his difficulties and well-preserved, socially appropriate behaviour in the presence of such severe intellectual impoverishment. It is an example of how degraded higher intellectual function may be on psychological examination in contrast to day-to-day or clinical impressions.

Case: OD

This 55-year-old telephonist was admitted for investigation of patchy memory loss of relatively sudden onset, apparently extending back some weeks. The only medical history was of hypertension which was well controlled by medication. Certain features of the history suggested a possible vascular cause for her difficulties and, after other examinations proved negative, aortic arch arteriography was performed. The major blood vessels were unusually tortuous, but freely patent and smooth walled. There was a smooth indentation in the posterior wall of the left internal carotid artery but this was thought to be of unlikely clinical significance.

It was difficult to obtain a history of recent events from the patient who stated that she did not know whether her memory was bad or not. Her family and friends were in no such doubt. Examination with the Wechsler Memory Scale rapidly confirmed the presence of a marked recent memory disorder which stood in contrast to the preservation of old information during the clinical interview.

WMS , Form I

Information	3	Digits Total	11
Orientation	4	Visual Reproduction	3
Mental Control	9	Associate learning	7 (4,0;4,0;4,1)
Memory Passages	1		
MQ 77			

There was some confusion of temporal orientation. She gave the year as twenty years before, but corrected this without significant difficulty and correctly gave the day and the month. Likewise she gave as the name of the Prime Minister that of a man who had held the office twenty years earlier. Once again, she gave the correct answer with little prompting. She received the maximum score for Mental Control and performed well on Digits Forward, but was able to retrieve only fragments of the Memory Passages and began to confabulate when pressed. She readily produced four of the easy associate pairs on the first trial but failed to improve on this and had produced only one difficult association by the third trial. Her attempts on Visual Reproduction were marked not only by poverty of recall but also by micrographia (Fig. 3.2). The latter feature was subsequently found in her writing.

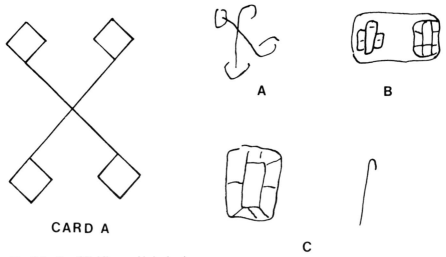

Fig. 3.2   Case OD. Micrographia in drawing.

To estimate her current level of intellectual functioning, subtests of the NHAIS were given:

Information	9	Letter Symbol	7
Comprehension	8	Block Design	4
Similarities	11	Object Assembly	3
Memory for Digits	10		

The level and quality of responses on the verbal subtests seemed consonant with her educational background. She described herself in this regard as a plodder. In contrast she had the greatest difficulty with the two problem-solving constructional tasks. She seemed unable to develop a strategy for solving any but the simplest Block Design problems and sometimes would select the correct face of a block only to place it wrongly, and seemed to be unaware of her error. No constructional deviations were noted. On Object Assembly she had no idea where to begin and the few pieces scored correct probably occurred by chance. At this juncture it was clear that there was a widespread intellectual difficulty rather than an isolated amnesic syndrome. Testing was incomplete when the patient was allowed to return to her home in the country for a short time. However, the case was labelled tentatively as one of presenile dementia.

Ten days later the patient was re-admitted for further investigation and the neuropsychological examination was extended:

Porteus Maze Test. OD took two trials to succeed on years VII and IX, passed on the first trial of years VIII and XI and failed all higher levels. The exceedingly poor performance (Mental Age of 9 years) seemed in keeping with the preliminary diagnosis.

Rey Figure. A complete figure was produced in a piecemeal fashion (Fig. 3.3). The recall at 3 minutes was devoid of detail and micrographic. When asked, the patient said she was aware that her drawing was much smaller than the model. It was decided to see whether the patient might improve her performance if she were provided with a strategy for going about the task. She was taken through a series of steps suggested by Lhermitte et al (1972). After this training and only a one minute delay there was not the slightest improvement in her recall.

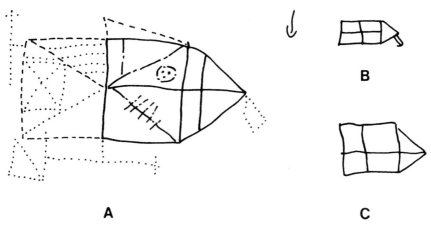

Fig. 3.3 Case OD. Rey Figure. A, Copy. B, Recall. C, After training.

Following this second examination it was apparent that the patient was much more intellectually reduced than appeared on clinical examination. Observation in the ward revealed that the patient's mood fluctuated from one of indifference to fatuous euphoria. Confirmation of the diagnosis was provided by an air encephalogram which showed 'some dilatation of the ventricular system with marked dilatation of the sulci'. Further confirmation of the widespread nature of the decline in higher functions was given by the speech therapy department who found a disorder of language which included mild visual-graphic naming difficulties with paraphasias, decreased verbal fluency and problems with reading comprehension. The therapist also remarked on the flippancy of some of the responses which was in keeping with her 'frontal' disinhibition shown occasionally in the ward. When examined briefly some ten months later there appeared to be no change in her condition. She was not seen again.

On discharge the most likely diagnosis was thought to be Alzheimer's disease. Exhaustive medical investigation had failed to reveal any other cause for the dementia.

Case: YK

The referring neurologist wrote succinctly about this 60-year-old man: 'This patient was sent to me with depression, anxiety and failing ability to teach. He has a past history of considerable social, physical and psychic disruption due to the Second World War. His CT scan shows considerable cerebral atrophy and I would be very grateful if you could run a neuropsychological examination upon him to give us an estimation of his cerebral horsepower because I think this is in fact worrying him—with good cause.'

YK had qualified and worked as a chemical engineer in Europe. In 1949 he emigrated to Canada where he taught high school mathematics until 1970, when he moved to Australia and continued this profession. He had noticed that he had become increasingly forgetful over the two years preceding his referral and was becoming unable to cope effectively with his teaching. At the age of 59 he took the opportunity offered to him of early retirement. At this stage his wife found it necessary to leave written instructions for him each day before she left for work or she would return home to find basic chores undone. She reacted by becoming upset and angry with his forgetfulness and this worried the patient.

During the preliminary interview YK showed an acute awareness of his reduced mental ability and realized that his reaction was compounding a condition of anxiety and depression stretching back to his horrendous experiences during the Second World War. His remote memory was well preserved and he gave a good chronological account of his life. He recounted the trauma of the concentration camp, telling of the daily horror, including a period when he was confined next to the gas chambers used for mass executions. His memory of more recent events appeared intact over a period of about six months before the interview. During this preliminary inquiry he volunteered information over his concern that his present decline was due to a hereditary condition, as he recalled his father having similar difficulties at a relatively early age. He became progressively more relaxed during these discussions and showed no overt signs of being unduly anxious during formal testing. The relatively simple material of the Wechsler Memory Scale, Form I allowed him some successes which appeared to reassure him further:

Information	6	Digits Total	11 (6,5)
Orientation	5	Visual Reproduction	7
Mental Control	8	Associate Learning	13.5 (6.1;5.2;6.2)
Memory Passages	7		
MQ 110			

Though the memory quotient might be described as being in the upper range of normal, it was thought to represent a considerable degradation from what might have been expected—his conversation and his occupational and educational (university) background would suggest a superior intellect. The pattern of performance is one we have seen quite early in the dementing process, namely, preserved orientation, immediate memory, and automatic mental operations with a nonspecific lessening of new learning.

Several performance subtests of the WAIS were given. These were selected in the knowledge of the history and CT scan findings, and our experience that much of the verbal portion of the WAIS may hold up well in cases of early intellectual decline, especially in literate subjects. There was a poor performance on the Digit-Symbol substitution test (SS,7) as might be expected. However, the patient had no observable difficulty with Block Design (SS,12) and his relatively poor showing on Object Assembly (SS,9) seemed to be due to a general psychomotor retardation with no qualitative features suggestive of constructional apraxia. On the Trail Making Test the slowing was evident more on the alternation series (Part B, 115 seconds) than on Part A (35 seconds) though there were no errors. At this stage it was felt that while intellectual impairment was present it was not of gross degree.

However, we have found that in the early stages of most forms of dementia, and particularly in Alzheimer's disease, intellectual decline is shown most clearly in tests of adaptive abilities of the 'frontal lobe' type. For this reason we always include these tests in such situations.

Austin Maze Test. YK grasped the nature of what he had to do and by the third trial appeared to be well on the way to success. A further seven trials resulted in no progress whatsoever and he became increasingly frustrated with a task which he sensed was well within his former ability. At this stage the test was abandoned in order not to distress the patient and since the common difficulty of error utilization had been demonstrated to the examiner's satisfaction. The performance had been characterized by repeated errors at the same choice points on trial after trial despite the patient's obvious awareness of the sites at which he went wrong.

Colour-Form Sorting Test. YK handled this test with ease. The test has subsequently been shown to be insensitive to early intellectual decline in intelligent subjects for whom it seems to represent a relatively automatic mental operation and thus not a true test of conceptual manipulation.

Rey Figure. YK produced a neat, well-ordered copy with maximum points but an extremely depleted recall after three minutes (Fig. 3.4).

In summary, at this stage, it was considered that the patient was showing signs of mild to moderate intellectual decline in keeping with the neurological evidence. There was no evidence of any attempt to exaggerate nor any evidence of a major effect on the tests from his anxiety and depression. Serial examination was recommended but the patient was not referred again until more than two years later.

On the second occasion the patient reported that his condition seemed to be much the same. His main subjective complaint was of his poor memory. He was still living at home and managed only the simplest of tasks with the aid of memoranda left by his wife each day when she went to work. Even some of these were forgotten despite her notes. At interview the patient presented as before though he appeared to have less insight and less concern. On examination he showed the same pattern of performance as before with a worsening in most areas.

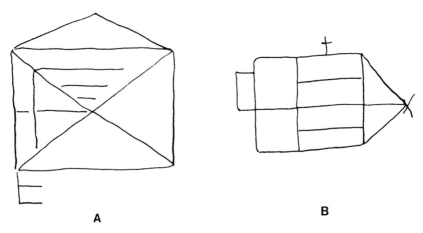

Fig. 3.4   Case YK. Rey Figure. A, Recall. B, Recall, two years later.

WMS. Form II

Information	6	Digits Total	11 (6,5)
Orientation	4	Visual Reproduction	3
Mental Control	6	Associate Learning	7 (2,0;4,0;4,2)
Memory Passages	3		
MQ 83			

A repetition of the WAIS performance subtests given two and a half years previously showed some decline in level and a now obvious difficulty with the more advanced items on the Block Design subtest. A number of other tests given before (but not reported) also showed a moderate lowering. The Austin Maze performance (B) is shown in comparison with the earlier testing (A).

Trial	1	2	3	4	5	6	7	8	9	10
Errors (A)	12	11	6	7	8	6	6	4	9	8
Errors (B)	20	18	19	18	11	12	17	10	7	10

Once again he expressed dissatisfaction that he could not improve beyond a certain point and asked to be allowed to stop. His performance was marred by the same qualitative errors as before.

Rey Figure. He obtained the maximum score for his copy and a very reduced recall though he scored a few more points than on the first occasion.

All in all, although some further decline had probably taken place, this had not progressed at the rate we have seen in other cases of what we assume to be Alzheimer's disease with comparable degenerative changes on CT scan. This case is closer to a number of others who have shown little progression after the impairment has come to light, and which one might label stable or non-progressive cerebral impairment rather than Alzheimer's disease. Unfortunately, little or no information exists on the neuropathology in such cases. The demonstration of the very slow progression in these cases has been supportive for those patients who fear not only that the condition is progressive but that it will also be rapidly so.

Case: RN

This 78-year-old former university professor was referred for investigation of deteriorating mental functions over the preceding three or four months. Up to that time he had been active but frail and it was known that he had continued some aspects of university teaching well into his seventies. In keeping with his background he was able to discourse intelligently about literary criticism and other matters relevant to his lifetime academic interests. On day-to-day matters, however, he was far from clear and, though co-operative, appeared mildly confused and sometimes wandered from the point. Physically, he was clearly weak.

The accompanying medical history showed him to have been in good health until some three years before when he was discovered to have hypotension. Four months before the present referral, secondary deposits of carcinoma had been found invading the lymph glands and surrounding tissue of the left axilla. Further investigation revealed a primary lung tumour which was inoperable. It was during these investigations that what was thought to be a mild mental impairment came to the fore. At first it was thought that his deteriorating mental state might be due to secondary carcinomatous deposits in the brain but no cerebral metastases were seen in the CT scan.

As the interview proceeded a memory defect became obvious. This included some difficulty with recalling remote events as well as a severe problem with recent memory. In fact, his ability to repeat the strongly overlearned material from his professional life gave a totally false impression of a preserved memory and intellect. He was unaware of the name of the hospital but knew, correctly, that it began with the letter 'A' and knew of its location.

He gave the year and month correctly but not the date. At times questions had to be repeated and later instructions needed stressing to maintain his attention and motivation. He was fully co-operative throughout, though the examination was conducted slowly because of his frail condition. The Wechsler scales were considered adequate to answer the question of the presence of dementia. The figures in parentheses represent scaled scores.

WAIS

Information	17(18)	Digit Symbol	0 (8)
Comprehension	17(19)	Block Design	0 (0)
Similarities	11(14)	Picture Arrangement	0 (0)
Digit Span	10(13)	Object Assembly	0 (4)

WMS, Form 1

Information	5	Digits Total	11 (6,5)
Orientation	3	Vis. Reproduction	3
Mental Control	5	Assoc. Learning	8 (3,1;4,0;5,1)
Memory Passages	7.5		
MQ 90+			

The quality of responses on Information and Comprehension clearly demonstrated the sparing of a good deal of his old information, while those on Similarities were obviously inferior for a man of his background. However, on the Performance items his intellectual deterioration became most apparent. He managed only a raw score of 19 on Digit-Symbol but clearly knew what to do. On Block Design he was unable to complete even the simplest item even when provided with extra help. On the Picture Arrangement subtest he picked up each card and spoke about it but could not integrate them at all into a series. One of his better efforts on the Object Assembly is shown (Fig. 3.5). The Wechsler Memory Scale confirmed the clinically apparent difficulty with recent memory.

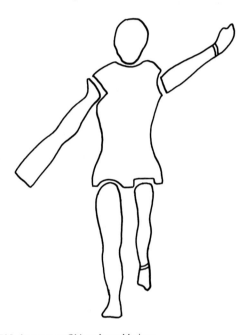

Fig. 3.5 Case RN. Attempt on Object Assembly item.

Two other tests were given at this examination:

Porteus Maze Test: Having failed two trials on year VIII, RN was given the five-year-old problem which he solved (only with some difficulty), and the test was abandoned.

Colour-Form Sorting Test: RN sorted the pieces into groups according to shape, commenting 'circles, triangles—can't remember, oblongs or squares. Squares I think'. He was then able to sort the pieces into the colour groupings. The preservation of the ability of formerly intelligent subjects to do this conceptual sorting in the face of obvious general intellectual impairment has been commented upon in the previous case (YK).

The psychologist reporting this case wrote 'RN has an adequate memory span (6 digits) but is having difficulty in coping with new learning and retention of new material. This is apparent for both verbal and visual material, but predominantly when the modality is visual. Old well stored information appears relatively intact and gives a verbal IQ of 138 but he has significant difficulties with visuo-constructive problem-solving tasks, and analysis and organization of complex visual material. *Pattern of deficits suggests involvement of right hemisphere functions,* [my italic].

This case is presented since it seems to represent the same type of simplistic inference that has been alluded to elsewhere (see Ch. 2) between poor performance on the non-verbal subtests and right hemisphere disturbance.

There is no doubt that RN performed very poorly indeed on visuo-spatial and visuo-constructive tasks. On the other hand there is insufficient novel, problem-solving material in the WAIS verbal subtests given to challenge this patient in the verbal sphere. Certainly his performance on Similarities is very much below those on the two 'Hold' tests of long stored information, viz. Information and Comprehension, and quite out of keeping with what would be expected from the context of his background. It is totally misleading to quote a Verbal IQ of 138 with the suggestion in the last sentence that there is relative sparing of left hemisphere (verbal) functions. The scores merely point to the relative insensitivity of measures of well stored information, especially in intelligent, literate individuals. Subsequent attempts to get this patient to solve verbal problems on the basis of novel information were all met with failure.

The air of preservation due to the patient's 'intelligent' conversation also meant that the referring physicians were surprised to hear that his intellectual decline was well advanced.

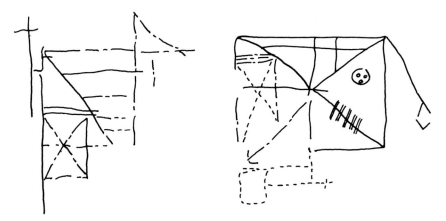

Fig. 3.6   Case RN. Two attempts to copy Rey Figure.

On a second occasion RN was asked to copy the Rey figure. Having begun to copy the figure (Fig. 3.6, left) he became dissatisfied with his efforts saying 'If I were doing this properly I should start with a rectangle and then add in the diagonals'. Despite this amount of insight his second attempt was also produced in a piecemeal fashion (Fig. 3.6, right). This was thought to represent an instance of the 'curious dissociation between knowing and doing' seen so frequently where pathological processes encroach on the frontal regions. His recall of the figure at three minutes (Fig. 3.7) bore little resemblance to the original. Further testing only served to confirm the presence a marked difficulty with new learning and all forms of problem solving irrespective of the type of material.

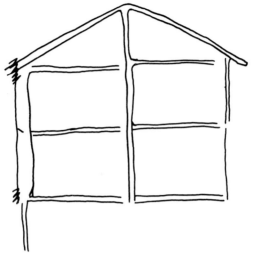

Fig. 3.7   Case RN. Rey Figure. Recall.

The nature of the dementing process was never discovered and no autopsy was possible when the patient succumbed to his carcinoma three months later.

The case represents a situation where the preservation of a store of sophisticated information at a level far beyond that seen in most intact people may give a misleading impression of relative mental preservation in formerly highly intelligent subjects. It is important when confronted with such a possibility to select a range of tests of adaptive behaviour in all spheres of mental activity to bring out the widespread nature of the intellectual decline.

Case: DY

This 49-year-old labourer living in a distant country town presented with a history of 'falls' which, his wife reported, extended back some eleven years. The episodes were poorly documented and apparently only occurred at lengthy intervals. After one of these episodes, four years previously, he was hospitalized and was apparently told that his condition was epilepsy. When he had two episodes at work in an eight week period he was started on sodium phenytoin and diazepam by his local physician. A month before his transfer to the department of neurology of a large city hospital he had suffered an episode of greater than usual severity. He started to shake, his legs went weak and he blacked out, waking up in the ambulance. Since then he had permanent weakness in the arms and legs and myoclonic jerking movements. The latter he reported to have suffered for two years, along with paraesthesia and numbness in the legs. His appetite had decreased, and he had lost 19 kg in that period. On admission he appeared to be well oriented, but his speech was monotonous, and he had a slow, stooped, broad-based gait. He was found to have considerable wasting, weakness and dystonia in all muscle groups, reflexes were depressed and he showed some spinothalamic distal sensory loss. Differential diagnosis included motor neurone disease, paraneoplastic disease and peripheral neuropathy.

CT scan revealed a moderate degree of cerebral atrophy, the EEG record was diffusely abnormal, and electromyography showed evidence of myopathy. Muscle biopsy supported a diagnosis of mitochondrial myopathy. These latter results were not available at the time of neuropsychological assessment.

At his first referral to the Neuropsychology Department the patient was still recovering from a generalized seizure, and therefore second and third examinations were carried out one and two weeks later. In view of the uncertainty as to the diagnosis, it was decided to sample cognitive functions with standardized tests. Though DY had had only basic schooling to the age of 13 he seemed of approximately average intelligence in general conversation. His performance on the Wechsler Memory Scale was unexpectedly poor.

First testing

WMS, Form I

Information	4	Digits Total	6(4,2)
Orientation	2	Visual Reproduction	4
Mental Control	5	Associate Learning	4.5(3,0;2,0;4,2)
Memory Passages	5		

M.Q. 64

It was felt that part of this poor performance might have been due to his recent seizure although he appeared alert and seemed to understand what was required of him on the simple material of the memory scale.

Several subtests of the NHAIS were attempted. He managed a score of 9 on Picture Completion but did not appear to understand what was needed on the Letter Symbol and Block Design subtests, so testing was abandoned. A tentative opinion was given that there might be a general lowering of intellectual function not solely accounted for by his preceding epileptic seizure. The ward staff evinced surprise that he might be suffering from 'dementia' since he had answered many questions on everyday matters adequately.

The patient's wife said that she considered her husband had been at least of average intelligence and her description of his history seemed to support this adequately.

She felt that he had become mentally slow for some time but thought that this was due to the undiagnosed disease which was causing his loss of weight, muscle twitching and falls. He had continued at work until a few weeks before his admission.

Second testing

There had been no seizures in the ensuing week and the patient appeared a trifle more robust. The findings of the special investigations were now to hand. There was little indication from his conversation that there was anything at all wrong with his mental functions and it was understandable that ward staff had been surprised at the suggestion of dementia. His performance on   motor tasks was hampered slightly by his hand tremor.

WMS, Form II

Information	4	Digits Total	7 (5,2)
Orientation	5	Visual Reproduction	7
Mental Control	5	Associate Learning	6.5 (3,0;5,0;3.1)
Memory Passages	11		

MQ 86

This represented a measurable improvement on the first examination but it was felt that there was still difficulty with new learning (Visual Reproduction and Associate Learning) and DY seemed totally unable to manipulate the digits to repeat them backwards, and he could not complete the serial addition task. At this stage he admitted on questioning that his memory had been troubling him for some time and he described a word finding difficulty.

WAIS (Scaled Scores)

Information	8	Block Design	3
Similarities	6	Picture Completion	10

While some of the poor test scores might have been accounted for by his restricted educational experience, his Block Design performance left no doubt that he had a serious acquired deficit. He managed to complete only two of the simpler designs (1 and 3). He was unable to solve either of the early embedded designs (2 and 4) even when given extra help. Despite much concerted effort on his part the test had to be discontinued without further success. The Picture Completion subtest produced a score thought to be close to the optimum but, qualitatively, his performance was marked by an obvious word-finding difficulty.

Colour-Form Sorting Test. While able to sort the pieces according to shape he could not be brought to recognize the principle of sorting by colour.

Porteus Maze Test. Mental Age 10.5 years. DY required two trials on years IX and X, three on year XII and was unable to succeed on year XIV although allowed five trials.

Associative Word Fluency
F-6; A-4; S-8

There was a discrepancy between the patient's conversational fluency and his marked difficulty in finding words to fit the letter categories. The increasing difficulty over elapsed time on each letter which has been noted with frontal lesions (Walsh 1987) was clearly evident. There was no comprehension difficulty of any marked degree as shown by a good score on the Token Test and DY readily grasped logico-grammatical relations.

Trail Making Test
Part A—120 seconds. Performed very slowly but accurately.
Part B—DY was in difficulties even on the sample but finally grasped what was required and proceeded with much difficulty and encouragement, after which he

made multiple errors; the test was abandoned at four minutes. He seemed unable to monitor what he was doing and constantly lapsed into a continuation of either the letter or number series.

After this examination it was considered that there was widespread intellectual fall-off of moderate to severe degree and the association of a dementing process in the presence of myoclonus and other neurological signs raised the possibility of Creutzfeldt-Jacob disease or one of its congeners despite the length of history. Despite further intensive investigations the diagnosis remained uncertain.

Third Testing

Because of the uncertain nature of DY's disorder, a videotape record was made of the neuropsychological examination two weeks later for future comparison. Apart from the features already described he was unable to complete any of the Object Assembly items even when told what the objects were and when the examiner began the construction. Testing was terminated with the copying of the Rey figure. In view of the poverty of this production (Fig. 3.8) it was thought pointless to ask the patient to attempt recall.

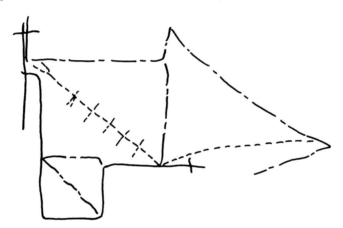

Fig. 3.8   Case DY. Rey Figure. Copy.

At discharge some weeks later the patient's epilepsy had responded well to sodium valproate and remained under control at review six months later though the myoclonus remained as before. There was no obvious further mental deterioration on clinical examination.

REFERENCES

Adams R D, Fisher C M, Hakim S, Ojemann R G, Sweet W H 1965 Symptomatic occult hydrocephalus with 'normal' cerebrospinal fluid pressure. A treatable syndrome. The New England Journal of Medicine 273: 117–126
Adams J H, Corsellis J A N, Duchen L W (eds) 1984 Greenfield's neuropathology, 4th edn. Arnold, London

Albert M S, Kaplan E 1980 Organic implications of neuropsychological deficits in the elderly. In: Poon L, Fozard J, Cermak L, Ehrenberg D, Thompson L (eds) New directions in memory and aging. Erlbaum, New Jersey

Baer P E 1972 Cognitive changes in aging: competence and incompetence. In: Gaitz C M (ed) Aging and the brain. Plenum Press, New York

Ball M J 1977 Neuronal loss, neurofibrillary tangles and granulovacuolar degeneration in the hippocampus with aging and dementia. A quantitative study. Acta Neuropathologica 37:111–118

Baltes P B, Willis S L 1979 The critical importance of appropriate methodology in the study of aging: the sample case of psychometric intelligence. In: Hoffmeister F, Muller C (eds) Brain function in old age. Springer-Verlag, Berlin

Benton A L 1977 Interactive effects of age and brain disease on reaction time. Archives of Neurology 34: 369–370

Benton A L Eslinger P J, Damasio A R 1981 Normative observations on neuropsychological test performance in old age. Journal of Clinical Neuropsychology 3: 33–42

Birren J E, Woods A M, Williams M V 1979 Speed of behavior as an indicator of age changes and the integrity of the nervous system. In: Hoffmeister F, Muller C (eds) Springer-Verlag Berlin

Blessed G, Tomlinson B E, Roth M 1968 The association between quantitative measurements of dementia and of senile changes in the cerebral grey matter of elderly subjects. British Journal of Psychology 114: 797–811

Blum J E, Jarvik L F, Clarke E T 1970 Rate of change on selective tests of intelligence: a twenty year longitudinal study of aging. Journal of Gerontology 25: 171–176

Bolton N, Britton P G, Savage R D 1966 Some normative data on the WAIS and its indices in an aged population. Journal of Clinical Psychology 22 184–188

Bolton N, Savage R D, Roth M 1967 The Modified Word Learning Test and the aged psychiatric patient. British Journal of Psychiatry 113: 1139–1140

Bondareff W, Baldy R, Levy R 1981 Quantitative computed tomography in senile dementia. Archives of General Psychiatry 38:1365–1368

Botwinick J, Storandt M 1974 Memory related functions and age. Thomas Springfield, Illinois

Brent R H 1979 Psychosocial variables in dementia and pseudodementia. American Journal of Psychiatry 136: 1613

Breslow R, Kocsis J, Belkin B 1981 Contribution of the depressive perspective to memory function in depression. American Journal of Psychiatry 38: 227–230

Brun A 1987 Frontal lobe degeneration of non-Alzheimer type: I Neuropathology. Archives of Gerontology and Geriatrics 6: 193–208

Brust J C M 1983 Vascular dementia—still overdiagnosed. Stroke 14: 298–300

Butler R N, Perlin, S 1983 Physiological-psychological-psychiatric interrelationships. In: Birren J, et al (eds) Human ageing: a biological and behavioural study. US Department of Health Education and Welfare, Bethesda, Maryland p 293–300

Caine E D 1981 Pseudodementia: current concepts and future directions. Archives of General Psychiatry 38: 1359–1364

Claveria L E, Moseley I F, Stevenson J F 1977 The clinical significance of 'cerebral atrophy' as shown by CAT. In: du Boulay G H, Moseley I F(eds) First European seminar on computerized tomography in clinical practice. Springer-Verlag, Berlin, p 213–217

Coughlan A K, Hollows S E 1984 Use of memory tests in differentiating organic disorder from depression. British Journal of Psychiatry 145: 164–167

Cronholm B C, Ottosson J-0 1961 Memory function in endogenous depression before and after ECT. Archives of General Psychiatry 5: 193–199

Dayan A D 1970a Quantitative histological studies on the aged human brain: 1 Senile plaques and neurofibrillary tangles in 'normal' patients. Acta Neuropathologica 16: 85–94

Dayan A D 1970b Quantitative histological studies on the aged human brain: 2 Senile plaques and neurofibrillary tangles in senile dementia. Acta Neuropathologica 16: 95–102

De Leon M J, Ferris S H, Blau I, George A E, Reisberg B, Kricheff I I and Gershon S 1979 Correlations between computerized tomographic changes and behavioural deficits in senile dementia. Lancet 2(8147): 859–860

De Leon M J, Ferris S H, George A E,Reisberg B,Kricheff I I, Gershon S 1980 Computed tomography evaluations of brain behaviour relationships in senile dementia of the Alzheimer's type. Neurobiology of Aging 1: 69–79

Donnelly E F, Murphy D L, Goodwin F K, Waldman I N 1982 Intellectual function in primary affective disorder. British Journal of Psychiatry 140: 633–636

du Boulay G H, Radu E, Thomas D J, Kendall B E 1979 Plain iothalamate-enhanced and xenon-enhanced CT in cerebral infarction. In: Price T R, Nelson E, (Eds) Cerebrovascular diseases. Raven Press New York

Faibish G M, Kimbell I 1977 Psychological correlates of severity of depression. In: Fann W E et al (eds) Phenomenology and treatment of depression. Spectrum, New York

Fields W S (ed) 1975 Neurological and sensory disorders in the elderly. Stratton Intercontinental, New York

Fisher C M 1968 Dementia in cerebral vascular disease. In: Toole J F, Sickert R G, Whisnant J P (eds) Cerebral vascular disease. Sixth Princeton conference. Grune and Stratton, New York

Folstein M F, Folstein S E, McHugh P R 1975 Mini mental state. Journal of Psychiatric Research 12: 189–198

Fox J H, Kaszniak A W, Huckman H M 1979 Computerized tomographic scanning not very helpful in dementia—nor in craniopharyngioma. New England Journal of Medicine 300:437

Freemon F R 1976 Evaluation of patients with intellectual deterioration. Archives of Neurology 33: 658–659

Friedman A S 1964 Minimal effects of severe depression on cognitive functioning. Journal of Abnormal and Social Psychology 69: 237–243

Gal P 1959 Mental disorders of advanced years. Geriatrics 14:224–228

Gallinek A 1948 The nature of affective and paranoid disorders in the light of electric convulsive therapy. Journal of Nervous and Mental Disease 108: 293–303

Goldin S, MacDonald J E 1955 The Ganser State. Journal of Mental Science 101: 267–280

Graham F K, Kendall B S 1960 Memory for Designs Test: revised general manual. Perceptual and Motor Skills 147–188

Gustafson L 1987 Frontal lobe degeneration of non-Alzheimer type: II Clinical picture and differential diagnosis. Archives of Gerontology and Geriatrics 6: 209–223

Hachinski V C, Iliff L D, Zilhka E, du Boulay G H, McAllister V L, Marshall J, Ross Russell R W, Symon L 1975 Cerebral blood flow in dementia. Archives of Neurology 32: 632–637

Hachinski V C, Lassen N A, Marshall J 1974 Multi-infarct dementia: a cause of mental deterioration in the elderly. Lancet 2: 207–210

Hagberg B 1987 Behaviour correlates to frontal lobe dysfunction. Archives of Gerontology and Geriatrics 6: 311–321

Hagberg B, Gustafson L 1985 On diagnosis of dementia: psychometric investigation and clinical psychiatric evaluation in relation to psychiatric diagnosis. Archives of Gerontology and Geriatrics 4: 321–332

Harrison M J G, Marsden C D 1977 Progressive intellectual deterioration. Archives of Neurology 34: 199

Heiss W D, Herholz K, Pawlik G, Klinkhammer P, Szelies B 1989 Positron emission findings in dementia disorders: contributions to differential diagnosis and objectivizing of therapeutic effects. Keio Journal of Medicine 38: 111–135

Hooper M W, Vogel F S 1976 The limbic system in Alzheimer's disease. American Journal of Pathology 16: 85–94

Hughes C P, Berg L, Danziger W L, Coben L A, Martin R L 1982 A new clinical scale for the staging of dementia. British Journal of Psychiatry 140:566–572

Inglis J 1957 An experimental study of learning and memory function in elderly psychiatric patients. Journal of Mental Science 103: 799–803

Inglis J 1959 Learning retention and conceptual usage in elderly patients with memory disorder. Journal of Abnormal and Social Psychology 59: 210–215

Jacoby R J, Levy R 1980 Computed tomography in the elderly: 2 Senile dementia: diagnosis and functional impairment. British Journal of Psychiatry 136: 256–269

Jacoby R J, Levy R, Dawson J M 1980 Computed tomography in the elderly: 1 The normal population. British Journal of Psychiatry 136: 249–255

Jarvik L F, Falek A 1963 Intellectual stability and survival in the aged. Gerontology 18: 173–176

Jellinger K 1976 Neuropathological aspects of dementias resulting from abnormal blood and cerebrospinal fluid dynamics. Acta Neurologica Belgica 76: 83–102

Johanson A, Hagberg B 1989 Psychometric characteristics in patients with frontal lobe degeneration of non-Alzheimer type. Archives of Gerontology and Geriatrics 8: 129-137

Kahn R L, Goldfarb A I, Pollack M, Peck A 1960 Brief objective measures for the determination of mental status in the aged. American Journal of Psychiatry 117: 326–328

Kamo H, McGeer P L, Harrop R et al 1987 Positron emission tomography and histopathology in Pick's disease. Neurology 37:439–445

Kaszniak A W, Garron D C, Fox J 1979 Dffferential effects of age and cerebral atrophy upon span of immediate recall in older patients suspected of dementia. Cortex 15: 285–295

Kaszniak A W, Garron D C, Fox J H, Bergen D, Huckman M 1979 Cerebral atrophy, EEG slowing, age, education and cognitive function in suspected dementia. Neurology 29: 1273–1279

Katzman R, Terry R D, Blick K L 1978 Recommendations on the nosology, epidemiology and etiology, and pathophysiology: communications of the workshop/conference on Alzheimer's disease. In: Katzman R et al (eds) Senile dementia and related disorders. Raven Press, New York

Kay D W 1977 Cognitive function and length of survival in elderly subjects living at home. Australian and New Zealand Journal of Psychiatry 11: 113–117

Kemper T L 1978 Senile dementia: a focal disease in the temporal lobe. In: Nandy K (ed) Senile dementia: a biomedical approach. Elsevier North Holland, New York

Kendrick D C, Parboosingh R-C, Post F 1965 A synonym learning test for use with elderly psychiatric subjects: a validation study. British Journal of Social and Clinical Psychology 4: 63–71

Kendrick D C, Post F 1967 Differences in cognitive status between healthy psychiatrically ill and diffusely brain damaged elderly subjects. British Journal of Psychiatry 113: 75–81

Kiloh L G 1961 Pseudodementia. Acta Psychiatrica Scandanavica 37: 336–351

Kiloh L G 1981. Depressive illness masquerading as dementia in the elderly. Medical Journal of Australia 2: 550–553

Klisz D 1978 Neuropsychological evaluation of older persons. In: Storandt M et al (eds) The clinical psychology of aging. Plenum Press, New York

Knopman D S, Christensen K J, Schut L J et al 1989 The spectrum of imaging and neuropsychologic findings in Pick's disease. Neurology 39: 362–368

Kral V A, Emery O B 1989 Long-term follow-up of depressive pseudodementia in the aged. Canadian Journal of Psychiatry 34: 445–446

Kramer N A, Jarvik L F 1979 Assessment of intellectual changes in the elderly. In: Raskin A, Jarvik L F (eds) Psychiatric symptoms and cognitive loss in the elderly. Halstead Press, New York

Levy R 1975 The neurophysiology of dementia. British Journal of Psychiatry Special Publication No 9: 119–123

Lezak M D 1976 Neuropsychological Assessment. Oxford University Press, New York

Lhermitte F, Derouesné J, Signoret J L 1972 Analyse neuropsychologique du syndrome frontal. Revue Neurologique 127: 415–440

Lhermitte F, Gautier J C, Derouesné C, 1970 Nature of occlusions of the middle cerebral artery. Neurology 20: 82–88

Lieberman M A 1965 Psychological correlates of impending death: some prelmnary observations. Journal of Gerontology 20: 181–190

McDonald C 1969 Clinical heterogeneity in senile dementia. British Journal of Psychiatry 115: 267–271

McHugh P R 1964 Occult hydrocephalus. Quarterly Journal of Medicine 33: 297–308

McHugh P R, Folstein M F 1979 Psychopathology of dementia: implications for neuropathology. Research Publications of Association for Research in Nervous and Mental Disease 57: 17–30

Mapother A, Lewis A 1937 Psychological medicine. In: Price F W (ed) A textbook of the practice of medicine, 5th edn. Oxford Medical Publications, London

Marie P 1901 Des foyers lacunaires de désintégration et de différents autres états cavitaires du cerveau. Revue de Médecine 21: 281–298

Marsden C D, Harrison M J G 1972 Outcome of investigations of patients with presenile dementia. British Medical Journal 2:249–252

Miller E 1973 Short and longterm memory in presenile dementia (Alzheimer's disease). Psychological Medicine 3: 221–224

Miller E 1975 Impaired recall and the memory disturbance in presenile dementia. British Journal of Social and Clinical Psychology 14: 73–79

Miller E 1977 Abnormal ageing: the psychology of senile and presenile dementia. Wiley, Chichester

Miller E 1978 Retrieval from longterm memory in presenile dementia: two tests of an hypothesis. British Journal of Social and Clinical Psychology 17: 143–148

Naeser M A, Gebhardt C, Levine H L 1980 Decreased computerized tomography numbers in patients with presenile dementia. Archives of Neurology 37: 401–409

Naguib M, Levy R 1982 Prediction of outcome in senile dementia–acomputed tomography study. British Journal of Psychiatry 140: 263–267

Neary D, Snowden J S, Bowen D M et al 1986 Neuropsychological syndromes in presenile dementia due to cerebral atrophy. Journal of Neurology, Neurosurgery and Psychiatry 49: 163–174

Neary D, Snowden J S, Shields R A et al 1987 Single photon emission tomography using 99mTc-HM-PAO in the investigation of dementia. Journal of Neurology, Neurosurgery and Psychiatry 50: 1101–1109

Neary D, Snowden J S, Northen B, Goulding P 1988 Dementia of frontal lobe type. Journal of Neurology, Neurosurgery and Psychiatry 51: 353–361

Nelson H E, McKenna P 1975 The use of current reading ability in the assessment of dementia. British Journal of Social and Clinical Psychology. 14: 259–267

Nelson H E, O'Connell A 1978 Dementia: the estimation of premorbid intelligence levels using the new adult reading test. Cortex 14: 234–244

Newton R D 1948 The identity of Alzheimer's disease and senile dementia and their relationship to senility. Journal of Mental Science 94: 225–249

Nott P N, Fleminger J J 1975 Presenile dementia: the difficulties of early diagnosis. Acta Psychiatrica Scandanavica 51: 210–217

O'Carroll R E, Gilleard C J 1986 Estimation of premorbid intelligence in dementia. British Journal of Clinical Psychology 25:157–158

Ojemann R G, Fisher C M, Adams R D, Sweet W H, New P F J 1969 Further experience with the syndrome of 'normal' pressure hydrocephalus. Journal of Neurosurgery 31: 279–294

Orrell M W, Sahakian B J, Bergmann K 1989 Self-neglect and frontal lobe dysfunction. British Journal of Psychiatry 155: 101–105

Palmore E B 1969 Physical, mental and social factors in predicting longevity. The Gerontologist 9: 103–108

Pearce J, Miller E 1973 Clinical aspects of dementia. Baillière Tindall, London

Perez F I, Rivera V M, Meyer J S, Gay J R A, Taylor R L, Matthew N T 1975 Analysis of intellectual and cognitive performance in patients with multi-infarct dementia; vertebrobasilar insufficiency with dementia and Alzheimer's disease. Journal of Neurology, Neurosurgery and Psychiatry 38: 533–540

Post F 1975 Dementia, depression and pseudodementia. In: Benson D F, Blumer D (eds) Psychiatric aspects of neurologic disease. Grune and Stratton, New York

Radue E W, du Boulay G H, Harrison M J G, Thomas D J 1978 Comparison of findings between patients with multi-infarct dementia and those with primary neuronal degeneration. Neuroradiology 16: 113–115

Rapaport D, Gill M, Schafer R 1945 Diagnostic psychological testing, vol 1. Year Book Publishers, Chicago

Raskin A, Jarvik L F (eds) 1979 Psychiatric symptoms and cognitive loss in the elderly. Halstead Press, New York

Risberg J 1987 Frontal lobe degeneration of non-Alzheimer type: III Regional cerebral blood flow. Archives of Gerontology and Geriatrics 6: 225–233

Roberts M A, Caird F I 1976 Computerized tomography and intellectual impairment in the elderly. Journal of Neurology, Neurosurgery and Psychiatry 39: 986–989

Robinson R A 1979 Some applications of rating scales in dementia. In: Glen A I M, Whalley L J (eds) Alzheimer's disease: early recognition of potentially reversible deficits. Churchill Livingstone, Edinburgh, p 108–114

Ron M A 1977 Brain damage in chronic alcoholism: a neuropathological, neuroradiological, and psychological review. Psychological Medicine 7: 103–112

Ron M A, Toone B K, Garralda M E Lishman W A 1979 Diagnostic accuracy in presenile dementia. British Journal of Psychiatry 134:161–168

Roth M 1955 The natural history of mental disorder arising in the senium. Journal of Mental Science 101: 281–301

Roth M 1981 The diagnosis of dementia in late and middle life. In: Mortimer J A, Schuman L M (eds) The epidemiology of dementia. Oxford University Press, New York

Roth M, Hopkins B 1953 Psychological test performance in patients over 60: 1 Senile psychosis and the affective disorders of old age. Journal of Mental Science 99: 439–463

Roth M, Myers D H 1975 The diagnosis of dementia. In: Silverstone T, Barraclough B (eds) Contemporary psychiatry. Headly Brothers, Ashford

Salmon E, Franck G 1989 Positron emission tomographic. study in Alzheimer's disease and Pick's disease. Archives of Gerontology and Geriatrics, Supplement 1: 241–247

Savage R D 1973 Old age. In: Eysenck H J (ed) Handbook of abnormal psychology. Pitman Medical, London, ch 18

Seltzer B, Sherwin I 1978 'Organic brain syndrome': an empirical study and critical review. American Journal of Psychiatry 135: 13–21

Shraberg D 1979 The myth of pseudodementia: depression and the aging brain. American Journal of Psychiatry 135: 601–603

Slaby A E, Wyatt R J 1974 Dementia in the presenium. Thomas Springfield, Illinois

Slater E, Roth M 1969 Clinical psychiatry, 3rd edn. Baillière Tindall, London

Smith S T, Kiloh L G, Ratnavale G S, Grant D A 1976 The investigation of dementia: the results in 100 consecutive admissions. The Medical Journal of Australia 2: 403–405

Smith W L, Kinsbourne M (eds) 1977 Aging and dementia. Spectrum, New York

Squire L R, Zouzounis J A 1988 Self-ratings of memory dysfunction in depression and amnesia. Journal of Clinical and Experimental Neuropsychology 10 : 727–738

Steinberg D E, Jarvik M E 1976 Memory functions in depression. Archives of General Psychiatry 33: 219–224

Strub R L, Black F W 1981 Organic brain syndrome: an introduction to neurobehavioral disorders. Davis, Philadelphia,

Szelies B, Karenberg A 1986 Disorders of glucose metabolism in Pick's disease. Fortschritte der Neurologie, Psychiatrie 54: 393–397

Todorov A B, Go R C, Constantinidis J et al 1975 Specificity of the clinical diagnosis of dementia. Journal of the Neurological Sciences 26: 81–98

Tomlinson B E 1977 The pathology of dementia. Contemporary Neurology Series 15: 113–153

Tomlinson B E, Blessed G, Roth M 1968 Observation on the brains of non-demented old people. Journal of Neurological Sciences 7: 331–356

Tsai L, Tsuang M T 1979 The Mini-Mental State Test and computerized tomography. American Journal of Psychiatry. 136: 436–438

Walton D 1958 The diagnostic and predictive accuracy of the Wechsler Memory Scale in psychiatric patients over age sixty-five. Journal of Mental Science 104: 1111–1118

Walton D, Black D A 1957 The validity of a psychological test of brain damage. British Journal of Medical Psychology 30: 270–279

Weinstein H C, Hijdra A, van Royen E A, Derix M M 1989 Determination of cerebral blood flow by SPECT: a valuable tool in the investigation of dementia? Clinical Neurology and Neurosurgery 91: 13–19

Wells C E 1977 Dementia, 2nd edn. Davis, Philadelphia

Wells C E 1979a Pseudodementia. American Journal of Psychiatry 136: 895–900

Wells C E 1979b Diagnosis of dementia. Psychosomatics 20: 517–522

Whitehead A 1973 Verbal memory and learning in elderly depressives. British Journal of Psychiatry 123: 203–208

4. Pseudoneurological disorders

The term 'pseudo-neurologic' was used by Matthews et al (1966) to describe a situation in which patients may present with symptoms and signs which are considered to be potentially of organic origin but who, after further examination or the passage of time, turn out to have psychiatric rather than neurological disorders. The situation is clearly summarized by Heilbrun (1962):

> The major clinical contribution which the psychologist could make would be to make valid inferences regarding brain states in persons where the symptoms are much more subtle and the ability of neurologists to agree considerably less than standard research methodology has required. A crucial study would be one in which the neurological group is made up entirely of subjects of whom the neurologists disagree as to diagnosis or are unable to make a diagnostic statement at all at the time the psychological measure is obtained, and for whom retrospective diagnosis is possible. To validly infer damage when the neurologist is scratching his head is a contribution; to do so when the patient's family can reach the same conclusion is not.

The term pseudoneurological thus refers to any pattern of disturbance which approximates a neurological one. Included under this term are three types of presentation:

1. Conversion reactions, where the symptomatology is in the sensory or motor spheres, e.g. hysterical blindness, anaesthesia or paralysis
2. Pseudodementia, where the symptoms approximate a generalized cognitive impairment (see Ch. 3)
3. Circumscribed disorders of higher mental function which mimic neuropsychological disorders, e.g. psychogenic amnesias, language disorders and dyspraxias.

Such a division is useful for didactic purposes but many cases present a mixture of features, e.g. Feinstein & Hattersley (1988) describe a case showing responses approximating the Ganser syndrome, dysprosody, and psychogenic amnesia.

CONVERSION REACTIONS

The earliest description of a pseudoneurological condition was that of hysteria. Unfortunately, this term carries a number of meanings both in the scientific and general literature. The complexity of the concept has been reviewed by Chodoff

119

(1974) but most would agree with Mayer-Gross et al (1954): '. . . the category of hysteria is essentially a clinical one to which a name can be given, but no logically satisfying definition'.

The characteristic symptomatic expression in hysteria is the conversion symptom or conversion reaction and any disorder in which such symptoms find a prominent place may be loosely termed conversion hysteria. We will adopt the term conversion reaction. Such reactions are 'characterized by bodily symptoms that resemble those of physical disease—for example, paralysis, anesthesia, blindness, convulsions, pathological blushing, fainting and headaches—but have no somatic basis' (Freedman et al 1976). As suggested in this definition, the manifestations are protean and may mimic almost any disease.

The term 'conversion' derives from the psychoanalytic formulations of Freud. In this theory 'conversion hysteria provides a defence against overintense libidinal stimulation by means of a translation or conversion of psychic excitation into physical innervation' (Freedman et al 1976). In the same publication, these writers describe conversion as 'an unconscious defence mechanism by which the anxiety which stems from an intrapsychic conflict is converted and expressed in a symbolic somatic symptom' (op. cit. p 1292). Thus the term 'conversion reaction' is intimately bound up with the widely (but not universally) accepted notion of unconscious motivation of which it is an indirect expression; but whatever the theoretical explanation, the core of agreement among different theorists is the acknowledgement that the observed bodily symptoms are psychologically and not organically determined.

Hysterical symptoms versus hysterical personality

Further clarification can be made by distinguishing between the manifestation of symptoms of an hysteric type and modes of behaviour which typify the hysterical personality. Chodoff (1974) points out that hysterical personalities may manifest conversion symptoms but 'this is by no means generally true. Conversely, conversion reactions are certainly not confined to hysterical personalities but occur in a large variety of personalities and clinical psychopathological settings. For example, conversion reactions occur at least as frequently in men as they do in women, whereas the diagnosis of hysterical personality is usually confined to women' (op. cit. p 1074). Leaving aside the contentious issues raised in the latter part of this quotation, the neuropsychologist will encounter conversion reactions more frequently in some situations than in others. They are perhaps most common in medico-legal suits over personal injury claims where financial compensation is a major issue and thus may be more common in men than in women in this situation. They are next most commonly encountered in neurological practice where they may occur alone or in company with neurological signs and symptoms of undoubted organic origin. In the latter situation they may be referred to as a 'functional overlay'. They are also commonly seen in wartime.

Psychoanalytic theory of hysteria

The psychoanalytic theory of hysteria also introduced a conceptual distinction between a primary and a secondary advantage or gain to be derived from the development of a conversion reaction. Primary gain in psychoanalytic theory is 'the gain to the ego resulting from the relief of instinctual pressures (drives) through the partial discharge of drive-energy that occurs with the formation and maintenance of neurotic symptoms' (Eidelberg 1968). In other words primary gain arises from partial solution of a conflict through the production of symptoms. These symptoms may then result in 'secondary' gain by providing a source of secondary gratification to the total personality. For example, the conversion symptoms may lead others to express concern, and provide attention. Such secondary gain, when pronounced, may provide a serious stumbling block to successful therapy.

Not all theorists subscribe to this distinction which has at its roots the longstanding conflict within the person from the early stages of psychosexual development. Some situations, e.g. paralysis or blindness appear to have a more immediate motivation and one which is closer to the surface, namely a scarcely concealed cry for removal from an overwhelming situation.

Hysteria as communication

Postanalytic writers have produced a somewhat different conception of the hysterical illness (Szasz 1961, Ziegler & Imboden 1962, Hollender 1972). The central theme of these theories which lends them a family resemblance is that the symptoms are a symbolic form through which the patient expresses his distress and cries for help. 'We have found it useful to consider the patient with a conversion symptom as someone enacting the role of a person with 'organic' illness, symbolically communicating his distress . . . by means of somatic symptoms' (Ziegler & Imboden 1962, p 284). Although still using the blanket term hysteria Hollender (1972, p 314) wrote '. . . we can define hysteria as a special message, sent when conventional forms of expression are blocked. It is the dramatization of a forbidden wish or impulse, its prohibition or some compromise between the two'. The second part of this explanation has strong psychoanalytic overtones. The author considers the symptoms to be a form of body language or pantomime which we must learn to interpret. Such interpretations are fraught with the same difficulties and dangers faced by analytic theory. Another basic problem is the fact that some distressed individuals choose to use this disguised form of communication. A possible clue to an explanation lies in the fact that symptoms of physical illness are socially acceptable. Chodoff (1974, p 1075) comments, 'The symptom is not to be understood in medical terms, but within the context of role and game theory. This function of the conversion symptom is historically derived from Charcot's legitimization of the sick role as a device whereby an individual transmits his needs and his emotional distress covertly through the socially accepted symbols of physical illness'. We will argue that this expression can be extended to the expression of distress through cognitive as well as physical deficits.

Hysteria versus malingering

When simulation becomes apparent to the observer the question often arises as to whether the patient's motivation is conscious or unconscious. Some neuropsychologists feel that malingering is more a matter for detectives than for psychologists. However, their expert opinions as to whether the person's symptoms and performances on tests conform with known disorders of brain function will be of help in providing a basis on which decisions can be made. For example, the neuropsychologist's statement that a certain pattern of behaviour and test results strongly indicates that the poor performances are not the result of neural damage, may have a major effect on courts' decisions. Although the literature suggests that most post-accident cases have a poor prognosis despite large monetary settlements, it still remains possible that the person may improve later either spontaneously or under future treatment whereas stable deficits based on neurological incapacity will not. This distinction between conscious and unconscious arises not only with conversion reactions but also in hysterical pseudodementia and the possibly related Ganser syndrome and what we have termed role enactments. This issue receives scant treatment in most textbooks of psychiatry.

Ganser syndrome versus Ganser symptoms

Goldin & Macdonald (1955) corrected some misconceptions raised by the translation of Ganser's early papers (1898, 1904). They point out that Ganser described not only approximate and ridiculous answers that were so dramatic as to draw the attention of the observer, but that these were interspersed with correct answers and inconsistent wrong answers when the same question was put. The present author finds some types of tests and questions more evocative of Ganser-like responses than others. It is certainly true that they are the exception rather than the rule.

Subjects also evince no surprise, irritation or resentment at puerile questions which would normally be an insult to their intelligence, e.g. 'How many legs has a dog?' (Enoch & Irving 1962).

Whitlock (1967) pointed to a considerable difference of opinion among psychiatrists as to where the Ganser syndrome should fall in the classification of mental disorders. This is still true though many will adhere to the DSM III categorization (American Psychiatric Association 1987). Leaving this question aside he commends Scott's suggestion (1965) that a distinction should be made between Ganser symptoms and the Ganser syndrome. The former are relatively common while the latter is extremely rare, 'It is suggested that a diagnosis of a Ganser syndrome should be restricted to patients who, following cerebral trauma or in the course of acute psychosis, develop clouding of consciousness with characteristic verbal responses to questions, and whose illness terminates abruptly with subsequent amnesia' (Whitlock 1967, p 28). This author feels that the clouding of consciousness clearly separates the syndrome from hysterical pseudodementia which occurs 'without clouding of consciousness in intellectually dull persons in social difficulties'. As mentioned above, Ganser-like and related symptoms occur at all levels of intellectual ability though they may be more common in the mentally dull group (Lishman 1978). They may occasionally be seen in children (Adler & Toyuz 1989). Certainly, not one of the cases reported later in the chapter occurred in a dull subject, suggesting mechanisms of symptom production which are independent of intelligence.

Ganser symptomatology may also be seen in conjunction with psychosis and with neurological disorders such as cerebral tumours, though this is rare. Thus, while such symptoms are most frequent in psychological states, they do not exclude organic disease. It is always wise to seek diligently for signs of neurological or neuropsychological deficit in all suspected cases.

What we earlier termed neurotic role enactments vary all the way from extravagant Ganser-like symptoms to quite sophisticated enactments which may deceive all but the most wary. In both presentations only some responses are of the approximation type, most responses being of the apparently random kind. Also, in both, the phenomenon of approximate answers is so bizarre that it has suggested simulation or malingering to many observers. Ganser himself felt that no simulation was involved but his opinion is not shared by all, especially in situations where obvious gain is to be had. Lastly, in separating off true Ganser syndromes, Whitlock's final point is crucial: abrupt termination with subsequent amnesia for recent events does not appear in cases of hysterical pseudodementia.

Malingering

To malinger, according to one dictionary, is to 'pretend, produce or protract illness in order to escape duty'. Jones & Llewellyn (1917) in their treatise on the subject commented: 'Malingering is but a species of deceit—that most common of human frailties, where self-interest, "the ruling passion of mankind", is concerned.' In this book they provide such a wealth of detail that one wonders that there was anything left to say.

Malingering is defined by DSMIII as the 'production and presentation of false or grossly exaggerated physical or psychological symptoms. The symptoms are produced in pursuit of a goal that is obviously recognizable with an understanding of the individual's circumstances rather than of his or her psychopathology.'

The essence of all such definitions is *conscious* simulation. This might suggest that there can be only two forms of behaviour, conscious and unconscious, a dichotomy greatly strengthened and encouraged by psychoanalytic theory of unconscious motivation in hysteria. The matter is not so simple. Henderson & Gillespie (Batchelor 1969) comment: 'Simulation is the voluntary production of symptoms by an individual who has full knowledge of their voluntary origin. In hysteria there is typically no such knowledge, and the production of symptoms is the result of processes that are not fully conscious' (op. cit. p 156). The last three words allow a gradation of motivation from fully conscious to fully unconscious or various admixtures of conscious and unconscious motives. The authors argue for a gradation of behaviour between conversion and simulation and agree with Kretschmer that the dichotomy 'conscious versus unconscious' will not serve to separate malingering from hysterical manifestations, 'for not all motives of the healthy mind are conscious, and not all hysterical ones are unconscious.'

Miller & Cartlidge (1972) were more sceptical about the distinction of conscious versus unconscious motivation. Speaking in the context of medico-legal claims for allegedly post-traumatic impairment they commented: 'Since the distinction rests in the last resort on the claimant's credibility and on the doctor's affirmation that he knows and understands accurately what is in the claimant's mind—and since the claimant is certainly not unaware that he is making a claim for financial compensation—the contention or belief that he is unaware of any connection between his claim and his behaviour can hardly be accepted at face value'; and further, the belief that in accident neurosis the patient is deceiving himself as well as hoping to deceive the observer seems a tenuous basis for the distinction.' Miller (1966) felt that he was unable to tell the difference between hysteria and malingering, and reminded his audience that, despite their long experience, judges may not be able to tell whether people in their courts are telling the truth or not. Miller also pointed out that 'these patients also quite often complain of loss of memory, a complaint which is at striking variance to the detail in which they describe the accident after a two and a half year period' (op. cit. p 73). In a similar vein Reed (1978, p 321) said that 'the answers depend on an ability to measure consciousness which we do not possess'.

Certainly such cogently expressed extreme views will form an indissoluble barrier between those of Miller's persuasion and, psychologists and psychiatrists who believe there is evidence, both clinical and experimental, for motivational forces below the level of conscious awareness; the debate seems likely to be with us for a long time to come.

Although outright malingering is difficult to prove and we accept that there is a range of awareness of motive (or self-deception), certain features may aid in the identification of the malingerer. Chief among these is the patient's attitude to his affliction. The patient with so-called conversion reactions appears emotionally unaffected. In the words of earlier writers they display 'la belle indifférence'. They are more than pleased to talk about their symptoms in untiring detail and are often egocentric and dramatic in their descriptions. The malingerer on the other hand is always less forthcoming, cautious and guarded, seeing the examination as a threat. Direct questions are met with evasions, and occasionally with hostility. Perhaps even more characteristic is 'an appearance of sustained gloom' (Miller & Cartlidge 1972).

The broader category of role enactments covers a range of attitudes between the two extremes though few appear guarded and, when they appear so, they may well have a strong component of malingering.

An adequately taken history is of paramount importance though this is not often available from either the patient, or the friend or relative whom the patient may offer in support of his case. Nevertheless Sim (1974) points out that interview with the patient may prove useful by its negatives:

... for they not uncommonly deny even the slightest evidence of the normal insecurities to which all men are heir. They would have us believe that they have an impeccable family history, a most secure home background, a complete absence of neurotic traits in childhood, a stable and most successful employment record, a happy married life and no history of illness even of a trivial nature, till the accident, when catastrophe overtook them. If all this were true, then the patient should be capable of recovering from the most extreme stress imaginable, and the relatively minor insult of the accident should hardly be noticed.

Malingering should always be suspected when the claim for disablement appears out of proportion to the severity of the injury and there is a hope for gain, usually

but not universally financial. However, despite the best of efforts it is likely for other reasons that much malingering goes undetected. An added reason for the diagnostic difficulty is that the two conditions, namely hysteria and malingering, are not mutually exclusive. 'In practice the hysteric is not infrequently a malingerer too...' (Mayer-Gross et al 1954). In a very real sense the diagnosis of malingering is one for detectives rather than medical professionals who may, however, be asked an opinion as to the likelihood of such being the case.

Role theory as a unifying framework

It can be seen that notions of role theory are either explicit or implicit in much of the modern discussion of conversion reaction. Such applications have been used even more widely in sociopsychological formulations of abnormal behaviour (Cameron & Magaret 1951, Ullmann & Krasner 1969). As such a formulation will be used in what follows in an attempt to draw together various types of pseudoneurological disorders, the central notions of role theory will be outlined briefly.

The role concept

The concept of 'role' is a complex one and any attempt to cover it briefly is bound to lessen the appreciation of its value as an explanatory concept. A long needed synthesis of the numerous approaches was provided by Biddle (1979). The organizing concept has been defined in a number of ways:

'A role is a patterned sequence of learned actions performed by a person in an interaction situation' (Sarbin 1954, p 225).

'1. A behavior repertoire characteristic of a person or position. 2. A set of standards, descriptions, norms or concepts held (by anyone) for the behaviors of a person or position' (Biddle & Thomas 1966, p 11-12).

Roles consist of those behaviors that are characteristic of a set of persons and a context' (Biddle 1979, p 58).

The behaviour of the person in the role was earlier called by this name, viz 'role behavior' (Newcomb 1950). More recently the term role enactment has come into general use.

'Role enactment includes, among other segments of behavior, gross skeletal movements, the performance of verbal and motoric gestures, posture and gait, styles of speech and accent, wearing of certain forms of dress...In short, role enactment embraces what may be called the mechanics of the role-taking process...(Sarbin 1954, p 232).

Expression of the role

Role enactment depends critically on the knowledge of role expectations (Parsons & Shils 1951), i.e. certain behaviours are expected of certain roles. 'These expectations include certain prescriptions (things the person must do), and certain prohibitions (things the person must not do) as well as a range of less strictly defined expectations (the things the person ought to do in that role). We will call the prescriptions and prohibitions associated with a given role, the role *expectations* for that role' (McGrath 1964, p 68). Of course, any individual may fulfil only incompletely the expectations he and others have for that role. It is obvious that a person cannot enact a role unless he possesses the necessary expectations. As in the dramaturgical role, enactments require both the acquisition of knowledge and practice in the role, the learning, reinforcement, and extinction which govern all other aspects of behaviour. The individual will be conscious of only some of these. Although widely accepted, the idea that roles are induced through expectations covers some situations but not others. In some instances the context will have a determining effect. Biddle (1979) cites the differences in role behaviours of an audience according to whether it occurs in the context of a church service, football match, or concert.

Finally, most role enactments are of an interactive, reciprocal, or dyadic nature, the behaviour of one person serving as a stimulus for others. 'Role enactments evoke complementary role enactments from others, a person who behaves in the 'sick' role, for example, is likely to be responded to by others enacting the role of 'dealing with sick people', a role that includes behaviors likely to reinforce some aspects of the sick role and hence maintain sick behavior' (Ullmann & Krasner 1969, p 92). This means that when the person has enacted the role and it has been reinforced it may be very difficult to shed. There is considerable evidence to show that if social reinforcement is applied in certain ways termed schedules of reinforcement by operant conditioning theorists, the behaviour may become particularly resistant to extinction. It does not seem necessary for the patient to be fully aware of the reinforcement for it to be effective. The patient becomes *entrapped* in the sick role and is unable to shift back to his former role. This 'role entrapment' is further supported by the fact that to discontinue the role is to cast doubt on its validity. Some techniques for treating conversion symptoms offer an opportunity for patients to opt out of the sick role. The method described by Pankratz (1979) for functional sensory disorders seems capable of being adapted to other forms of pseudoneurological disorder (see below).

Evolution and shaping of roles

In the repeated examinations which form part of a very common, context for pseudoneurological disorders, namely, post-traumatic situations, one is in a position to observe another general characteristic of role enactments. This is the phenomenon of *shaping*. The role enactment may occasionally arise fully developed, but careful serial observation will often reveal that certain aspects of the original enactment will lessen or disappear, while others may become more prominent or quite new features arise. Some of this process whereby the enactment approximates more closely to an accepted organic syndrome is a function of subtle, and not so subtle, cues provided by the examiner. The process is closely akin to what Orne has called 'the demand characteristics' of the situation (Orne 1962, Orne & Scheibe 1964). Speaking of the behaviour of subjects in a social psychology experiment, Orne & Scheibe (op. cit. p 3) defined the demand characteristics as '...those cues, both implicit and explicit, that communicate to the subject *what is expected of him* in the experimental situation' [my italic]. They demonstrated the strength of these cues by manipulating them

experimentally to produce significant behavioral changes in their subjects even where the subjects were unaware of the influence of many of the situational variables on their behaviour. While it is not possible to eliminate demand characteristics from a situation, awareness of their effects may help in not reinforcing symptoms more than can be avoided.

The awareness of demand characteristics may even be exploited in diagnostic assessment. Certain test situations have stronger demand characteristics than others, prompting subjects to display their disability. An example is the 15 item memory test of Rey (1964). Several examples occur later in this chapter.

Some sick role enactments appear to be based on a process of modelling; where this is suspected it is advisable to look carefully into the patient's past history. The model may be a close relative or may arise from the patient's professional life. The ability to simulate symptoms (consciously or unconsciously) seems positively correlated with the patient's degree of medical sophistication. Ziegler et al (1960) described two physicians, two nurses, and two neurologists' secretaries who expertly simulated complicated disease entities. These authors point out that the 'existence of patients who are "expert simulators" is vivid evidence that conversion symptoms conform to the patient's imageries or ideas about a suspected disease'.

The patient's own prior experience is a further powerful source of information (Fallik & Sigal 1971). A patient who has suffered from a disorder himself may prolong the symptoms or reintroduce them on a subsequent occasion, e.g. a patient who has suffered from transient aphasia may enact a language disturbance more or less successfully at a later time.

However, despite these observations the present author is impressed with the large number of occasions on which he has observed the most primitive enactments produced by quite sophisticated individuals as if such persons were, by the very flamboyance of their professed symptoms, *bringing themselves under the notice of* skilled professionals. Such disguised cries for help should be considered seriously before reinforcement renders them too difficult to treat.

HYSTERICAL PSEUDODEMENTIA

This topic has been covered in the previous chapter but case examples are provided at the end of the present one.

CIRCUMSCRIBED PSEUDONEUROLOGICAL DISORDERS

The third class of pseudoneurological presentation consists of those instances in which patients choose to express their disabilities in terms of just one psychological process, other so-called higher mental processes remaining intact. Since the patient is more likely to have more information about disordered memory than, for example, about the aphasias or dyspraxias, psychogenic amnesia is more common than disorders of other functions.

PSYCHOGENIC AMNESIA

Complaints about memory number among the most frequent manifestations of the sick role enactment. They take a number of forms. Sometimes they are profound and global covering immediate, recent and remote material. On other occasions they are circumscribed, affecting only certain discrete periods or certain themes. The profound loss of memory for a considerable span of time is usually strikingly inconsistent with the preservation of other psychological functions. Amnesic disorders are prevalent in post-traumatic presentations, sometimes arising de novo some time after the injury, often a minor head injury, and at other times appearing as a prolongation and exaggeration of symptoms experienced in the early post-traumatic period. Charcot described such a temporal delay between cause and effect in hysteria as the 'period of meditation'. Miller and Cartridge (1972) are suspicious of the man with a very long retrograde amnesia after head injury and are convinced that such claims are often fabricated. Such a position is supported by the rarity of such cases deemed in the literature to be of organic origin. It should be remembered that severe amnesia on an organic basis is usually accompanied by confusion or marked cognitive impairment.

Theory and practice

Amnesia provides perhaps the best example of how background knowledge could be employed to decide between organic versus malingered or enacted symptoms. The salient point is to recall that in either of the two main categories of non-organic conditions the fitting of the enacted symptoms to the presented disorder must be a function of the individual's conception of the disorder. Thus it should not be impossible for examiners with detailed neuropsychological knowledge to determine if the pattern proffered matches that described in the literature and experienced by them. On the other hand, psychologists who are unfamiliar with the details of neuropsychological syndromes and who rely heavily on level of test performance are unlikely to detect these individuals.

To take an example in some detail not all mnemonic functions are equally compromised even in severely amnesic patients. Quite early in the modern study of amnesia it became apparent that some aspects of learning, particularly the learning of perceptual and motor skills, was preserved in some patients with extremely severe memory disorders of differing aetiologies (Milner 1962, Corkin 1965, Talland 1965, Starr & Phillips 1970, Kinsbourne & Wood 1975, Brooks & Baddeley 1976, Cohen & Squire 1980, Cohen & Corkin 1981, Moscovitch 1982) and this has become extended into other areas of acquiring new information and skill (Milner et al 1968, Warrington & Weiskrantz 1974, 1978, 1982; Huppert & Piercey 1976, Parkin 1982, Volpe & Hirst 1983, Cohen 1984, Graf et al 1984, Grossi et al 1984, Schacter et al 1984). Even the learning of complex skills for the use of computers has been shown to be preserved (Glisky et al 1986, Glisky & Schacter 1988). Brandt et al (1985) remind us that 'the naive malingerer is presumed not to know this and so 'overplays' the role, performing worse than true amnesics.' Recognition memory is a particularly simple test for the malingerer since the quite spectacular preservation of this form in many amnesics is not likely to be part of the body of knowledge of the enactor.

A recent review (Schacter 1987) covers a considerable amount of this evidence that the amnesic patient 'can acquire and retain new factual information, even though they do not explicitly remember when, where, and how they acquired the new facts.' The neurological cases showing 'learning' include those caused by head injury, viral encephalitis, and vascular lesions, as well as the Korsakoff disorder.

'Hysterical' amnesia

A particularly striking but relatively uncommon type of psychogenic amnesia takes the form of profound, pervasive retrograde amnesia in the presence of an unaltered ability to register and retain ongoing information. This form of psychogenic or functional amnesia is relatively uncommon and usually considered to be related to emotionally traumatic material:

> Amnesia is commonly of a circumscribed series of events in the patient's memory. It is as if part of this life has dropped out, although the hysteric may not be aware of the gap in his recollection until it is pointed out to him. This amnesia usually hides some incident about which the patient has felt guilty, and has forgotten what it would be painful for him to remember. . . . In some cases the amnesia is for the whole life up to a certain recent point. The patient may forget his own identity, the names and faces of friends, even his wife and children. The amnesia is always for something with which a strong emotion has become associated.

There has been a good deal written about phenomena related to hysterical and psychogenic amnesia, particularly with regard to the notion of so-called 'unconscious' motivation, i.e. that not only has the patient forgotten certain material but, because of mechanisms such as 'repression', he is of his own volition unable to bring it back into consciousness. This interpretation has been glibly repeated in books and articles ad nauseam.

On the other hand there are those (e.g. Bronks 1987) who believe that credence in psychogenic amnesia may have been sustained by the credulity of observers and this writer points to the experience of Sir Julian Symonds, reported by Merskey (1979), of at least half a dozen cases of claimed memory loss in what is generally termed an hysterical fugue. These cases were assured that their disclosures would remain confidential and that others would be told they had been cured by hypnotism and so forth. All of these cases were able to retrieve their 'lost' memories often telling, as one might have surmised, dramatic stories.

As Lishman (1987, p 31) comments: 'Amnesias of this severity do not occur in organic states unless at the same time there is abundant evidence of disturbance of consciousness or of severe disruption of cognitive functions generally. . . . Psychogenic amnesia is suspected when from the outset profound difficulty with the recall of past events is coupled with normal ability to retain new information . . .'

Little is know of the precise cognitive characteristics in hysterical amnesia, since such examinations are not carried out or not reported. Similarly Lishman (1978, p 44) writes that a 'delayed curve of forgetting, which during the course of some days or weeks leads to complete extinction of important and significant material, is likewise sometimes seen in psychogenic but not in organic amnesia'. Where psychogenic amnesia appears without relation to cerebral trauma it is generally retrograde, rarely anterograde.

NEUROPSYCHOLOGICAL ASSESSMENT

Poor test performance by pseudoneurological patients results from two main causes. The first might be thought of as a by-product of a psychological disorder while the second represents the patient's attempts to enact his disorder through the vehicle of test responses.

Nonspecific test effects

Under the first type of response would be those where the patient centres his attention on himself and his troubles to the exclusion of other matters including his participation in the test situation. Such observations are sometimes made by psychologists in medico-legal claims for injury damages. Unfortunately, some of them then go on to make inferences that poor test scores reflect neural incapacity, without paying attention to the fact that the patient was not giving of his best at the time of assessment.

Prime examples of non-specific factors are seen in depressed patients. Lishman (1978, p 571) remarked:

> The problem appears to have its roots . . . in the general psychomotor retardation which accompanies depression and in the withdrawal of interest and attention from the environment. The patient becomes slow to grasp essentials, thinking is laboured and behaviour becomes generally slipshod and inefficient. Events fail to register, either through lack of ability to attend and concentrate or on account of the patient's inner preoccupations. In consequence he may show faulty orientation, impairment of recent memory, and a markedly defective knowledge of current events.

At the other end of the scale is the extreme distractability of the hypomanic patient.

Such general psychological factors will have a widespread adverse effect on a large number of tests. There are also certain specific features of some psychological disorders which may effect some tests but not others, e.g. the thought disorder of some schizophrenic patients may reflect itself in idiosyncratic responses on certain verbal and conceptual tasks. For these reasons it is important for neuropsychologists to be familiar with the response patterns and deviations of psychiatric patients as well as those of normal and neurological patients.

Enactment in the test situation

The second type of response, namely that arising from enactment, may also take a variety of forms. The examples given below by no means encompass the entire repertoire but they should sensitize the psychologist to the importance of qualitative observations.

The most readily suspect patient is one whose enactment consists of getting it all wrong, i.e. failing on all tests in an indiscriminate manner. Chesterton's fictional detective, Father Brown, himself a master of shrewd observation, remarked about an attempt to mislead or deceive: 'The man who wrote that note knew all about the facts', said his clerical companion soberly, 'He could never have got 'em so wrong without knowing about 'em. You have to know an awful lot to be wrong on every subject—like the devil . . . I mean a man telling lies on chance would have told some of the truth'(Chesterton 1970).

Another characteristic feature in the cognitive examination of pseudoneurological cases, which makes no neurological sense, is the inconsistency of performance with regard to level of difficulty of the material. One of our post-accident cases failed on the six-year-old level of the Porteus Maze test while passing the adult level with ease. This failure cannot be based in neural incapacity. It is as if the person is saying 'I have difficulties but I do not want you to think that I am stupid'.

Symptom and syndrome validity

In 1961 Brady and Lind introduced a two-alternative forced-choice technique to evaluate hysterical blindness, and such logic has been widely used since for so-called conversion symptoms and feigned disorders of several kinds (Grosz & Zimmerman 1965, Theodor & Mandelcorn 1973, Pankratz 1975, Fausti & Peed 1975, Pankratz 1979, 1983; Pankratz, Binder & Wilcox 1987, Binder & Pankratz 1987, Pankratz & Paar 1988). It can be assumed that the patient who consistently does *significantly worse than chance* must (consciously or unconsciously) be detecting the stimuli. 'A score below the norm should make the clinician suspicious, but a score below chance is evidence of faking' (Binder & Pankratz 1987). In his numerous papers Pankratz (1979) has referred to this procedure as 'symptom validity testing'. 'Symptom Validity Testing detects deception because patients subjectively feel that giving correct answers half the time is not consistent with their disability'.

Of course, individuals may vary in their degree of intellectual sophistication and insight into what they feel the examiner expects of them. To cover this contingency Miller (1986) increased the complexity of the forced choice procedure.

An extension of this logic of checking the patient's responses against expectation can be extended readily into the sphere of the higher cognitive processes. Moreover, it is almost unheard of to meet uniformly poor performance in all areas of function in neurologically based disorders, even of the most widespread kind. Even patients with advanced Alzheimer's disease with whom one is unable to converse may surprise by effortlessly reading aloud words presented to them on cards.

The many ways of getting it wrong vary from patient to patient, some being more readily detected than others. Following a minor head injury, a patient (JS) was referred to us by a psychologist colleague as having a very short attention span, only three digits forward on the Digit Span Test, and the psychologist felt that this was at the basis of her difficulties in rehabilitation. When we repeated this task she did in fact pass on three digits but fail on four. Instead of ceasing at two failures we continued to increase the length of the series up to eight digits. While the patient continued to 'fail' it became apparent that this was generally because she reversed the last two digits (see below). Thus, on the eight digit series she could be said to have at least a digit span of six. Later she in fact succeeded in getting the first eight correct in a series of ten! These observations led to the successful exploration by the psychologist concerned of psychological factors which became the focus of treatment leading to successful readjustment. Acceptance of a diagnosis of learning difficulty based on traumatic brain injury in such cases merely serves to strongly reinforce failing behaviour until it becomes impossible to eradicate.

DigitSpan

Stimulus	Response
7 4 2 9 6	7 4 9 6
8 5 1 6 4	8 5 1 4 6
8 4 2 7 5 1	8 4 2 7 1 5
7 2 9 5 3 6	7 2 5 3 6
7 4 8 2 5 9 1	7 4 8 2 5 1 9
8 3 9 6 1 5 2	8 3 9 6 1 2 5
6 4 5 8 1 3 2 7	6 4 5 8 1 3 7 2
4 7 5 2 8 1 6 9	4 7 5 2 8 1 9 6

This patient, like so many others, construed failure as 'not passing'. It would be a pity if psychologists followed suit.

Other patients will fail by adding something that was not given (Case XD, p 145), some will give near misses, while others again will be bizarrely wide of the mark (Case IX, p 133).

A check of symptom validity should thus begin with observation of qualitative features at the item level. Notes should always be taken as observations are made. In the more subtle cases suspicion as to role enactment may only arise after the examination has concluded.

Apart from the item level, there are also opportunities to check the pattern of responding within a test or subtest. A not uncommon situation involves failing easy items while passing more difficult ones. Here psychometrically seduced practitioners will commit '*the sin of summation*', i.e. they will average over the test (as suggested in the manual) reporting a level of performance in terms of the normative data which is quite unrepresentative of the patient's capacity. It should be obvious that from the neural point of view, ability to perform the difficult in any sphere should encompass the ability to perform the simple. Once again causes other than dead or sick brain cells should be sought.

One of the most useful facets of the clinician's frame of reference is, of course, a knowledge and personal experience of just how patients with known neuropsychological disorders perform on the tests in question, e.g. Case VR (p 144) fails on the paired associate learning test in a manner which is quite uncharacteristic of all forms of organic amnesia.

Next, and most important of all, pseudoneurological cases will present patterns from the sundry tests which will not resemble those of the numerous, well documented neuropsychological syndromes, i.e. *they will not make neuropsychological sense*. In experimental tests Goebel (1983) showed that normal subjects could not produce convincing patterns on the Halstead-Reitan battery, and even more sophisticated nurses with some neurological experience fared little better in their attempts to fake credible patterns of disordered performance (Hayward et al 1987). One might term this approach '*syndrome validity testing*'. A detailed knowledge of such syndromes is necessary in order to check possible similarities in a quite specific way as they emerge although, in our experience, the exhibition of a standard set of cognitive measures will usually provide enough material for expression of the patient's enactment without specific hypothesis testing. In some situations recourse might be had to objective measures of exaggeration such as those derived by Clayer et al from Pilowsky & Spence's (1983) Illness Behaviour Questionnaire (Clayer, Brookless & Ross 1984, Clayer, Brookless-Pratz & Ross, 1986).

Finally, the words 'in the test situation' have been included purposely in the present section heading. Many subjects show an interesting dissociation between their performance when they construe something to be a 'test' and when the same material is given to them in an informal setting which I have dubbed 'coffee-break testing'. It arose over a patient who failed consistently on certain aphasia tests whether administered by the speech pathologist or the neuropsychologist. Having prepared certain conversational topics in which the failed type of language item was embedded it was easily demonstrated that the patient responded normally outside the test situation. It is helpful to push the test material aside sometimes to check in a less formal approach the consistency of the person's responses. Lest individuals object that we are deceiving the patient, one should point out that the exercise is to understand the nature of the disability so that appropriate therapy can be instituted. It does patients with psychologically based disorders no good to be treated as though they have neurological problems.

The case extracts which follow have been much abbreviated to permit a range of examples to be included.

CASE EXAMPLES

Possible organic confusional state

Case: IX

This 33-year-old woman had come to Australia with her family when she was eight years of age. She completed her ninth year of school at 15 years of age and had several unskilled factory jobs before her marriage. At the time of referral she had been a housewife for nine years and had three children. Her husband reported that there had been a gradual change in her behaviour which had worsened in recent weeks. He described her as being increasingly confused and professing to be unable to understand what to do in everyday situations. For example, she would stand at the traffic lights expressing bewilderment, saying that she was unable to tell when to cross the road. She sometimes acted as though she was disoriented in time and expressed fear about her failures in simple matters. It seemed clear that she was drawing her family's attention to her deficiencies. She was admitted for observation to the psychiatric ward of a large public hospital where she was found to be very garrulous and, although her English was fluent and generally competent she occasionally used words inappropriately. During the physical examination Mrs X failed to identify her fingers correctly. She responded incorrectly to questions about right-left orientation and failed on the simplest of arithmetical calculations.

The examining psychiatrist was convinced that her problem was essentially psychiatric in nature but the presence of possible finger agnosia, right-left disorientation, acalculia and dysphasia raised the question of an associated 'Gerstmann syndrome' and he sought a neuropsychological evaluation to clarify the diagnosis.

Neuropsychological assessment

At interview IX appeared alert but talked incessantly, constantly apologized for her performance, calling attention to her failures, and frequently sought direction and approval. She was unable to give a coherent account of her recent history but she admitted that she had not been coping as well with her housework as she had done previously. Occasionally she tended to use words, especially long words, inappropriately, though not in the way of those unfamiliar with the language. Her errors had a bizarre quality unsuggestive of dysphasia. It was decided to begin the examination with a general exploration of her language and intellectual functions.

Boston Aphasia Examination

IX wrote in a large, childish hand which was perfectly legible. Reading comprehension and colour naming were good. In reading aloud she made one verbal paraphasia and several verbal and literal paraphasias on a sentence repetition task, e.g. 'the bown (brown) swallow captured a bump (plump) worm'. Asked to repeat 'fifteen' she replied 'number', for 'purple' she answered 'colour', and for 'what' she answered 'colour'. Her perfectly normal repetitions of a number of other words clearly indicated that she understood the nature of the task. Her responses had more of the quality of Ganser-like expressions than paraphasias.

An exploration of some intellectual abilities was then conducted with subtests of the *WAIS:*

Information	7	Digit Symbol	6
Comprehension	2	Picture Completion	6
Arithmetic	3	Block Design	5
Similarities	8		
Digit Span	4		

This exceedingly poor set of performances had certain characteristics more in keeping with a role enactment than with an acquired neurological deficit. On the Comprehension subtest where she barely scored, all her answers were ill formed or imperfectly explained. On some items she merely restated the question and appeared perfectly content to do so. Her performance was markedly at variance with her responses in ordinary conversation. These characteristics were observed on other tests although it was felt that she was approaching her anticipated level on Similarities.

On the Performance subtests given there were qualitative features not suggestive of cerebral impairment. All responses were correct but her exceeding slowness resulted in poor scores. Testing with the *Wechsler Memory Scale*, Form I added further weight to a psychogenic aetiology:

Information	3
Orientation	5
Mental Control	6 (3,3,0)
Memory passages	3
Digit Span	7 (4,3)
Visual Reproduction	2
Associate Learning	9 (4,0;6,0;6,1)

Asked the name of the Australian Prime Minister she replied 'Sir Isaac Newton'! Despite her prior slowness on the WAIS items she gained full points for counting backwards and reciting the alphabet. However, she failed to produce even one correct addition on the third component of Mental Control. Her attempts at Visual Reproduction are shown in Figure 4.1.

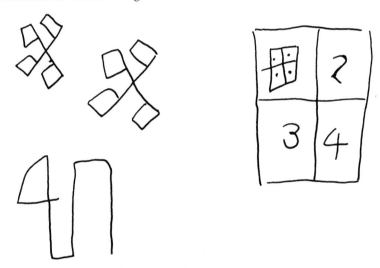

Fig. 4.1 Case IX. Attempts at Visual Reproduction.

On the second card she stopped drawing after completing the top left hand square. When asked what went in the others she paused, then filled in the numbers shown. The Rey Figure prompted another approximation with which she appeared to be well satisfied (Fig. 4.2) despite the fact that it took her six and a half minutes to produce it. After three minutes delay IX produced only the two external crosses in her attempt at recall. These elements were in the approximately correct positions on an otherwise blank page.

The last formal test given was the *Colour-Form Sorting Test* and the patient

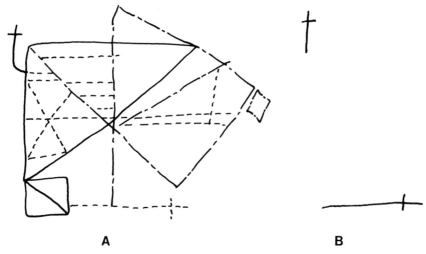

A   **B**

Fig. 4.2   Case IX. Rey Figure. Copy and recall.

surprised the examiner by sorting and correctly verbalizing both categories with ease.

Finally, IX was re-examined for the signs that had raised the question of a possible Gerstmann syndrome. While she failed on tests of finger naming and right-left discrimination, she did so in an unconvincing manner, e.g. failing to identify her left hand with her eyes open and strong visual cues in the form of several rings on her 'ring' finger. Hécaen and Albert (1978) argued that patients with organic disorders can often use such cues effectively. The 'acalculia' was obviously not based on organic impairment. The patient's responses were extremely rapid and at times simply incorporated parts of the original statement, e.g. 'If a man buys seven two-cent stamps and gives the clerk a half dollar, how much change should he get back?' Answer: 'Seventy two cents'. In fact, in clinical testing outside the formal assessment her response to the question 'How many cents are there in a dollar?' her reply was '99'. Thus this patient evinced both types of Ganser-like responses, namely missing by an inch and missing by a mile. Both have the same significance.

An unusual case of dyslexia and dysgraphia

Case NQ

This 36-year-old qualified nurse was the front seat passenger in a stationary car parked on a country road when it was struck from behind by another vehicle. She remembered her father speaking to her just before the impact and apparently did not lose consciousness though she fainted a short time after and awoke to find somebody removing the car door to get her out. She had pain in the hip and the back of her head and was unable to stand. She was taken to a nearby motel to rest but the next day was admitted to the local hospital following a period of vomiting. She remained in the hospital for two weeks, then moved to her sister's house in a nearby town. During this period she complained of posterior headache, neck pain, faintness and intermittent double vision. These symptoms lessened somewhat in intensity but remained prominent. It was considered that there had been aggravation of a pre-existing hyperextension injury to her cervical spine. This was now accompanied by 'an emotional response to her injuries with chronic depression and mild hysteria'. This state of anxiety and secondary depression accompanied by tension headaches was still much in evidence a year after the injury.

Two years after the event NQ was retired from her nursing post not having worked in the interim. Shortly after this she had a successful cervical fusion with improvement in some of her physical symptoms but no change in her psychiatric state. At times she complained of pains in nearly every part of her body with numbness and weakness in her arms and legs, all symptoms being intermittent and responding temporarily to treatment, only to recur or be replaced by others. The opinion of psychiatrists and neurologists was that her troubles were largely psychological in nature.

Finally, some five years after the accident she was referred for neuropsychological evaluation to clarify a disorder of reading and writing. This had emerged several months after the accident while she was attending a rehabilitation centre and, while there, was treated for nine months by a speech therapist with no improvement. Her writing contained various different types of errors. She drew the examiner's attention particularly to the frequent transposition or reversal of order of letters in a word, and remarked that this was worse for numbers. When asked by her neurologist to write a few spontaneous sentences she produced the following in a fluent hand:

'Today si Wesdnes Toromar si Thusday—Lunhc at Jane' afterwards to Susans ni ?
The neurologist felt that this writing disorder did not have a neurological basis, an opinion shared by a clinical psychologist who had seen her previously. Nevertheless her psychiatrist encouraged her to continue remedial reading and writing classes with a private tutor.

Neuropsychological assessment

The patient was fluent in conversation and showed no difficulty in auditory comprehension. Her conversation was sophisticated and she discoursed widely on her worldwide travels. On discussing her reading and writing difficulty she produced a story book suitable for the second year school-child and a lined exercise book in which she was doing her remedial writing. These were in the style of a young child using the widely spaced lines as a guide.

On dictation of 'the quick brown fox jumped over the lazy dog' and 'he shouted the warning' she wrote the material shown in Figure 4.3.

The strange looking symbols at the top right are her version of her date of birth: 9.3.36. In the mirror this reads from right to left 9/3/1396. The short passage of dictation contains the elements seen generally in her writing, viz letter reversals, letter and word substitution, letter omissions and phonetic spelling (ova for over). At no time did she show the slightest concern over her difficulties even while evincing great difficulty if reading aloud from the child's book. Here she failed to read simple words such as 'you' and introduced *reversals* such as pronouncing the word 'animal' as

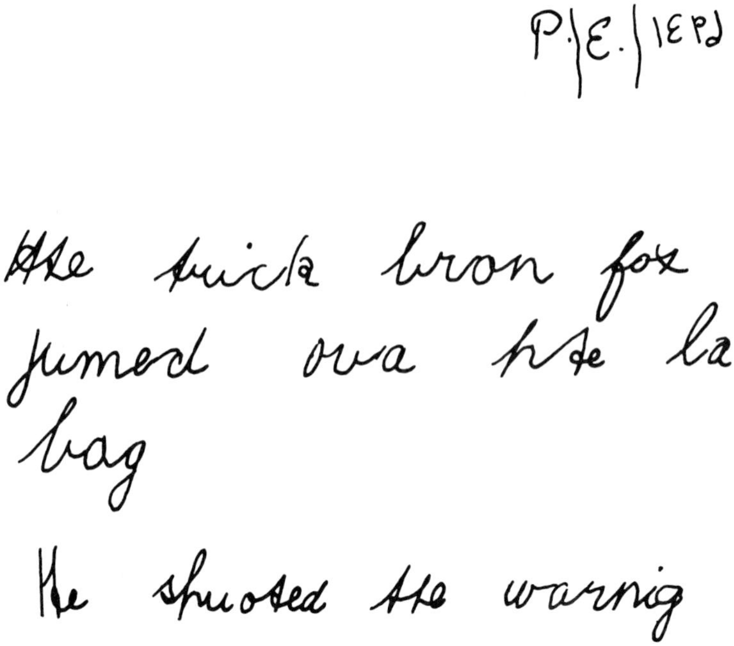

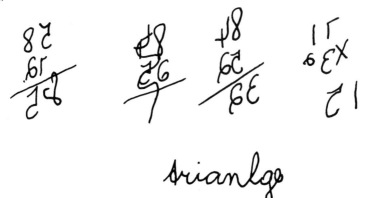

Fig. 4.3 Case NQ. Example of writing.

'aminal'. On this occasion she also introduced one or two reversals in her spontaneous speech.

At this stage the neuropsychologist felt that this was not an organically based language disorder but an enactment which he felt had been strongly shaped and reinforced by both speech therapist and remedial teacher. The dyslexia and dysgraphia stood in sharp contrast to the almost complete absence of signs in other language modes, a situation which fails to find support in the literature on the dyslexias. The number reversals were clearly shown in three computations from the dysphasia screening test (Russell et al 1970). These were 85−27; 48−25; 17x3 (Fig. 4.4).

Fig. 4.4 Case NQ. Number reversals.

If her workings are examined in a mirror, a number of inconsistencies emerge.

During the examinations she showed a characteristic 'belle indifférence', and her reading and writing difficulty stood in stark contrast to her conversational speech and understanding of the spoken word. An examination of other cognitive functions revealed no signs of impairment. On the Milner pathway of the Austin Maze she flagrantly disregarded the rules on the first trial but when chided about this she went on to learn the pathway rapidly and without further rule breaking.

The opportunity to compare her present state with that *several months after the accident* was provided by a psychologist who had carried out psychological assessment for the purpose of advising the patient about retraining, since her spinal problem rendered her unable to pursue her nursing career. The cognitive examination was unremarkable, all tests being at around the expected bright normal level as we had found more recently. What was remarkable was the presence in the file of a piece of creative writing which the psychologist had asked her to do during the early sessions. Unlike her later childish efforts, her handwriting was in a free flowing hand with no spelling mistakes or transpositions. The subject matter, which was self-selected, showed a sensitivity and imagination quite out of keeping with her recent productions. It was thus apparent that there was a considerable time lag between the motor accident and the development of the 'language disorder'.

The opinion was given that the reading and writing disorder was an hysterical enactment and the fact that this had been strongly reinforced over a long period seemed to point to a poor prognosis. This case of a circumscribed neuropsychological disorder parallels in most respects the exhibition by other patients of conversion symptoms, i.e. it differs only in the area of function through which the patient 'chooses' to express whatever difficulties lie at its base.

Post-traumatic neurosis

Case: KX

This 32-year-old electrical mechanic had held a responsible job before sustaining a minor head injury in which he was said to have lost consciousness but was conscious on arrival at the emergency department of general hospital a short time later. He had a haematoma of the scalp, and tenderness and minor bruising of the right side of his body. Examination was normal and he was discharged home within a few hours. Liability to the accident was admitted by the other party.

Though KX returned to work within two weeks of the event he had numerous somatic complaints and finally stopped work two years after the accident because he felt that he could no longer cope. He was seen by numerous doctors, all of whom considered that his condition had little or no basis in physical injury. Since the accident he had been depressed and complained of constant headaches. After leaving work, attempts were made to rehabilitate him over a period of a year without success. However, examinations by speech therapists and a clinical psychologist now suggested that 'he has cortical deficits which seemingly were not diagnosed or treated following the accident'. These opinions were markedly divergent from those of several neurological specialists and at the end of failed attempts at rehabilitation an effort was made to settle his claim for damages. To assess the claim for possible brain impairment a neuropsychological examination was requested.

Perusal of reports from the rehabilitation centre noted the following among his numerous failures: poor visual memory, neglect of use of the left arm and hand, imperfect understanding of spoken instructions, slow oral sentence completion with many failures, slow and confused reading, simple subtractions poor and failure to retain information. On psychometric testing at the rehabilitation centre he had scored 87 and 100 on the WAIS VIQ and PIQ. This was considered to be below his pre-accident level but comments were made about his tendency to give up when the items became difficult. On the Porteus Maze test his mental age was said to be 7½ years!

At our neuropsychological examination KX complained that his memory was poor and had worsened despite a year of therapy. With the suggestion of a 'cortical deficit' causing language dysfunction the neuropsychologist was careful to include a range of grammatical constructions from simple to complex in the preliminary interview, where the effect of the accident was discussed. He showed not the slightest difficulty, but when confronted with basic 'tests' of language he made the most elementary blunders. There were no paraphasias or other qualitative difficulties characteristic of dysphasia. This discrepancy between everyday and test behaviour is typical of pseudoneurological states (McEvoy & Wells 1979, Wells 1979a). A repetition of the Porteus Maze test produced a failure on the seven-year-old level (Fig. 4.5) but steady pressure elicited passes at most subsequent levels including the Adult maze, successfully completed in three trials.

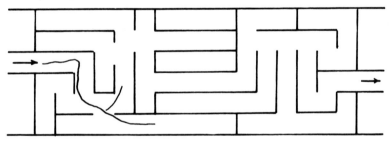

Fig. 4.5   Case KX. Failure on Year VII, Porteus Maze Test.

Discontinuation at earlier failed levels (according to normal test instructions) would no doubt have produced a low Mental Age as described by the previous examiner. Passing the more difficult items made it clear that the reason for failure did not result from neural incapacity. Considering the general lack of co-operation shown throughout the testing KX obviously had intact the abilities necessary for this task.

Testing of general intellectual abilities produced responses in keeping with the patient's background, apart from numerous 'don't know' responses with an occasional odd statement of qualification after a correct reply, e.g. having explained that Michelangelo was an artist, KX asked subsequently whether the artist was still alive. Throughout the standardized tests he showed the pattern of failing on some very easy items while passing some of the most difficult, which is almost pathognomonic of pseudoneurological cases. Despite his description earlier of a visual memory difficulty he reproduced the designs of the WMS Visual

Reproduction subtest fluently and in complete detail. He also showed ability to learn new verbal associations readily though he recalled little of prose material.

As the examination was extended, nothing of a qualitative or quantitative nature emerged which would support the presence of brain impairment, as might have been expected considering the nature of his injury. Finally, he was given the *Fifteen Item 'Memory' Test* of Rey (1964) cited in Lezak (1976). 'The principle underlying it is that the patient who consciously or unconsciously wishes to appear impaired will fail at a task that all but the most severely brain damaged or retarded patients perform easily'. Lezak (1983) suggested that malingering should be considered in individuals who deny being able to remember at least 9 of the 15 items, a criterion supported by a study of acutely disturbed psychiatric patients and intellectually deficient patients (Goldberg & Miller 1986).

Our patient's effort is shown (Fig. 4.6) in comparison with that of a patient with long-standing epilepsy and mental retardation (VIQ 74. PIQ 77). Not only did KX do poorly, his performance was quite suspect. (The numerals against his responses denote the order in which he made them.) Note that the evocation of 'a' did not cause him to complete the letter series.

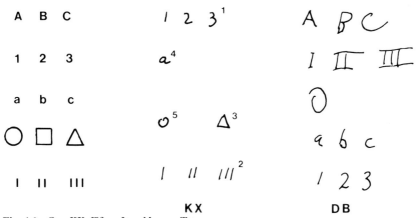

Fig. 4.6   Case KX. Fifteen Item Memory Test.

There were many similar features in this case which illustrated that failures on tests of language, memory and other functions may be produced in a way quite uncharacteristic of neurologically induced brain impairment. Furthermore, the history of late onset and worsening of symptoms with time is quite the reverse of that encountered after traumatic brain injury, where considerable recovery takes place over time even in severe cases. Any case which goes contrary to this 'law of recovery' should be suspect of having a large psychological component.

Case: VR

This 33-year-old university educated school teacher sustained a mild head injury when a cupboard fell over on him at work. He was said to have been unconscious for 15 minutes though this was never verified. Certainly he was recorded as being fully conscious on arrival at hospital within the hour. Neurological examination and skull

X-rays were normal. He surprised the staff by claiming that he could recall nothing in the preceding ten years, conveying this information in Arabic which had been his native language. He had been highly fluent in English having learned the language prior to coming to live in Australia and having taught in English for some years.

Over some two weeks the retrograde amnesia shrank to remain constant at about one and a half years. He said the return of his memory was aided by the use of diaries he had kept and by his family taking him to places he had visited previously. During this relearning period he was surprised to discover that he had been married and was distressed when he learnt that he had been divorced three years before.

After the injury he was troubled with numerous somatic complaints. These included severe headaches and loss of sensation and paraesthesia in his feet. He had a number of episodes each lasting a few minutes when he had total loss of vision in his left eye. Investigations suggested that his symptoms were probably functional in nature. On the day the patient was to return to work he said he had lost sight temporarily and as a result crashed his car into the fence on his way out.

VR was born in the Middle East where he was educated and was looked up to by his peers because he represented his country in international sporting competitions. He said his family were very close and that he did well at school. He completed tertiary education in his homeland and came to Australia at the age of 24 following which he completed his teacher training and entered his present position which he enjoyed.

One year after his arrival he married an Australian girl and thereby incurred the wrath of his parents who felt that he should have consulted them. However, when his parents joined him in Australia two years later they had adjusted to the idea of his marriage. He said the marriage was a happy one although there was some sexual maladjustment due to his wife's allegedly prudish ideas. The marriage had broken up three years before when his wife left him for a younger man. He blames this on the fact that she had some sort of nervous upset following a back injury. He had not had any girlfriends before he met his wife and since she left him he has not considered remarriage or developed any close relationship until fairly recently.

The hospital records showed that he had been treated several times in the preceding years for minor ailments such as epigastric pain, all of which were thought to be due to anxiety. Two weeks after the head injury his doctor wrote:

He presented as a fit-looking young man with flamboyant mannerisms who was angry at what he claimed was the poor treatment he had had at the hospital and was full of blame for the various people he had seen since his head injury. He tended to relate his story in a rather dramatic manner and frequently went into great detail about relatively trivial aspects of the history. At times he seemed quite paranoid. He wondered if the mirror in the room was a two-way mirror so that other people were watching him and seemed unreasonably sensitive about what he perceived was the attitude of the doctor he had seen the day before. His affect was labile but mainly angry and anxious. He was also mildly depressed.

Formal examination revealed no evidence of hallucinations, delusions or other phenomena suggestive of psychosis. He was correctly oriented and was said to perform well on tests of short-term memory though the details were not specified. His thought content was mainly directed towards his amnesia and how he was coping with his headache which he attributed directly to the accident.

The opinion was expressed that his amnesia was dissociative, i.e. hysterical in origin and that the headache, loss of vision, and other symptoms were also psychogenic. At this stage a neuropsychological examination was sought 'to exclude brain damage'. It was then four weeks after the injury.

In the interview preceding assessment the psychologist noted that VR made no reference to rapid forgetting, difficulty with new learning or other problems recounted so typically by patients after head injury. The patient concentrated his complaints solely on his retrograde amnesia which remained at over a year.

Wechsler Memory Scale, Form I

Information	5	Digits Total	10 (5,5)
Orientation	4	Visual Reproduction	11
Mental Control	2	Associate Learning	5.5 (3,0; 3,0; 3,1)
Memory Passages	5.5		
MQ 72			

This grossly deficient performance for a man of university education was out of all proportion to the severity of the injury and the general behaviour of the patient during testing. Despite being attentive, alert, and well oriented he was unable to manage the simple automatic mental operations of counting backwards and serial addition. He gave only the gist of each of the prose passages although he could give the fullest of detail of recent events in general conversation. He repeatedly failed to improve on five digits forwards though he managed five backwards with ease. The remaining subtests will be described in more detail.

On Visual Reproduction he performed well on Cards A and B while on Card C he produced the unusual response shown (Fig. 4.7). The left-hand figure approximated roughly to the presented design whereas the right-hand figure, while essentially correct, included the two arrows and stick figures.

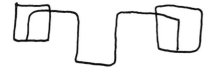 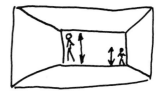

Fig. 4.7   Case VR. Reproduction of Card C Wechsler Memory Scale.

He commented that this was a drawing of the Ames distorted room, a reference to one of a series of perceptual illusions described by Kilpatrick (1961) which are often included in elementary courses in psychology. VR seemed to want to convey that he, too, had studied psychology. He thus demonstrated that not only could he hold the given visual information, he could also carry other material simultaneously in memory without disturbing the original.

The responses to the Paired Associate learning task are set out in Table 4.1 in detail since they present qualitative features seen frequently in pseudoneurological cases.

Table 4.1   Paired Associate learning—Case VR. Responses on three trials

		Patient's responses		
Cue	Response	Trial 1	Trial 2	Trial 3
North	South	South	South	South
Fruit	Apple	Pear	Inch	Flower
Obey	Inch	Disobey	Mother	Inch
Rose	Flower	Flower	Flower	Flower
Baby	Cries	Mother	Mother	Mother
Up	Down	Down	Down	Down
Cabbage	Pen	Rocks	Inch	Inch
Metal	Iron	Building	Labourer	Crush
School	Grocery	Students	Inch	—
Crush	Dark	Cabbage	Iron	Metal

Though the overall score was very poor there was an absence of the pattern usually found in organic amnesias, where the accent is on difficulty with new learning. Thus the organic patient, almost independent of the aetiology, reawakens all or most of the old or logical associations by the third trial, often being able to produce a number of them on the first trial. On the other hand, such patients find the acquisition of new verbal associations very difficult and lose them easily. This dissociation between old and new associate pairs is highly characteristic of organic amnesias. VR failed to display this pattern, managing to repeat only three old (easy) associations and one new one by the third trial. It was noteworthy that this patient, who did so badly on such a learning task had absolutely no subjective complaint of recent memory disorder. Once again, the performance on formal testing is out of proportion to the severity of the injury and is typical of pseudoneurological patients.

Rey Figure. VR produced a complete copy in a slow deliberate way in a poorly organized sequence, deleting several incorrect lines in the process. After a delay of three minutes he produced the recall shown (Fig. 4.8).

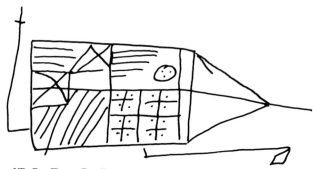

Fig. 4.8   Case VR. Rey Figure. Recall.

Having subdivided the main figure into four, he filled in all but the right lower quadrant, paused for a minute or so and then proceeded to fill in the blank space with what is essentially the Card B design from the Wechsler Memory Scale given some time before. This was also considered to be in the nature of a role enactment where the subject produces an 'incorrect' response but lacks the sophistication of knowing how the organic patient goes wrong.

Other tests added nothing further to suggest that more extensive examination would be more productive and it was left to the treating psychiatrists to request examination later. We learned that these symptoms later resolved but it is unlikely that the patient will remain symptom free. No doubt his dissatisfaction with our hospital will have led him to seek assistance elsewhere.

Neurological lesion with functional overlay

Case: XD

This 38-year-old shoe machinist was working at her trade when she developed slurred speech during her coffee break. The right side of her face appeared to sag and she became alarmed when the coffee she was drinking ran out of the side of her mouth. She did not lose consciousness and her walking was unaffected. In fact, she walked a considerable distance to a doctor's surgery only to find that she could not be seen. Her husband drove her to hospital where a neurological examination revealed a mild paresis of the right side of her face, left arm and leg, and other signs suggestive of a pontine infarct. This diagnosis was confirmed several days later by a CT scan. The arm and leg paresis cleared rapidly but the facial palsy remained in evidence. Other signs were variable and the neurologist felt that most of these were not organic in origin. The patient was emotionally labile and at the end of two weeks was referred to the Neuropsychology Unit with a diagnosis of 'resolving pontine infarct with functional overlay', with a request to assist in confirming or refuting the latter part of this diagnosis. There were symptoms of a neurological kind which the neurologist felt could not be explained on an anatomical basis.

Neuropsychological assessment (two weeks after infarction)

XD gave a coherent and detailed account of the events of the day of her infarct and since. Her affect appeared appropriate and though she dabbed at her eye with her handkerchief, this was soon seen to be unilateral lachrymation, a legacy of her neurological episode. She admitted to no emotional difficulties before or since the event and applied herself to the tests with apparently full co-operation. Because of the known pathology in the posterior (vertebrobasilar) circulation which also supplies the hippocampal regions via its main terminal branches, the left and right posterior cerebral arteries, the examination began with the *Wechsler Memory Scale*, Form I:

Information	6
Orientation	5
Mental Control	0
Memory Passages	5
Digits Total	5 (3,2)
Visual Reproduction	2
Associate Learning	12.5 (3,0; 6.2; 6,3)

MQ 66

Several unusual features could be seen in this performance. The overall performance produced a quotient quite out of keeping with the excellence of her memory at interview. The pattern of subtest performance was quite unlike any of the known organically based amnesic disorders. Despite perfect scores on Information and Orientation, XD scored zero on Mental Control as follows:

1. 20 19 17 16 14 13 11 9 8 7 6 4 3 2 1 (30 seconds)
2. ABCDEFGHI (pause) LMNOPQ (pause) U (pause) Z (22 seconds)
3. 1 4 7 12 16 19 23 27 31 (60 seconds)

On the verbal memory tasks, despite performing poorly on Digit Span and producing only rudiments of the prose passages, she was able to cope with the more searching Associate Learning task up to the standard one might have expected. Attempts on Visual Reproduction had a Ganser-like quality with some approximation to the presented designs and an unusual quality unsuggestive of either an amnesic or a graphic disorder (Fig. 4.9).

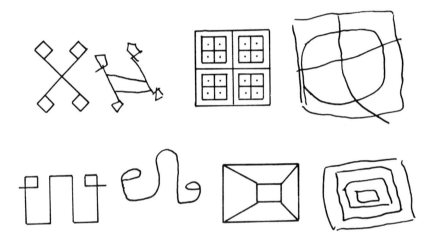

Fig. 4.9   Case XD. Visual Reproduction, Wechsler Memory Scale.

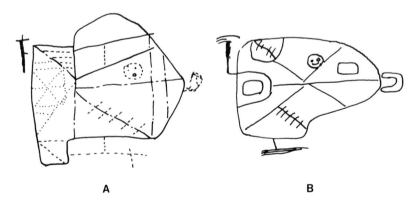

A   B

Fig. 4.10   Case XD. Rey Figure. Copy and recall.

The WMS was followed by the *Rey Figure* since the hypothesis of functional overlay was now receiving strong support and it was thought that further graphic material might allow the enactment to be documented further. This proved to be the case. The productions (Fig. 4.10) were unlike any type of amnesic or executive disorder of neurological origin.

Naylor Harwood Adult Intelligence Scale. The following subtests were given to sample her intellectual abilities:

Comprehension	10	Letter Symbol	5
Similarities	10	Block Design	8
		Object Assembly	4

The two verbal subtests seemed to be consonant in level and quality of response with her background. Interpretation of the Performance scores was made difficult by uncertainty about the presence of any residual visual problems of a neurological nature which had been present early in the illness. The fact that the patient passed on some of the more difficult Block Designs while failing on the easier ones supported, once again, a psychogenic hypothesis for at least one major factor depressing the scores.

The *Colour-Form Sorting Test* was carried out without difficulty.

Finally, the patient was given the *Porteus Maze Test*, years VIII to XIV. Her Mental Age score of 9 years was not thought to be a valid representation of her ability. There were no qualitative features of the type seen with frontal lobe damage and once again a perceptual difficulty seemed unlikely.

During this examination XD complained of a word-finding difficulty and was referred to the Speech Therapy Department. The opinion given at this stage was that there was, at most, only equivocal evidence of neuropsychological dysfunction and that most of the observations strongly supported a major psychogenic component. She was discharged from hospital to attend as an outpatient for occupational therapy and psychiatric help.

Second examination (3 1/2 months after infarction)

She was quiet and co-operative and gave a clear account of what had been happening to her. The chronology was accurate. An attempt was made to check the 'psychogenic' hypothesis. An oral Digit Span test produced the following set of responses:

Examiner	Patient
2 8 6 1	2 6 1
5 3 9 4	5 3 9 10
7 4 2 9 6	7 4 6
3 9 2 6 1	3 9 6 1
4 7 1 8 6	4 7 (pause) 10 6

The *Knox Cube Test* (see Appendix) was then given:

	Examiner	Patient
Practice	1 1 2 3 4	1 2 3 4
	1 4 3 2	1 4 .. 2 3
	4 1 2 3	4 1 .. 3 2
	2 1 4 3	1 2 .. 4 3
	3 1 4 2	1 4 3 2
	2 4 1 3	2 4 3 1
Practice 2	1 2 3 4 1	1 2 3 4 1
	1 3 1 2 4	1 4 3 2 1
	4 3 2 3 1	1 2 3 4 1 3 1
	3 2 4 3 1	2 3 4 .. 1 3—test abandoned

Practice items were passed with ease but she failed all other items.

We have found this simple test very useful in such situations. Patients who are enacting will invariably get the practice items correct since they seem to construe from the test instructions that these items are not to be counted in the scoring. The 'pregnant pauses' (..) are also characteristic. The reader should remember that patients who have correctly given the first two of a four item series immediately reduce the available degrees of freedom. If they are not careful (pause) they might get the item correct by mistake!

As the assessment proceeded the only failures which came to light served to confirm the diagnosis of a pseudoneurological disorder and, as the patient was already under psychiatric care, further examination was deemed unnecessary.

Non-organic memory disorder

Case: QW

This 60-year-old woman was admitted for neurological investigation following episodes of alterations in her conscious state. The history was given by her husband and daughter who had witnessed several of the attacks. The description included apparent lowering of consciousness during which there was an inability to move or communicate, and flickering of the eyelids was observed.

Her husband reported that at the beginning of the spells she looked pale, and would them slump back into her chair with eyes closed for about 20 minutes. She woke up speaking quietly and having difficulty choosing her words. At one stage drooping of the left side of her face was noticed. She had never fallen or injured herself and there were no involuntary movements nor any incontinence. There had been eight episodes, all identical, in the four months preceding admission. They occurred at various times of the day although several were noted to have occurred just before a meal.

The patient herself said she experienced a feeling of extreme tiredness at the onset, noted that her speech was thick and slow, and would then usually make her way to bed to either fall asleep or lose consciousness. She would wake to find her legs weak but no other aftermath. She said she shuffled about for several hours before returning to her normal state.

She was described as a capable housewife who led an active social life which included regular golf, a sport at which she was quite competent. She also assisted her husband, who was a busy public official, by taking phone messages.

The medical history included nothing of neurological interest. Her only other recent complaint was of periodic numbness of the face unrelated to the episodes being investigated. She had enjoyed good health otherwise in recent years.

Neurological examination showed no clinical evidence of epilepsy or narcolepsy and the consultant psychiatrist felt that there might be an element of anxiety but that there was no sign of major psychiatric disturbance. Physical examination was normal apart from a blood pressure of 190/100. EEG examination was normal but CT scan revealed moderate dilatation of the right lateral ventricle without midline shift, and slight atrophy of the overlying cortex. She was then admitted for ventriculography to see if a cause could be found for the mild unilateral hydrocephalus. The results suggested the presence of partial obstruction of the right interventricular foramen. However, at no stage could an obstructive lesion be visualized. On the basis of these findings, ventriculoscopy and installation of a shunt were performed. Immediately after operation QW developed what was described as an acute confusional state. It was thought originally that her symptoms might be due to an 'acute brain syndrome'; the presence of a gross memory deficit even raised the outside possibility, in one member of the neurosurgical team, of inadvertent operative damage to the fornix or related structures. However, there seemed little likelihood of this.

When seen by the neuropsychologist ten days postoperatively QW was alert and was in no distress. She gave her age as 37 years and that of her daughter as 39. Asked the name of the hospital she replied that it was a maternity hospital and, questioned further on this, said she must be going to have a baby. She gave many other bizarre answers without any show of emotion and became evasive when pressed over inconsistencies in her replies. Every single question was answered incorrectly whether it pertained to recent or remote events. The neuropsychologist gave his opinion that the cognitive disturbance did not have a neurological basis. Discussion with ward staff confirmed that she clearly remembered events over 24 hours or more though she invariably gave incorrect answers when asked direct questions. The patient's family were concerned that the mental impairment had been produced by the neurosurgery and, unfortunately, a psychiatrist called in by the family tended to support this diagnosis. With some question of litigation in the air it was decided to document her intellectual capacity with formal testing.

The patient began the session by asking the examiner to remind her to take her cigarette lighter when leaving as she now had a very bad memory. The relevance of this will become clear later.

Wechsler Memory Scale, Form I

Information	0	Digits Total	8 (5,3)
Orientation	1	Visual Reproduction	0
Mental Control	5	Associate Learning	7.5 (5,0; 5,0; 5,0)
Logical Memory	4		

MQ 63

This performance was quite out of keeping with her ward behaviour. It contained random and inconsistent statements given with a smiling air of indifference. At all times she was extremely attentive and denied any awareness of having made mistakes. Her responses on serial addition of threes were: $1-4-7-13-16-22-25-31-34-37$. This 'dropping out of responses' (10, 19, 28) was thought to represent a pseudoneurological reaction. One of the sure ways to fail is to give only some of the correct responses. Her Visual Reproduction responses also supported a pseudoneurological hypothesis (Fig. 4.11). Even patients with quite severe organically based amnesic syndromes tend to produce much of the basic information from the first two cards.

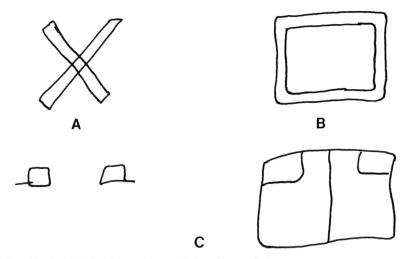

Fig. 4.11   Case QW. Visual Reproduction, Wechsler Memory Scale.

The drawings were thought to represent QW's idea of an incorrect response. A visual difficulty seemed unlikely also, as the basis for such a poor performance and a perfect score was returned on the Albert Test of Visual Neglect (Albert 1973).

Colour-Form Sorting Test. The patient was unable, or unwilling, to proceed beyond placing all the pieces together in a complex assembly.

Porteus Maze Test. Year VIII was passed but year IX was failed, even when five trials were allowed.

Rey Figure. This proved most illuminating. Her first copy contained many of the correct elements but some were incorrectly related to the total figure (Fig. 4.12 left). The examiner withdrew this effort and asked her to draw it again with more care.

She produced a second copy (Fig. 4.12 right) also with errors of relationship, two of which she spontaneously corrected.

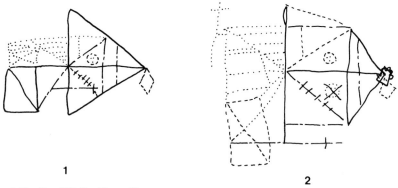

Fig. 4.12   Case QW. Rey Figure. Two attempts to copy.

The examiner felt that further drawings would probably result in copies which, unlike those of organic patients, would be different from one another.

Finally, after a further three minutes delay she produced Figure 4.13 with an air of confidence and stated that she was sure hers was just like the original. Such a 'creation' seemed totally in keeping with a role enactment formulation.

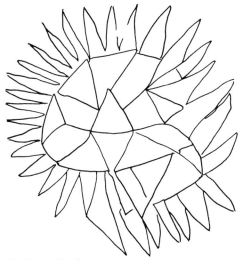

Fig. 4.13   Case QW. Rey Figure. Recall.

At the end of this two hour examination, during which her concentration never flagged, QW chided the examiner for not reminding her about her cigarette lighter, not realizing that this was at variance with her display of seemingly gross memory deficit throughout the testing.

After a period of psychiatric care in another hospital this patient returned home where she was able to manage the running of her home and prepare meals for her husband and herself although she complained of patchy memory and her husband felt that she was not fully recovered. The neurosurgical team who reviewed her two months after operation wrote as follows: 'She is bright and fluent and logical in her conversation and it is only when directly challenged by testing that any abnormality appears'. The following extract of the hospital record provides an example:

'Repeat after me the following digits: 2,4,3,5,1,8'.
Reply: '2,4,3,5,1,8'.
'Repeat after me: 2,4,3,5,1,8,0,2'.
Reply: '2,4,5,1,8,0, (pause) 3
'No, that's not it, we have trouble in the middle and the end—let's go over it again: 2,4,3,5,1,8,0,2'.
Reply: '2,4,3,5,1,8,0,4'.
'No, that's not it—try again: 2,4,3,5,1,8,0,2'.
Reply: '2,4,3,5,1,8,0,5—I think'.
Another example: 'What is the year' (correct answer, 1979)
Reply (given unhesitatingly): '1969'.
'No—try again'.
Reply (again without hesitation): '1959'
'Let's try 1979'.
Reply: '*Yes, it must be because next year is 1980*'.

Several months later neuropsychological assessment showed improvement in most areas of functioning though there were still aberrant responses which lowered some test results. At this time it was learned that QW had had a similar episode years before following an abdominal operation, and had also developed hysterical deafness after being upset at a social function. This illustrates that not only may the vehicle or type of symptom through which the expression takes place vary from patient to patient but also within the same patient.

Post-traumatic neurosis

Case: HY

This 40-year-old woman referred herself for advice regarding the effects of a prior head injury, the result of a motor vehicle accident. She was the driver of a car which ran off a country road and hit a tree some 16 months before. She said she had lost consciousness for about half an hour and had been disoriented for about two weeks. There was no confirmatory evidence available at the time of interview. The history, extracted from her with difficulty, was sparse. She had attended a rehabilitation centre where she claimed they had found 'subtle memory and visuospatial problems' (her terms).

One of the salient features which she omitted was that the acute management of her head injury and orthopaedic problems had been at the hospital where the interview was being conducted. Later inspection of the records showed that she was an inpatient for five weeks before being transferred to a rehabilitation centre. The reason for her stay appeared to be purely orthopaedic. There had been no report following her admission of any signs suggestive of significant head injury, e.g. no evidence of post-traumatic amnesia.

HY had qualifications both in nursing and as a teacher, with a degree encompassing a good deal of psychology, and had been on her way to a professional conference when she had her accident.

She remained an inpatient in rehabilitation for about two months and then a further two months as an outpatient. The chronology was hard to extract from her and she appeared mildly depressed though generally co-operative. She was also vague about the psychosocial problems for which she said she was attending a private psychiatrist once a week and would not elaborate.

Her main cognitive complaints were also hard to pin down. She said she functioned now at a lower level, and that she had failed at work experience (working with the visiting teacher at the rehabilitation centre). She added that she had had trouble with the health authorities and the accident board, failing to get certificates to them on time. At the time of her self-referral, apart from weekly therapy, she was attending part-time college courses twice each week.

Assessment by a clinical psychologist began with a standard intellectual evaluation:

WAIS-R (age scale scores)

Information	17	Digit-Symbol	11
Comprehension	16	Picture Completion	14
Arithmetic	15	Block Design	15
Similarities	14	Picture Arrangement	14
Digit Span	13	Object Assembly	16
VIQ 130		PIQ 122	

These measures appeared to be consonant with her educational and occupational background. There were no indications of a qualitative nature suggesting neuropsychological deficits. In view of her stated difficulties several tasks specifically relevant to her complaints were then given.

WMS, Form I

Information	3	Digits Total	6 (3,3)
Orientation	5	Visual Reproduction	3 (2,0;0,1)
Mental Control	0	Associate Learning	9 (4,0; 5,1; 5,1)
Memory Passages	4 (4.5,3)		
MQ 64			

Despite having performed very well on digit span in the context of the intelligence test, HY managed only three digits forward when told that her memory would now be tested in some detail. Also, despite complete control of many difficult items on the WAIS-R, she scored zero on the routine tasks of Mental Control and performed badly on virtually everything else. Thus there was a striking difference between the intelligence test measures and the memory scale performance. We then told her that we would test her memory further.

Supraspan Digit Learning. Ignoring the fact that she had scored seven forward earlier, we explained that we would repeat a short series until she managed to repeat it correctly. Her responses were as follows, the relative length of her pauses being indicated by the number of dots:

Series given—748259
Consecutive trials:
.7...2....8....3...............
..7....8....2....9......4......
....7.8...5...9......2.........
.....7...8....5....9.........
...7...... 8...2.......5.........9
...7.....2.....8....5...... 9

After six trials it seemed pointless to continue. The examiner was convinced that the number 4 would not be produced again even if a large number of trials were to be given. The span difficulty stood in stark contrast to the amount of material HY could deal with when it was not construed as being a *memory* test.

Rey Figure. Copy score 17/36. Recall score 13/36. (Fig. 4.14)

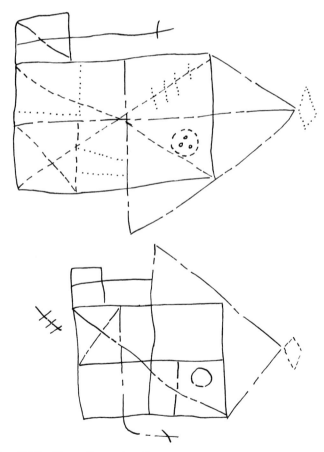

Fig. 4.14   Case HY. Rey Figure. Copy and recall.

Like several of the cases earlier in this chapter, HY's copy and recall were quite unusual being qualitatively different both from the normal and from sundry forms of neuropsychological disorder that make this a difficult test for some neurological patients. It also provides a very productive vehicle for enactment.

It seemed that the deviant responses which HY produced were meant to reflect her claimed 'subtle memory and visuospatial disturbances'. If these were real they would have declared themselves time and again on the earlier intellectual examination from which they were strangely missing.

Rey's Fifteen Item Test. The poverty of response is combined with a very strange order of procedure which is indicated in Figure 4.15 by the added arrows and numbers (row 1 was done first from left to right, row 2 was done next from right to left, and so on).

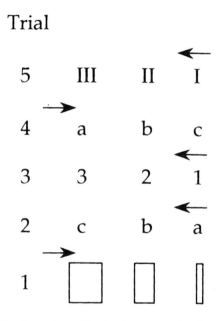

Fig. 4.15   Case HY. Fifteen Item Memory Test showing bizarre order of reproduction.

Following the examination she did not return for three months despite the fact that she had been given no feedback about her performance on the tests. At this interview the neuropsychologist said that in his opinion there was little or no indication that her present state was due to residual brain damage, a view which was also the opinion of the rehabilitation psychologists despite her earlier statement at the original interview. She was advised that, apart from her present psychiatrist who was apparently getting nowhere, she might seek help from another rehabilitation psychologist.

Extracts from this rehabitation psychologist's report following interview and examination are as follows:

She finds that she has difficulty with art and technical things that are 'spatial' or have 'perspective'. As a 'creative person' she has difficulty sewing and knitting. She has home help twice a week. She complained in the following terms of poor concentration, long-term and short-term memory. She said she had difficulty in organizing herself, gets lost and has trouble with information overload. She feels very tired, is slow in everything she does and has headaches. She has had her eyes tested and there was nothing medically wrong but her eye movements were slow and information was getting in but not coming out as it should.

In terms of personality she felt she now does not have 'the get up and go' she once had. She was always active, bright and never ruffled by anything. Now she has difficulty tolerating noise, and gets tired and agitated when there are a lot of people around her. She says she cries frequently. She had a depressed air and generally spoke slowly and softly . . .

There followed a report sheet with details of testing, including the following:

Visual Recognition Memory. Shown ten pictures of familiar objects and then asked to select them from 20, she made numerous errors—both false positives and false negatives.

Warrington Recognition Memory for Words. She scored 29/50 (less than the 5th centile). This is a fine example of the poorer than chance concept mentioned under 'Symptom and syndrome validity' earlier in this chapter.

Colour-Form Sorting Test. On this conceptually simple test she managed only the sorting by colours, without any qualitative features that there was a difficulty in shifting response set.

Benton Visual Retention Test She scored *none* correct with 23 errors.

Rey Auditory Verbal Learning Test. HY managed to learn only five words over the five trials (4,4,4,5,5).

WAIS Block Design subtest. She was unable to construct any of the designs correctly. She made some attempts but said that she was unable to see that they were incorrect. This stood in stark contrast to an age scaled score of 15 on Block Design for the previous psychologist.

The rehabitation neuropsychologist wrote in conclusion:

Clearly the results from our tests are consistent with your own findings of exaggeration of symptoms to a degree which is completely inconsistent with her ability to cope in daily life. Her slowness in speech during testing contrasted with her normal speech presentation when she wanted to discuss the results. She was anxious to undertake a program with us but I felt obligated to inform her that our programs are not suited to her needs. She appeared to be upset by this, wanting to argue at length about issues such as how we could possibly make this judgment after a brief assessment. As you know our program is cognitively oriented and we do not feel that our expertise lies in treating post-traumatic psychological disturbances such as she is experiencing.

This is a striking but by no means rare example of an intelligent professional person who nevertheless presents quite crude response deviations in her enactment of the sick role. In this case her background contained quite an exposure to psychology at a tertiary level and in professional day to day contacts.

THE OTHER SIDE OF THE COIN

There are occasions when symptoms might appear to be psychiatric even where there is known neurological damage. At times this may lead to a misclassification of 'functional overlay' especially where the symptoms do not appear to fit readily into our knowledge of commonly occurring neuropsychological syndromes. The following case illustrates that it may be difficult at times to classify the case in any simple scheme. Neuropsychologists will provide a useful service if they can supply information which helps to clarify the probable basis of the patient's symptoms.

Query functional or organic

Case: XZ

A private neurologist referred this 28-year-old truck driver with the following detailed information:

> He complains of an inability to drive following a moderately severe head injury in January and my question is whether his complaint is organically based. He was involved in a motor car accident about seven months ago. I do not have the full details of his injuries, but I believe he sustained a skull fracture and was unconscious for three or four days. He dates his visual symptoms back to the time of his injury and claims they were present when he left hospital. Mostly he complains of a lack of clarity or brightness, though more recently he has also mentioned that his 'side vision' is deficient. I am not certain if he first noticed this before his visual field defect was detected. It is noteworthy that his visual difficulties make driving impossible though they do not bother him at any other time. Thus he can read, watch television, find his way about and recognize objects as formerly, though he is totally unable to return to his former work as a driver. When asked what prevents him he mentioned that he becomes confused by the white lines in the centre of the road, fails to appreciate oncoming traffic and finds approaching headlights unpleasantly bright. He informs me that he has had two near accidents while attempting to drive. His inability to drive stands in stark contrast to his complete lack of any of the multitudinous symptoms so often encountered after head injuries. He is a right-handed man whose visual acuity without correction is 6/7.5 in both eyes. His near vision without correction was size two type on the Moorfields chart. He made only one error in twelve with each eye on the Ishihara plates. There is a congruous left lower quadrantic homonymous field defect which extends from the horizontal to about 30 degrees below it and spares fixation. The borders of this field seem to be constant when plotted with a variety of colours or sizes of target suggesting a vascular aetiology. A CT scan performed in June showed two almost symmetrical areas of reduced density in both occipital poles which are presumably areas of atrophy. A CT scan done elsewhere after the accident was said to be normal. I have not seen the picture myself. I am troubled that this man's disability seems out of proportion to his demonstrable deficits, but concerned that I may be missing a subtle visuospatial problem.

The patient was co-operative throughout the testing and was well aware that some doctors might consider that he was inventing or exaggerating his symptoms, as he admitted he found his visual problems difficult to describe to others. We have met such difficulty frequently in patients with proven lesions of the occipital lobe. Before beginning to examine his perceptual functions specifically we thought it wise to gain some background information on his other intellectual abilities and to exclude some of the more common sequelae of head injury.

On the *Wechsler Memory Scale* his quotient was 112. The only depressed score was on Visual Reproduction. Several subtests of the *WAIS* were also given during this screening examination:

Information	14	Picture Completion	11
Similarities	13	Block Design	7
Digit Span	15	Object Assembly	6

The level and quality of response on the three verbal subtests were above that anticipated from his occupational history. Though he had had a high school education he said he preferred manual work. His recognition and naming of objects on the Picture Completion subtest were excellent and he had little difficulty in finding many of the missing items. However, he had difficulty on the later items of Block Design (6,8,9,10) where visual decomposition must precede re-assembly, but succeeded on item 7 where a block by block strategy will suffice (see Ch. 1). He managed to complete three of the four Object Assembly problems with extra time but was having obvious difficulty.

The dissociation between performance on visuospatial and other tasks tended at this stage to support the presence of a neurologically based deficit. The possibility of a deficient visual memory raised by the Visual Reproduction subtest was then examined with the Benton Visual Retention Test.

BVRT. On administration A he scored only five correct with 10 errors but was a little better on the multiple choice form (11 out of 16) indicating support for a visual memory problem as well as other difficulties. There was no evidence of difficulty related to the quadrantanopia, such as more problems with certain parts of the field than with others, and he encountered no difficulty with the Albert test of Visual Neglect (Albert 1973) and the Benton Judgment of Line Orientation Test (Benton et al 1978), scoring 27 out of a possible 30 on the latter. He was able to make a fair copy of the Rey Figure (Fig. 4.16) but his poor recall at three minutes lent further support to the possibility of a visuospatial defect in the sphere of memory.

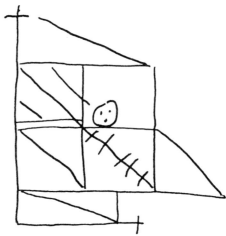

Fig. 4.16   Case XZ. Rey Figure. Copy and recall.

Porteus Maze Test. XZ took one trial for years VIII to XI but three each for the more visually complex items XII, XIV and Adult. There were none of the impulsive or perseverative errors of the frontal lobe type but he said he found it difficult to sort out the lines. He had difficulty in learning the Milner pathway on the *Austin Maze* which was abandoned on the 16th trial after he had failed to eradicate his last three or four errors over the preceding nine trials and was becoming frustrated at what he felt should have been a relatively simple task for him.

An interim report was made at this time as the patient had to leave the city temporarily. It was felt that the problem had been sufficiently explored but the following points were made:

1. The consistency of his performances suggested strongly a subtle but nonetheless disruptive deficit of visuospatial function including visuospatial memory.

2. There was nothing in his performance to support the notion that the patient was generating his symptoms, consciously or unconsciously.

3. Consideration should be given to an experimental investigation of the nature of his difficulty, particularly with serial examination using tests which might approximate the perceptual skills needed in driving.

4. Arrangements should be made, if the deficit remained stable, for training for other employment since the patient was highly motivated to return to work.

We felt convinced, as ever one can be in such a situation, that this was not a case of exaggeration or functional overlay but an area of genuine lack of knowledge of the effects of lesions in certain locations. Unfortunately, we lost sight of the patient but heard that he was able to return to driving about a year later.

REFERENCES

Adler R, Toyuz S 1989 Ganser syndrome in a 10 year old boy: an 8 year follow up. Australian and New Zealand Journal of Psychiatry 23: 124–126

Albert M L 1973 A simple test of visual neglect. Neurology 23: 658–684

American Psychiatric Association 1987 Diagnostic and statistical manual of mental disorders, 3rd edn. American Psychiatric Association, Washington

Batchelor I R C 1969 Henderson and Gillespie's textbook of psychiatry, 10th edn. Oxford University Press, London

Benton A L, Varney N R, Hamsher K 1978 Visuospatial judgement: a clinical test. Archives of Neurology 35: 364–367

Biddle B J 1979 Role Theory: expectation, identities and behaviors. Academic Press, New York

Biddle B J, Thomas E J 1966 Role Theory: concepts and research. Wiley, New York

Binder L, Pankratz L 1987 Neuropsychological evidence of a fictitious memory complaint. Journal of Clinical and Experimental Neuropsychology 9: 167–471

Brandt J 1988 Malingered amnesia. In: Rogers R (ed) Clinical assessment of malingering and deception. Guildford Press, New York, ch 5, p 65–83

Brandt J, Rubinsky E, Lassen G 1985 Uncovering malingered amnesia. Annals of the New York Academy of Science 444: 502–503

Bronks I G 1987 Amnesia: organic and psychogenic. British Journal of Psychiatry 151: 414–415

Brooks D N, Baddeley A D 1976 What can amnesic patients learn? Neuropsychologia 14: 111–122

Cameron N A, Magaret A 1951 Behaviour pathology. Houghton, New York

Chesterton G K 1970 The wisdom of Father Brown. Penguin Books, Harmondsworth, Middlesex, p 49

Chodoff P 1974 The diagnosis of hysteria: an overview. American Journal of Psychiatry 131: 1073–1078

Clayer J R, Brookless C L, Ross M W 1984 Neurosis and conscious exaggeration: its differentiation by the Illness Behaviour Questionnaire. Journal of Psychosomatic Research 28: 237–241

Clayer J R, Brookless-Pratz C L, Ross M W 1986 The evaluation of illness behaviour and exaggeration of disability. British Journal of Psychiatry 148: 296–299

Cohen N J 1984 Preserved learning capacity in amnesia: evidence for multiple memory systems. In: Squire L R, Butters N (eds) Neuropsychology of memory. Guildford Press, New York p 83–103

Cohen N J, Corkin S 1981 The amnesic patient HM: learning and retention of a cognitive skill. Society for Neuroscience Abstracts 7: 235

Cohen N J, Squire L R 1980 Preserved learning and retention of pattern-analyzing skill in amnesia: dissociation of 'knowing how' and 'knowing what'. Science 210: 207–209

Corkin S 1965 Tactually guided maze learning in man: effects of unilateral cortical excisions and bilateral hippocampal lesions. Neuropsychologia 3: 339–351

Eidelberg G L (ed) 1968 Encyclopaedia of psychoanalysis. Collier–Macmillan, Toronto, p 329

Enoch M D, Irving G 1962 The Ganser syndrome. Acta Psychiatrica Scandanavica 48: 213–222

Fallik A, Sigal M 1971 Hysteria: the choice of symptom site. Psychotherapy and Psychosomatics 19: 310–318

Feinstein A, Hattersley A 1988 Ganser symptoms, dissociation, and dysprosody. Journal of Nervous and Mental Disease 176: 692–693

Freedman A M, Kaplan H 1, Sadock B J 1976 Modern synopsis of comprehensive textbook of psychiatry, 2nd edn. Williams and Wilkins, Baltimore

Ganser S J M 1898 Über Einen Eigenartigen Hysterischen Dämmerzustand. Archiv Für Psychiatrie und Nervenkrankheiten 30: 633–640. Translated by Schorer C E in British Journal of Criminology 1965 5: 120–126

Glisky E L, Schacter D L 1988 Long-term retention of computer learning by patients with memory disorders. Neuropsychologia 26: 173–178

Glisky E L, Schacter D L, Tulving E 1986 Learning and retention of computer-related vocabulary in memory-impaired patients. Journal of Clinical and Experimental Neuropsychology 8: 292–312

Goebel R A 1983 Detection of faking on the Halstead-Reitan neuropsychological test battery. Journal of Clinical Psychology 39: 731–742

Goldberg J O, Miller H R 1986 Performance of psychiatric inpatients and intellectually deficient individuals on a task that assesses the validity of memory complaints. Journal of Clinical Psychology 42: 792–795

Goldin S, MacDonald, J E 1955 The Ganser state. Journal of Mental Science 101 : 267–280

Graf P, Squire L R, Mandler G 1984 The information that amnesic patients do not forget. Journal of Experimental Psychology: Learning, Memory and Cognition 11: 501–518

Grossi D, Fasanaro A M, Modaferri A, Busciano G A 1984 Residual verbal learning capacity: two patients with amnesia caused by a left occipital lesion. Acta Neurologica (Napoli) 6: 215–221

Grosz H, Zimmerman J 1965 Experimental analysis of hysterical blindness. Archives of General Psychiatry 13: 225–260

Hayward L, Hall W, Hunt M, Zubrick S R 1987 Can localised brain impairment be simulated on neuropsychological test profiles? The Australian and New Zealand Journal of Psychiatry 21: 87–93

Hécaen H, Albert M L 1978 Human neuropsychology. Wiley, New York

Heilbrun A B 1962 Issues in assessment of organic brain damage. Psychological Reports 10: 511–515

Hollander M H 1972 Conversion hysteria. Archives of General Psychiatry 26: 311–314

Huppert F A, Piercey M 1976 Recognition memory in amnesic patients: effects of temporal context and familiarity of material. Cortex 12: 3–20

Jones A B, Llewellyn L J 1917 Malingering or the simulation of disease. Heinemann, London

Kilpatrick F P 1961 Explorations in transactional psychology. New York University Press, New York

Kinsbourne M, Wood F 1975 Short–term memory and the amnesic syndrome. In: Deutsch D D, Deutsch J A (eds) Short–term memory. Academic Press, New York

Lezak M D 1976 Neuropsychological Assessment. Oxford University Press, New York, p 476f

Lezak M D 1983 Neuropsychological Assessment, 2nd edn. Oxford University Press, New York

Lishman W A 1978 Organic psychiatry: psychological consequences of cerebral disorder. Blackwell, London

Lishman W A 1987 Organic psychiatry: psychological consequences of cerebral disorder. 2nd edn. Blackwell, London

McEvoy J P, Wells, C E 1979 Case studies in neuropsychiatry. 2: Conversion pseudodementia. Journal of Clinical Psychiatry. 40: 447–449

McGrath J E 1964 Social psychology: a brief introduction. Holt Rinehart and Winston, New York

Matthews C G, Shaw D J, Kløve H 1966 Psychological test performances in neurological and 'pseudo-neurologic' subjects. Cortex 2: 244–253

Mayer-Gross, W Slater, E Roth M 1954 Clinical psychiatry. Cassell, London

Merskey H 1979 The analysis of hysteria. Baillière Tindall, London

Miller E 1986 Defecting hysterical sensory symptoms: an elaboration of the forced choice technique. British Journal of Clinical Psychology 25: 231– 232

Miller H 1966 Comments on accident neurosis. Proceedings of the Medico-Legal Society of Victoria 10: 71–82

Miller H, Cartlidge N 1972 Simulation and malingering after injuries to the brain and spinal cord. Lancet 1: 580–585

Milner B 1962 Les troubles de la mémoire accompagnant des lésions hippocampiques bilatérales. In: Passovant P (ed) Physiologie de l'hippocampe. Centre de la Recherche Scientifique, Paris

Milner B, Corkin S, Teuber H-L 1968 Further analysis of the hippocampal amnesic syndrome: 14 year follow-up study of H M. Neuropsychologia 6: 215–234

Moscovitch M 1982 Multiple dissociations of function in amnesia. In: Cermak L S (ed) Human memory and amnesia. Lawrence Erlbaum, Hillsdale, New Jersey, p 337–370

Newcomb T M 1950 Social psychology. Dryden Press, New York

Orne M T 1962 On the social psychology of the psychology experiment. American Psychologist 17: 776–783

Orne M T, Scheibe K E 1964 The contribution of non deprivation factors in the production of sensory deprivation effects: the psychology of the panic button. Journal of Abnormal and Social Psychology 68: 3–12

Pankratz L 1979 Symptom validity testing and symptom retraining: procedures for the assessment and treatment of functional sensory deficits. Journal of Consulting and Clinical Psychology 47: 409–410

Pankratz L 1983 A new technique for the assessment and modification of feigned memory deficit. Perceptual and Motor Skills 57: 367–372

Pankratz L, Binder L M, Wilcox L M 1987 Evaluation of an exaggerated somatosensory deficit with symptom validity testing. Archives of Neurology 44: 798

Pankratz L, Fausti S A, Peed S 1975 A forced choice technique to evaluate deafness in the hysterical or malingering patient. Journal of Consulting and Clinical Psychology 43: 421–422

Pankratz L, Paar G H 1988 A test of symptom validity in assessing functional symptoms. Zeitschrift für Klinische Psychologie, Psychopathologie und Psychotherapie 36: 130–137

Parkin A J 1982 Residual learning capacity in anmesia. Cortex 18: 417–440

Parsons T, Shils E (eds) 1951 Toward a general theory of action. Harvard University Press, Cambridge, Massachusetts

Pilowsky I, Spence N D 1983 Manual for the Illness Behaviour Questionnaire (IBQ), 2nd edn. University of Adelaide

Reed J L 1978 Disorders of conscious awareness. Compensation neurosis and Munchausen syndrome. British Journal of Hospital Medicine 19: 314–321

Rey A 1964 L'examen clinique en psychologie. Presses Universitaires de France, Paris

Russell E W, Neuringer C, Goldstein G 1970 Assessment of brain damage: a neuropsychological key approach. Wiley, New York

Sarbin T R 1954 Role theory. In: Lindzey G (ed) Handbook of social psychology. Addison-Wesley, Massachusetts, ch 6

Schacter D L 1987 Implicit expressions of memory in organic amnesia: learning of new facts and associations. Human Neurobiology 6: 107–118

Schacter D L, Harbluk J L, McLachlan D R 1984 Retrieval without recollection: an experimental analysis of source amnesia. Journal of Verbal Learning and Verbal Behavior 23: 593–611

Scott P D 1965 The Ganser syndrome. British Journal of Criminology 5: 127–134

Sim M 1974 Guide to psychiatry. Churchill Livingstone, Edinburgh, p 499

Starr A, Phillips L 1970 Verbal and motor memory in the amnesic syndrome. Neuropsychologia 8: 75–88

Szasz T S 1961 The myth of mental illness. Hoeber, New York

Talland G A 1965 Deranged Memory. Academic Press, New York

Theodor L H, Mandelcorn M S 1973 Hysterical blindness: a case report and study using a modern psychophysical technique. Journal of Abnormal Psychology 82: 552–553

Ullmann L P, Krasner L 1969 A psychological approach to abnormal behaviour. Prentice-Hall, London

Volpe B T, Hirst W 1983 Amnesia following the rupture and repair of an anterior communicating aneurysm. Journal of Neurology, Neurosurgery and Psychiatry 46: 704–709

Warrington E K, Weiskrantz L 1974 The effect of prior learning on subsequent retention in amnesic patients. Neuropsychologia 12:419–428

Warrington E K, Weiskrantz L 1982 Amnesia: a disconnection syndrome? Neuropsychologia 20: 223–248

Wells C E 1979a Pseudodementia. American Journal of Psychiatry. 136: 895–900

Whitlock F A 1967 The Ganser syndrome. British Journal of Psychiatry. 113: 19–29

Ziegler F J, Imboden J B 1962 Contemporary conversion reactions. 2: A conceptual model. Archives of General Psychiatry 6: 279–287

Ziegler F J, Imboden J B, Meyer E 1960 Contemporary conversion reactions: a clinical study. American Journal of Psychiatry. 116: 901–909

5. Adaptive behaviour and head injury

OUTCOME OF SEVERE HEAD INJURY

Despite the large number of studies dealing with the relatively long-term outcome of severe head injury (Miller & Stern 1965, Fahy et al 1967, Bond 1975, Jennett 1976, Jennett et al 1976, Levin et al 1979, 1982, 1987, Lewin et al 1979, Najenson et al 1980, Broe et al 1981, Jennett et al 1981, Tate et al 1982, Brooks et al 1986, 1987, 1989) there are few which do not have serious limitations. Many of these are imposed by the nature of the problem but there are correctable methodological shortcomings. Most of the difficulties and deficiencies are discussed by Levin and colleagues in the extensive coverage in two companion volumes (Levin et al 1982,1987). Among the medical factors are problems with the reliable documentation of severity, exclusion of other causes of brain impairment, and lack of comparability due to examinations being carried out at different time intervals in different studies. Adequate longitudinal studies are virtually nonexistent. From the psychological perspective, difficulties are posed by the employment of insensitive measures, the lack of estimates of premorbid functioning, the almost total reliance on group data, problems with repeated measures and the lack of control subjects where applicable.

Measures of severity

Two principal measures of severity have been employed, viz length of coma and length of post-traumatic amnesia.

Coma

The usefulness of employing length of coma as a measure of severity against which to correlate clinical and social sequelae was lessened by the variable and uncertain ways in which coma was defined in the early studies. This situation has been improved by the widespread adoption of the Glasgow Coma Scale, a simple standardized chart of eye opening, motor response and verbal response (Teasdale & Jennett 1974).

Post-traumatic amnesia (PTA)

This measure was introduced by Russell & Nathan (1946) following an earlier study by Russell (1932). This used the length of time from injury to the time the patient

163

became aware that he had regained consciousness. It corresponds to the time when the patient begins to retain a stable record of ongoing events. The definition by Russell & Nathan (op.cit.) and the minor modification by Russell & Smith (1961) combines the length of unconsciousness with the period when the patient is awake and responding but not consolidating memories, i.e. coma plus the period of anterograde amnesia. Artiola i Fortuny et al (1980) attempted to provide an objective assessment of PTA. This simple quantitative procedure correlated well with independent estimates made by experienced neurosurgeons. A new version of the Oxford scale, now termed the Westmead PTA Scale, which has high inter-rater reliability and has proven easy to use in clinical practice has been under trial for several years in Australian hospitals with encouraging preliminary results (Shores et al 1986). This scale demonstrated in a two year follow-up study that such measures of PTA are superior to duration of coma in predicting outcome (Shores 1989). The Westmead scale differs from the Galveston Orientation and Amnesia Test (Levin et al 1979) in that, in the former, both correct orientation and the ability to recall newly learned information are required to define the emergence from post-traumatic amnesia.

A detailed discussion of the relative merits of the two major measures, namely length of coma and PTA, is provided by Levin et al (1982) though there are few direct comparisons available. One of these (Brooks et al 1980) found that duration of coma as measured by the Glasgow Coma Scale bore little relation to cognitive outcome as measured by psychological tests, whereas duration of post-traumatic amnesia significantly predicted cognitive performance. Newcombe (1982) warns that the complexity of factors involved means that there will be no simple relationship between PTA and severity of defect. While a convincing general trend may be apparent in group data, there are bound to be exceptions in both directions, some individuals with lengthy PTA having little impairment, while others having shorter PTA are left with considerable deficit.

Psychological deficit

A simple classification of post-traumatic deficits is that of Broe et al (1981). Three broad classes of difficulty are recognized:

1. Physical deficits in the form of motor and sensory dysfunction
2. Cognitive deficits which include perceptual, intelligence and memory disorders
3. Organic psychosocial deficit.

They define organic psychosocial deficit as follows: '... such patients may be impulsive, emotionally labile, disinhibited, aggressive, irresponsible and as a consequence of their impairment have lost insight into their emotional response. So while physically and cognitively well recovered ... [these] patients experience deficits which have adverse effects on their interpersonal relationships and return to employment.' (op.cit. p 95). Other experienced workers such as Lezak (1978a,b) have described these changes in some detail and stress the enormous strain which they place on family relations. Lezak nicely terms this group the 'characterologically altered brain injured.'

In recent years there has been an accumulation of evidence that the cognitive and psychosocial deficits make a greater contribution to lasting disablement after head injury than physical disabilities (Bond 1975, Bond & Brooks 1976, Heiden et al 1979, Broe et al 1981). Though there may be some difference in what different writers would group under such terms as cognitive change, behavioural change or psychosocial change, the message is the same:

> The physical problems of language deficits, weakness, spasticity and ataxia have responded more successfully to rehabilitation treatment. The residual cognitive deficits (impaired recent memory, decreased intelligence, and behavioural changes) have interfered more than physical factors with independence in activities of daily living. The residual problems of decreased insight, judgement, impaired thought organization and apathy limit social adjustment. In patients disabled with a moderate or severe disability, cognitive dysfunction has contributed more than physical problems to the residual disability. Social re-integration (including leisure activities, return to work), however, is primarily dependent on recovery of these cognitive functions; physical parameters play a far smaller role as an ultimate determinant of social restoration (Bond 1975 p 193).

In a 12 to 18 month follow-up of 60 survivors after severe head injury (defined as seven days or more of hospitalization as a result of the injury), Broe et al (1981) found that 38 had no physical defect. However, a total of 27 patients of this group who 'would be assessed on a standard neurological examination as having made a good recovery from their head injury' had evidence of organic psychosocial deficit with or without cognitive impairment. Studies specifically addressed to social outcome are in strong agreement (Oddy et al 1978a,b, Oddy & Humphrey 1980).

In many cases, changes in both cognition and personality are dependent on damage to the frontal lobes. They frequently coexist and are difficult to disentangle in the individual patient. The common combination of a 'behavioural' change such as the inability to inhibit inappropriate responses, coupled with 'cognitive' changes such as the inability to plan and eradicate errors, often dooms all attempts at rehabilitation to failure.

The main reason for making adaptive behaviour the focus of this chapter is the far reaching effects which such changes have on the individual's ability to benefit from therapy and to utilize those abilities of perception, memory, praxis and so on which have been largely spared by the injury. 'When these defects compromise the patient's ability to formulate goals, to plan or to execute a course of action, they render the patient socially dependent regardless of how well he might perform on formal tests or a mental status examination.' (Lezak 1981). Allied to this is the fact that the defects may be subtle though devastating and be overlooked or underestimated unless appropriate methods of evaluation are employed. 'Investigation of possible behavioral changes after brain damage depends to a great extent on the hypotheses in question and the experimental procedures devised to test these hypotheses.' (Stuss, 1987). This author tested the hypothesis that if the frontal lobes were injured, subtle deficits due to frontal dysfunction might be discovered in closed head injury patients who appeared to be recovered. This was the case and this point is strongly underlined in what follows. For an appreciation of the very wide range of factors which might be effected the reader should consult Stuss and Benson (1986).

Intellectual recovery

'Considering the major implications of intellectual deficit for postinjury functioning, relatively few studies dealing with this question have been reported.' (Levin et al 1982, p 23).

While this statement is patently true there are also serious shortcomings in those studies which have attempted to relate measures of cognitive performance to severity of head injury. Because of its well deserved popularity in general, much of our available data is based on studies using the WAIS.

The general tenor of studies using this scale is somewhat surprising. Even cases with severe damage show considerable improvement over time, especially if only the quantitative summarizing measures are used (Bond, 1975, Mandelberg & Brooks 1975, Brooks & Aughton 1979). Several studies report the greater sensitivity of the Performance IQ compared with the Verbal IQ measure in the form of greater reduction and slower recovery (Kløve & Cleeland 1972, Mandelberg & Brooks 1975, Levin et al 1979). The first two studies showed eventual recovery to levels comparable with the VIQ and to a normal or near normal level. Such studies would be encouraging if the WAIS measures could be taken to mean return to effective cognition, a conclusion which must be in doubt in view of the cases in this text describing the presence of 'normal' levels of performance (expressed by the intelligence quotients) in the presence of clearly demonstrable pathology with associated neuropsychological deficits. A number of recent articles warn that the intellectual consequences of head injury may not be reflected adequately in standard tests of intelligence (Miller 1979, Newcombe & Artiola i Fortuny 1979, Newcombe 1982, Walsh 1982).

Some of the problem lies in the nature of tests used. Quite independently, recent writers (Russell 1980, Newcombe 1982) have reminded us of the distinction made by a number of writers in the 1940s between two general forms of intellectual abilities (Hebb 1942, 1949; Cattell 1943). Cattell (op.cit.) termed the two characteristics as 'fluid' and 'crystallized.' 'Fluid ability has the character of a purely general ability to discriminate and perceive relations between any fundamentals, new or old ... crystallized ability consists of discriminatory habits established in a particular field, originally through the operation of fluid ability, but no longer requiring insightful perception for their successful operations.'

If this concept is applied to the Wechsler Scales it will be apparent that they measure a good deal of crystallized ability, especially on the Verbal subtests. Since well stored information and developed skills are known to be relatively resistant to all forms of cerebral impairment, the findings with such tests are not surprising. The greater sensitivity of the Performance IQ is partly a result of the need for fluid ability in some of the subtests though even these may not be adequate to reveal quite significant defects of adaptive behaviour. In 1944 Wechsler defined intelligence as *the aggregate or global capacity of the individual to act purposefully, to think rationally and to deal effectively with his environment'* [my italics]. While decades of experience with countless intact individuals in all walks of life would appear to support the correlation between Wechsler quotients and levels of effective behaviour, it is also apparent that the scale does not reflect the individual's *current* ability in the three major attributes mentioned in the definition. It is an everyday occurrence to find head-injured patients, as well as patients with other forms of brain lesion, who rate dismally in all three areas which renders them occupationally and socially incompetent but who, nevertheless, score in the average or even superior levels on this test battery.

Another obvious feature which has not received attention in examination of WAIS data in head injury is the contribution of slowed information processing. The presence of such a deficit, so clearly shown by Gronwall and her colleagues for patients with less severe injuries (Gronwall 1976, Gronwall & Sampson 1974, Gronwall & Wrightson 1974,1975), suggests that such an approach would be productive in more serious cases. The principal test used by this group is the Paced Auditory Serial Addition Test (PASAT) based on a visual paradigm of Sampson (1956). The subject is required to attend to a lengthy series of digits presented at different rates on a tape recorder, adding the second digit to the first, the third to the second and so on. For example, the subject's responses to the series 3-8-7-4-9 should be 11-15-11-13. The test provides an excellent measure of improvement which is simple and repeatable.

Clearly it is important to distinguish the relative contributions to poor performance on timed tests of both general factors such as information processing as well as specific neuropsychological deficits.

Finally, the concept of fluidity seems to be closely allied to that of adaptive behaviour so that even in the absence of the neuropathological evidence cited it would seem reasonable to incorporate such measures in every examination of closed head injury.

Outcome scales

The Glasgow group under Jennett has provided standardized criteria of recovery in the form of an Outcome Scale (Jennett & Bond 1975) but even in its extended form (Jennett 1981) it is far too coarse to be of significant value in the individual case as anything more than an approximation. Levin et al (1982) point out the difficulties posed by the fact that individuals vary so widely in premorbid levels of educational, occupational and social competence. As stressed elsewhere, deficit measurement implies comparison with the individual's own prior level of performance, and group norms cannot be used in any way as a satisfactory yardstick, no matter how complete the scales may be. It was pointed out in Chapter 3 how difficult it is to estimate premorbid cognitive ability from postmorbid testing. It is even more difficult to estimate retrospectively prior levels of social, occupational, and behavioural competence. Rating scales for charting the progress of severely head-injured patients in a rehabilitation setting are reviewed by Rappaport et al (1982) who also provide a promising Disability Rating Scale.

PATHOLOGY OF HEAD INJURY

The most common cause of craniocerebral injury is the rapid acceleration and deceleration of the head which occurs in motor vehicle accidents. Even where the skull is not fractured, the brain may sustain a wide variety of pathological lesions. These include both generalized or diffuse lesions scattered throughout the brain with or without localized damage such as contusion, laceration or haemorrhage. With this complexity of pathology, clinico-anatomical correlation might seem to be an unproductive exercise. However, the presence of residual neuropsychological deficits of memory and adaptive behaviour in many so-called recovered patients, and the proven relations between these disorders and lesions of the frontal and temporal regions of the brain, tempt one to draw a causal relationship between the major locus of damage in closed head injury and such deficits. Before considering this possibility readers should consult sources which convey the complexity of the pathology (Strich 1969, Adams 1975, Gurdjian 1975).

The advent of the CT scan offers an opportunity to correlate the major focus of localized pathology and behavioural change in the individual case. So far, no systematic study of this kind has been reported. The role of the CT scan is summarized well by Levin et al (1982) but even this is unlikely to be sensitive to the diffuse microscopic lesions which occur in severe head injury. Nevertheless, the CT scan often provides dramatic confirmation for the local character of some lesions (see case UX). Even more promising is the newer method of magnetic resonance imaging (MRI). Although much more restricted because of the costly installation and technical factors, it has already demonstrated that areas of cerebral dysfunction can be detected which are not revealed by CT scan even where repeat scans are taken (Wilberger et al 1987, Hadley et al 1988). MRI also correlates well with neuropsychological assessment (Levin et al 1989), and improved appearance in magnetic resonance scans parallels neuropsychological improvement (Levin et al 1987). Neuropsychological outcome seems more related to late than early scans (Wilson et al 1988).

Briefly, cerebral damage may be defined as primary or secondary. Primary lesions are associated with the trauma itself. The principal forms are contusion, laceration or haemorrhage, though there is often a mixture of all three, and contusion and laceration cannot be distinguished on clinical grounds. Secondary lesions arise after the event and their detection will largely determine the outcome. They include ischaemia, anoxia, oedema and brain distortion due to intracerebral bleeding. The remainder of the discussion centres on local contusion with or without laceration.

Mechanism and sites of cerebral contusion

The exact mechanisms of production of contusional lesions is still debated though there is general agreement about the use of two descriptive terms. 'Coup' injuries refer to damage beneath the site of impact, while 'contre coup' injuries refer to lesions at some distance from the site. The mechanics of head injuries have been the focus of numerous studies using inert models, animals and man (Holburn 1943, Lindenberg & Freytag 1960, Rowbotham 1964, Gurdjian et al 1966, Ommaya & Gennarelli

1974). Lindenberg & Freytag pointed out that the Académie Royale de Chirurgie in Paris in 1766 offered a prize 'établir la théorie des contrecoups dans les lésions de la tête et les conséquences qu'on peut en tirer.' The matter is still not resolved.

Though there is disagreement about what mechanical stresses produce the damage, there is no such disagreement about their location. Courville (1942) observed that the greatest zone of brain contusion following head injury was not invariably opposite to the impact. 'Essentially identical lesions of the subfrontal and anterior temporal regions result from contact of either the frontal region or the occipital region of the moving head...and the fact that neither gross coup nor contrecoup lesions occur in the occipital region...suggests that the anatomic relation of the brain and the portion of the skull proximate to it is essentially responsible for the nature and distribution of the lesion.' Speaking of the sudden deceleration of the head in motor vehicle injuries Jamieson (1971) likened the movement of the brain within the skull to the movement of objects within the motor vehicle: 'The soft brain then travels onward and crashes into the built-in dashboard that each of us owns, the knife-like sphenoidal ridges (complete with anterior clinoid projections), together with an unyielding fascia of front wall of middle fossa and a windscreen of rough orbital plates and frontal bone.' In modern motor accidents with high velocity deceleration the damage to the anterior portion of the temporal lobe and sometimes the frontal lobe may be so great, including subdural haemorrhage, brain contusion/laceration and intracerebral bleeding, that it has been termed the 'exploded pole' (Bottrell & Stewart, cited in Hooper 1966). The fronto-temporal concentration of contusional injury has been confirmed frequently (Gurdjian et all 1943, Courville 1945, Gurdjian et al 1955, Lindenberg & Freytag 1957, Hooper 1966, 1969). Figure 5.1 provides a composite sketch from these sources.

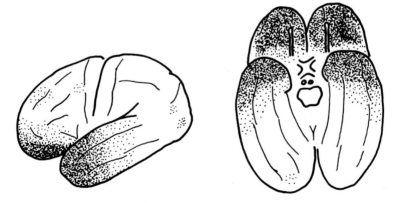

Fig. 5.1 Composite drawing of the areas most frequently contused in closed head injuries.

In the series of Gurdjian et al (1943) of 191 contusions found in 72 autopsied cases, 160 were in frontal (68) and temporal regions (92), with 72% of the frontal lesions being in the inferior portion.

A good deal of this evidence comes from more serious cases with a short survival period. However, improved methods of acute neurosurgical care means that we have seen more survivors with severe contusion/laceration injuries in recent years. While most of these will have obvious clinical signs, the case of UX below attests to the fact that some could escape detection because they are physically intact. Much less severe damage can produce the adaptive difficulties outlined below and it is our experience and that of others (Levin & Eisenberg 1979) that residual impairment will occasionally be found in patients with relatively mild injuries. Once again we are using the 'method of extreme cases' in our exposition.

ADAPTIVE BEHAVIOUR AND THE FRONTAL LOBES

For behaviour to be effective it must meet environmental conditions. It must be appropriate, modifiable, energized or motivated and be free from disruptive internal influences. Effective behaviour requires an anticipatory relationship to the goal in the form of planning. It requires the ability to monitor ongoing actions so as to effect change should deviations from the plan occur, and the effectiveness of action must finally be checked against the anticipated outcome and any necessary adjustments made. In the broadest sense we may speak of behaviour which fulfils these requirements as adaptive behaviour. Most, if not all, of these necessary conditions for effective behaviour are dependent upon the integrity of the frontal lobes, and converging lines of evidence suggest that one can conceive of at least three qualitatively different modes of behaviour as related to three major areas of frontal cortex and their connections. These areas are (1) the dorsolateral cortex, which is concerned with the preparation and execution of action; (2) the medial frontal cortex, which mediates self-initiated action and sustains behaviour at an appropriate level; and (3) the basal or basomedial cortex, which appears to be related to the flexible control of excitation and inhibition and the emotional control of behaviour.

The complexity of the so-called frontal lobe syndrome can now be appreciated since individual cases will show a wide variety of combinations of the dysfunctions related to the different areas. The presence of relatively pure cases of the sub-syndromes, i.e. their dissociation from one another, provides a strong argument for the separation of functions within the vast territory in front of the central sulcus.

Dorsolateral frontal cortex

This area of cortex may be usefully subdivided into three major sub-zones (prefrontal, premotor and motor) and two specialized areas (Broca's area and frontal eye fields) (Fig. 5.2).

The prefrontal cortex appears to be related to the ideational or intellectual control of action, and damage to this area will result in ineffectual behaviour. Disruptions to its functions are dealt with in detail below for two important reasons. Firstly, it is commonly the site of damage with closed head injuries, and secondly, its effects may be subtle, though pervasive and disruptive, and thus may be easily overlooked unless appropriate methods of assessment are used. Dysfunction in this region of the brain produces serious impediments to effective rehabilitation.

The premotor cortex plays a role in motor organization especially with complex movements where it may serve as a zone of complex integration (Derouesné 1973).

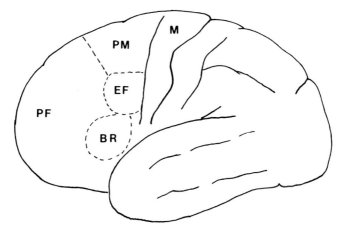

Fig. 5.2   Dorsolateral frontal cortex. BR, Broca's area; EF, frontal eye fields; M, motor cortex; PF, prefrontal cortex; PM, premotor cortex.

Much of our scant knowledge of this zone derives from the writings of Luria (1969, 1973) who conceived of it as an intermediary between the ideational aspects of planned action in the prefrontal region and the implementation by movements effected by activity of specific areas of the motor cortex.

The two specialized areas within the dorsolateral cortex are Broca's area and the frontal eye fields. The exact extent of these two areas is uncertain. Broca's area is usually considered to include Brodmann's cytoarchitectonic area 44 and part of area 45. Traditionally it is considered as a vital part of the cortical zones subserving language. Lesions in this area and the subjacent white matter characteristically produce a non-fluent form of dysphasia.

The frontal eye fields extend forward from the motor cortex concerned with facial movements. They are centred in area 8 but also take in part of the adjacent areas 9 in front and 6 behind. Their location and functions are described by Crosby et al (1962) and Warwick & Williams (1973). The strategic siting of the frontal eye fields between the prefrontal cortex and the motor cortex raises the speculation that they may be concerned in the complex visual scanning and perceptual integrative difficulties shown by some frontal patients mentioned below.

In describing different aspects of the intellectual changes accompanying prefrontal damage any division of function is bound to be arbitrary. Three aspects will be selected for discussion in the context of observations on commonly used tests.

Planning, learning, and related matters

Clinical observations of patients with significant frontal lobe lesions have reported planning difficulties since the classical description in 1848 of the post-traumatic behaviour of Phineas P. Gage (see p 177). An early study of the first two cases of large frontal lobe resection for tumour described the most obvious effect as an 'impairment of those mental processes which are requisite to planned initiative'. (Penfield & Evans, 1935).

The earliest test to show consistent loss with frontal lobe damage was the Porteus Maze Test (Porteus & Kepner 1944, Porteus & Peters 1947, Porteus 1958, 1959, 1965). This relationship has been confirmed on a large number of occasions. However, in our experience, failure on this test is as often due to an inability to inhibit a response tendency as it is to inadequate planning. While we frequently observe failure on this test in patients with prefrontal lesions, we have noted that there are numerous exceptions. These seem to be mainly persons of above average intelligence. Few if any of these exceptional cases are able to cope with the more 'abstract' Austin Maze where the visual perceptual support of the Porteus problems has been removed.

Error utilization and imperfect learning. The more abstract maze problem as exemplified by the Milner pathway (Milner 1965) brings out a number of related difficulties. Most observers were aware of the uncritical attitude which frontal patients showed to their own actions, especially their own errors. Luria and his co-workers (Luria & Homskaya 1964, Luria et al 1964) considered this to be due to an inadequate evaluation of the patient's own action which did not arise from a failure to appreciate or fully comprehend the nature of the instructions. Konow & Pribram (1970) subsequently described a patient who not only clearly recognized her own errors and those of others but remained unable to utilize this information to modify her subsequent course of action. This distinction between error recognition and what Konow & Pribram termed 'error utilization' is a crucial one. Since that time we have seen a large number of individuals, most of them following closed head injury, with this deficit as a result of frontal contusion, even when many measures of cognitive ability have obviously returned to the premorbid level. Such patients often provide the frontal lobe paradox of a person with seemingly preserved or restored intelligence who fails to cope with the demands of their occupation or profession.

The subtlety becomes more apparent when it is observed that many of these patients, when faced with the Austin Maze problem, make a relatively small number of errors at the outset and decrease these over the first few trials. However, further trials show little further improvement and even after reaching an errorless trial they are apt to make errors on subsequent trials. This deficit of *imperfect learning* may be seen not only in traumatic frontal damage but also after alcohol related damage and other forms of frontal pathology.

If this imperfect learning deficit is clearly observable six to nine months after injury the prognosis for full recovery is poor. It often accounts for inexplicable errors in the workplace, and such errors are particularly difficult for employers to understand when the worker can clearly verbalize what he should do, i.e. shows the 'curious dissociation between knowing and doing'. (Teuber 1964) Unless appropriate examination is made this deficit may be easily overlooked.

The imperfect learning difficulty is often played down in cases of medico-legal dispute over the degree of monetary compensation after head injury. On the basis of a learning performance with a small number of residual errors many a patient has been said to be almost completely recovered. The question should then be posed as to what constitutes an adequate criterion of learning. A reasonable answer to this would be to recognize that most life situations of consequence require the corresponding programmes of behaviour to be stable and error free. '*Near enough is not good enough*' should be written up in all rehabilitation centres. The importance of detecting this deficit when one imagines the consequences of making even a small number of errors in many of life's situations, e.g. baking a cake, operating a machine or flying a jet aircraft, requires a constant reminder to therapists. Of course, errors do not occur in situations where old, well-tried stereotypes will suffice, but will become apparent in new learning or in adapting old programmes of learning to new situations; it is surprising how much change and adaptation is needed in what at first may appear stereotyped operations.

In the rehabilitation situation patients are often considered to be capable of adequate new learning since they are capable of following the directions of the educator and can give oral or written proof of understanding what has to be done. This is a situation where another person's frontal lobes are guiding the behaviour. The difficulty comes when this exterior frontal guidance system is withdrawn. The patient then demonstrates an inability to carry through the 'learned' behaviour in an appropriate manner; even well-drilled sequences of behaviour demonstrate their inertness since the person is unable to emit even a slightly modified version of the programme to suit similar but not identical circumstances. The danger in teaching such patients specific programmes of action is to assume that they will be able to generalize. *The crucial test of recovery of patients who have shown frontal lobe signs after injury is to ascertain whether they are capable of self-guided as opposed to impressed learning.*

IQ measures and effective intelligence. Again, in medico-legal settings it is often claimed that the person with IQ measures preserved at 'an above average level' cannot be seriously incapacitated. We point out that these measures denote what the person would normally be capable of should the frontal lobes be intact. In layman's terms, he has an intellectual capacity that he is unable to put to effective use. For the same reason we have often advised against the simple use of IQ measures as part of selection of patients for rehabilitation. Of two equally intelligent people, one with a post-injury IQ of 135 but with prefrontal damage, is a poor prospect; the other, with a post-injury IQ of 96 associated with perceptual, constructional or other 'non-frontal' difficulties, may still be trained to work effectively, albeit in a lowered capacity.

A further learning difficulty seems to result from a lack of organization of the material to be learned. This can be seen in the disappearance or fragmentation of the serial order effects from lengthy serial learning. The Rey Auditory Verbal Learning test shows a lack of the normal primacy and recency effects, the responses coming in a haphazard order from trial to trial. This results in inefficient learning and, as pointed out by Luria (1973), a *plateau effect*, whereby an increasing number of trials does not lead to increased item retention.

Conceptual behaviour, mental set, and perseveration

The earliest thinking about the role of the frontal lobes ascribed to them the capacity for abstract thinking (for a review, see Walsh 1987). A good deal of the support for this contention came from the difficulties shown by frontal patients on conceptual tasks such as the Colour-Form Sorting Test (Goldstein & Scheerer 1941) and the

Wisconsin Card Sorting Test (Grant & Berg 1948, Milner 1963). On these tests Walsh (1960) and Milner (1964) pointed to examples where patients were able to enunciate principles of categorization suitable to the situation, but were nevertheless unable to use this verbalization as a guide to action—another example of the 'curious dissociation' already mentioned. In addition such patients show a difficulty in changing response set and even after changing such set are likely to respond on future occasions not according to the newly acquired principle or rule but to some previously well established set, despite the fact that they recognize it as inappropriate and, like case BC (Ch. 1), are frustrated when they find themselves doing so. In Milner's words *they are unable to inhibit customary modes of responding*. It may well be that much of the difficulty that frontal patients find with these tasks is not so much a matter of disruption of an intellectual process as an interference with the voluntary control of inhibition, a deficit which is more related to the basal or orbital cortex than to the dorsolateral.

In support of a real intellectual component to the difficulties of frontal patients are the numerous instances which reveal difficulty in assuming an attitude to a hypothetical situation. This difficulty forms part of a shift from a conscious and volitional mode of behaviour based on abstract thought processes, to a concrete determination of behaviour by aspects of the present situation. For this reason frontal patients have been described as 'stimulus-bound.' In turn, this seems related to the tendency of the patient to show little concern with the past and future, an alteration which has been construed as a 'personality' change.

Complex integration and problem solving

Frontal problem solving difficulties are readily demonstrated on visuo-constructive tasks such as block-design copying. This may take the form of difficulty with preliminary analysis as in the '2–4–6–8' phenomenon described in Chapter 1, or difficulty in integrating the blocks to form the pattern even if they have been chosen correctly. Luria & Tsvetkova (1964) have shown clearly that these constructional difficulties may be affected at any point in the process of solution.

Patients who show an analytical or integration difficulty on block design copying, rather than a visuo-spatial difficulty, usually demonstrate deficient problem solving in other areas such as mathematics. There is significant loss, not of known arithmetical operations, but of the logical analysis and redintegration necessary for solution. Patients may also be able to solve problems for which they have a ready made solution though they may fail with an heuristically simpler problem, i.e. one for which they must generate a new solution—yet another example of the frontal difficulty in dealing with novelty of all kinds. The text of Luria & Tsvetkova (1967) deals with the topic in detail. Some examples are given in the case examples below.

The word finding test. A little known but useful test of integration of ideas is Reitan's Word Finding Test (Reitan 1972). This is one of the few tests which directly approaches problem solving in the verbal mode. Most other verbal tests measure abilities which have been acquired in the patient's past. The patient is asked to discern the meaning of a nonsense word through its verbal context. The items have five sentences each providing information about the 'hidden' word. The subject must integrate information from two or more sentences to reach the solution. Our experience suggests that it is a sensitive test for left (and bilateral) frontal damage in keeping with Rzechorzek's (1978) findings in a small number of unilateral frontal tumours. One of Rzechorzek's patients, with a left frontal tumour, demonstrates the difficulty on the following test items:

Item 13 (Grobnick = thirteen)
  1. Grobnick is often considered to be unlucky—'opal'.
  2. A few people maintain that grobnick is lucky for them—no response.
  3. By actual count, there are grobnick full moons each year—'eclipse'.
  4. You still hear grobnick referred to as a baker's dozen—'dozen'.
  5. Except for misdeals, you will receive grobnick cards in a bridge hand—'lucky cards'.

Item 14 (Grobnick = roof)
  1. Every house has a grobnick—no response.
  2. Grobnicks are constructed in different shapes, but the purpose is the same—no response.
  3. It would be quite uncomfortable to live in a house which didn't have a grobnick—'door'.
  4. A leak in a grobnick is usually detected during a heavy rain—'pipe or gutter'.
  5. Some people are very happy if they have food in their stomach and a grobnick over their head—'a hat or scarf'.

The common difficulty of frontal patients is the inability to abstract information from particular instances to achieve an integration or convergence which will satisfy each of the statements. It is part of the total complex process which Goldstein termed 'taking up the abstract attitude'. (Goldstein & Scheerer 1941).

Picture sequence integration. A similar difficulty of integration may be seen on the Picture Arrangement subtest of the WAIS. In this test the subject is given in random order a number of cartoon-like pictures which, when placed in the correct sequence, will tell a logical story. The frontal patient often tends to describe each picture as separate rather than as part of an integrated series and may on occasions be quite satisfied to leave the cards in the presented random order. This latter tendency was shown to be more common with frontal than non-frontal lesions particularly on the right side (McFie & Thompson 1972) although patients with lesions elsewhere, particularly in the right temporal region, also perform poorly on this task. As with most psychological tests the responses are determined by a number of factors.

Performance of frontal patients on Picture Arrangement bear a remarkable similarity to Luria's (1973) description of the difficulties of such patients when asked to elucidate the theme of a picture containing a good deal of detail. His description of the processes involved suits both situations precisely. 'To understand the meaning of such a picture the subject must distinguish its details, compare them with each other, formulate a definite hypothesis of its meaning and then test this hypothesis with the actual contents of the picture, either to confirm or to reject it and then resume the analysis.' (op. cit. p 213–214). Experimental studies of visual search and eye movements when confronted with complex visual material raise the possibility that encroachment of the lesion on the frontal eye fields may account for at least part of the inefficient searching strategies employed.

Frontal amnesia. This term was coined by Barbizet (1970) to account for the difficulties of some frontal patients on certain memory and learning tasks. Other writers have pointed to the qualitative difference between these frontal disorders and those associated with temporal lobe lesions (Luria et al 1967). Simple registration and recall of both visual and verbal material is largely unaffected by frontal lesions. The frontal difficulty comes to the fore when the subject is confronted with novel material, particularly when it is lengthy or complex. It is best to consider it as a difficulty in the intellectual organization of material for the process of committing it to memory, rather than as an amnesic difficulty. It may thus be assisted by an external agent organizing the material for the patient so that the 'amnesia' is overcome for that particular piece of learning. 'The evidence seems to suggest that frontal lesions suppress the programs that govern the execution of the mental strategies that bring recall and memorization into play during the operation of any new task, whether it be the resolution of a problem or the learning of a piece of poetry' (Barbizet 1970, p 87). This explanation is almost identical to that given by Luria in many of his works.

If planning and organization are, as it were, the vehicle for registration and recall, then 'frontal amnesia' will become apparent on tasks where the subject has to impress organization on the material. We find the Rey Figure and the Rey Auditory Verbal Learning Test useful for this purpose. The lack of organization in the copying of the Rey Figure which leads to poverty of recall was exemplified in Case AE (Ch. 1). Similar results have been described by others, e.g. Messerli et al (1979). The lack of organization is reflected on the RAVLT in the form of an unsystematic order of recall from trial to trial, with loss of the primacy and recency effect normally present in learning; and in a plateau in the learning curve, which may be only one or two units above the immediate memory span which is itself normal in such cases.

Basal and basomedial frontal cortex

This area is situated above the floor of the anterior cranial fossa. As already described it ranks among the most frequently damaged areas of the brain. A good indicator of such basal damage is the presence of anosmia (loss of smell) due to damage to the olfactory bulb and tract which lie on the inferior surface of the frontal lobe (see Case UX).

Disinhibition

The hallmark of basal frontal damage is loss of control of inhibition. This forms a central part of the personality changes which are such a source of disability. The description of the classical case of Phineas Gage by his physician Dr Harlow might fit any of the numerous victims of motor vehicle accidents today. This efficient and capable foreman was injured in 1848 when a tamping iron was blown by an explosive charge through the frontal region of his brain:

He is fitful, irreverent, indulging at times in the grossest profanity (which was not previously his custom), manifesting but little deference to his fellows, impatient of restraint or advice when it conflicts with his desires, at times pertinaciously obstinate yet capricious and vacillating, devising many plans for future operation which no sooner are arranged than they are abandoned for others appearing more feasible. His mind was radically changed so that his friends and acquaintances said that he was no longer Gage (quoted by Kimble 1963).

This pattern of behaviour, even in a moderate degree, creates a good deal of the psychosocial deficit which so incapacitates the severely head injured patient and poses such a burden to his relatives, friends and therapists. However, lesser degrees of inhibition control may interfere seriously with the cognitive activities of the patient and thus pose a serious bar to adaptive behaviour, even when social control appears adequate. Careful history taking in these minor cases will often uncover profound social disinhibition in relation to alcohol consumption and in many of these individuals this sensitivity to alcohol remains throughout life.

An adequate control of inhibition is a basic requirement of intellectual processes requiring selectivity, i.e. where a decision has to be made between competing hypotheses or response tendencies. Selection of the appropriate response demands concurrent suppression or inhibition of the inappropriate. Patients with basal frontal damage find it difficult to suppress customary modes of responding. This explains much of their difficulty on tasks like the Wisconsin Card Sorting Test. Another test which brings out this difficulty is Part B of the Trail Making Test where the subject has to constantly switch between the two well established series of numbers and letters. In every item of the series 1–A–2–B–3–C ... the subject has to suppress the next of one series while selecting the correct one of the other. In fact this is an instance of continual shifting of response set. The frontal patient has a constant battle to prevent these stereotyped series from running on and thus may be exceedingly slow on the alternate series of Part B whereas he has no difficulty with the single series of Part A. In more serious cases the patient is to inhibit some of the responses, e.g. 1–A–2–B–3–C–D, or 1–A–2–B–3–4–5. As in other situations the patient may be fully aware of what has to be done.

Loss of selectivity may be seen on vocabulary tests which require the patient to define words. The frontal patient will respond to some association aroused by the word to be defined rather than to the word itself. Since the examiner may be unaware of the patient's personal association aroused by the stimulus, some of the definitions may take on an idiosyncratic flavour. Luria et al (1967) have noted this tendency to produce extraneous associations in a patient with a left frontal tumour. In severely damaged cases the responses are given on the basis of the sound of the word rather than of its meaning, the 'clang' association. Such patients are invariably disinhibited in other ways, e.g. they are unable to inhibit verbal responses which are socially undesirable. The following vocabulary responses are from a patient cited in Walsh (1987):

DESIGNATE	'Blow up something.'
REMORSE	'Man is overcome with stone, rocks, everything.'
FORTITUDE	'Where all the soldiers are all going back to the fortitude because all the Indians attack.'
TIRADE.	Here the patient gave a long rambling description of disaster at sea, shipwreck, etc. and finished by announcing with a great guffaw 'and this was all about a tirade wave'.

Many of this patient's other responses were perfectly acceptable definitions and on return to some of the stimulus words he showed that he clearly understood the meaning. Further examples of deviant vocabulary responses are given later in this chapter in Case VP (p 198).

While utilizing the 'method of extreme cases', as an explanatory method, it is wise to remember that many patients designated as fully recovered will have this selectivity deficit in a less obvious form, which may nevertheless have serious consequences in their occupation or profession.

Personality change

The organic psychosocial deficit exemplified by loss of inhibition and insight is only part of an extremely complex set of changes subsumed under personality change, and readers should acquaint themselves with the large and complex literature on the subject. The earlier review of psychiatric sequelae of head injury by Lishman (1973) is still well worth consulting and can be extended by recent work such as McClelland (1988) Head injuries after all take place in individuals with diverse premorbid personalities and there are bound to be enormous variations in individuals' reactions to the sense of their own cognitive, social and occupational downgrading as a result of damage to the central nervous system. Though personality change is commonly mentioned in the literature there has been a remarkable dearth of attempts to look at the problem in a quantitative way and to study change over time. The Glasgow group have addressed the issue recently (Brooks & McKinlay 1983, Brooks 1988). Some of the changes obviously have a direct relationship to physical brain injury while others are, in one sense or another, reactive.

Depression, anxiety and irritability so often accompany lesions in any part of the cerebrum that they must be to a large degree reactive rather than a product of specific neural damage. Lezak (1978a) outlines how disruptive the subtle sequelae of brain damage such as perplexity, distractability and fatigue may be.

Finally, there is a set of changes, which Walsh (1960) termed modification of the personality, that will be frequently found in association with damage to the frontal lobes and not with damage elsewhere; for example, loss of ego-continuity, which will have important consequences for the patient's adjustment to life. The importance of trying to ascertain which features are reactive and which are based in irreparable brain damage is that the former may be favourably influenced by therapeutic intervention while the latter will not.

Medial cortex

This area is less often damaged than the other two cortical subdivisions with the result that its functional roles are less well known. It is supplied by the anterior cerebral arteries and damage due to spasm of these arteries associated with regional cerebral aneurysms (or their surgery) is the main source of our knowledge of its clinical syndromes. Such bilateral spasm may lead to a state marked by adynamia and amnesia, and often impotence in the male patient. Similar functional changes can be seen with midline frontal tumours. While *selective* damage to the medial frontal cortex is not seen with closed head injury because of the latter's protected location, damage may occur in severe frontal injury where the functional deficits become imbedded in a 'complex frontal lobe syndrome'.

Adynamia

In the relatively pure case of medial damage, patients may show a peculiar anergia or passivity in which they appear to be unable, voluntarily, to initiate and sustain activity. The problem is one of self-regulation of arousal or motivation since they may respond appropriately to external stimulation especially if this is repeated. However, they lapse back into inactivity when the external source is removed. It can be seen that this form of behaviour could readily be construed as a psychological condition of resistance, apathy or even depression. Patients who work well enough under the therapist's direction may be found at the same stage in the task at hand when the therapist returns some time later.

Adynamia will vary in degree ranging from akinetic mutism to a minor lack of drive akin to that of 'lazy' people. Once stable it forms one of the most serious impediments to rehabilitation and one which may be overlooked or misunderstood. In traumatic cases, since there are always other cognitive and psychosocial deficits, the outlook is particularly poor. At present no therapy seems to be of lasting help.

LATERALITY AND THE FRONTAL LOBES

Although brain lesions following head injury tend to be bilateral there are instances where there is an asymmetry of the lesions. This raises the question as to whether there is evidence to suggest a dissociation of function between the frontal lobes in line with the general evidence demonstrating hemispheric asymmetry of function. The evidence in support of frontal lobe lateral specialization is suggestive but far from established.

Milner (1971) described patients with frontal lobe lesions as having difficulty with the temporal ordering of events. Superimposed on this was a material specificity, patients with left frontal lesions having difficulty with verbal recency-tasks and those with right frontal lesions having difficulty with nonverbal tasks.

Perhaps the best established relationship is that of disturbance of verbal fluency with left frontal lesions.

Verbal fluency

The assessment of fluency is a complex issue. Decrease in fluency is associated with lesions in the medial aspect of the frontal lobes, where it forms part of a general adynamia (see Ch. 6). Decreased verbal output, often effortful in nature, is associated with lesions in the region of Broca's area, while basal lesions may lead to interference with selectivity. To date, no study has addressed itself to a clinico-anatomical analysis of these different deficits on standard tests of fluency. Nevertheless, decreased verbal fluency remains one of the principal arguments in favour of frontal asymmetry of function.

Milner (1964) compared patients with left frontal, right frontal and left temporal lobectomies on Thurstone's test of written verbal fluency. The poorest performance was by the left frontal group. Since there was a marked difference between the left frontal and left temporal groups the result cannot be due solely to involvement of the left (language) hemisphere. These findings have been confirmed and extended by others (Benton 1968, Ramier & Hécaen 1970). The most commonly used test is one of spoken word fluency where the subject has to give in sixty seconds as many words as possible beginning with a particular letter.

Our own clinical experience supports the notion that there are different mechanisms present in individual cases. Perret (1974) thought that the basic difficulty with left frontal lesions lay in the fact that for successful performance the patient must suppress the habit of using words according to their meaning. The contention that this is an example in the verbal mode of the general tendency of frontal patients to have difficulty in novel situations is strengthened by the fact that the same patients also had difficulty with the Stroop test (Stroop 1935) where one response tendency is pitted against another. The subject has to name the colour in which each of a series of words is printed, the word itself being the name of a colour, e.g. BLUE printed in red, GREEN printed in blue.

Possibly related to the same mechanism is our observation, and that of Zangwill (1978), that patients may begin fluently, only to find increasing difficulty with the passage of time. This can be noted by dividing the sixty second time into four segments. In many cases virtually all responses will have ceased in the first two or, at most, three segments. It is as if the effort involved generates reactive inhibition which impedes the activity. Finally, gross loss of inhibition can be seen in the breaking of rules such as giving capitalized words and in the ready production of coarse or obscene words out of keeping with the patient's prior usage, and in the failure to suppress words beginning with the correct sound but starting with another letter, e.g. 'circumference' and 'psychology' in the 'S' series.

While there is strong support for a simple association of verbal fluency with the left frontal lobe, only one study suggests a complementary role for the right frontal lobe. Jones-Gotman & Milner (1977) described a difficulty in generating a range of different non-verbalizable drawings (design fluency) in patients with right frontal lesions. This remains to be confirmed.

Finally, we have noted a consistently poor performance of our left frontal patients on the Colour-Form Sorting Test as well as poor verbal fluency. The association of these two disabilities argues strongly for left frontal dysfunction whatever the pathology. We had also formed the clinical impression that our right frontal patients performed worse on the Austin Maze Test than patients with lesions in other locations, but this is now seriously in doubt following the spectacular case of WS who blew out his right frontal lobe in an explosion and performed at a very high level on this test (see Walsh 1987, ch 10).

AMNESIA

Disorders of memory are among the most consistent findings with trauma to the head. These traumatic amnesias have been the subject of special clinical studies by Russell and his colleagues (Russell 1932, 1935, 1971; Russell & Espir 1961, Russell & Nathan 1946, Russell & Smith 1961). This work has been furthered by more recent studies employing psychometric and experimental methods (Brooks 1972, 1974a,b, 1975, 1976; Hannay et al 1979, Lezak 1979a). Nevertheless, much remains to be done.

One of the difficulties posed is the fact that the term traumatic amnesia covers a diversity of disorders. Barbizet et al (1965) examined 39 severely head injured patients six to eighteen months after trauma. Nearly three quarters had significant residual memory disturbance. Ten had global or mixed memory disturbance, nine had predominantly cortical amnesia, and ten had amnesia with characteristics suggestive of localized damage in the axial formations, i.e. general or Korsakoff-like amnesia. Thus, studies which contain a heterogeneous collection of disorders will be both difficult to interpret and perhaps misleading to use as a basis for rehabilitative measures.

Since temporal lobe damage is a most common pathological feature and amnesia a common clinical finding, there are those like Jennett (1969) who find it tempting to assume a causative relationship in the light of the well substantiated role of temporal lobe structures in memory. Even in cases of amnesia after penetrating missile wounds there have been reports of a correlation between damage to the axial and mesial structures and the presence of a general amnesic syndrome (Bender et al 1949, Russell & Espir 1961, Whitty & Zangwill 1977, Hillbom & Jahro 1969, Lehtonen 1973), though the incidence of such amnesia is very low.

In line with statements in earlier chapters it is of paramount importance to use neuropsychological findings from the literature to elucidate the nature of the disorder in the individual case. Studies such as that of Kear-Colwell & Heller (1980) which confirm the clinical experience that tests of recent memory (WMS Associate Learning, Logical Memory) are more sensitive than other memory tests in cases of head injury, do not mean that one pathophysiological mechanism is responsible. The variable nature of the pathology means that there will often be an admixture of memory disturbances of different types, e.g. it is not uncommon to have what appears to be a mild general amnesic syndrome compounded by the presence of the complex learning difficulty termed frontal amnesia. Test performance is also likely to be affected by attentional and motivational disorders.

The reason for introducing this note is that because of the common association of temporal and frontal pathology a combination of memory and adaptive disorders is very common and both sets of disorders may form serious impediments to performance in everyday situations.

In order to assess the possible interaction with other dysfunctions the examination of memory in traumatic cases should aim at an appreciation of:

1. the adequacy of immediate apprehension of material
2. the specificity (i.e. verbal or nonverbal) versus the generality of the disorders
3. any bias introduced by the sense modality of presentation
4. the rate of forgetting as well as the rate of acquisition
5. the sensitivity to interference
6. the capacity of the individual to order the material
7. the role of incidental versus focussed memory
8. the effect on long-stored information.

A thorough examination of this type will greatly aid an evaluation of concomitant disorders of adaptive behaviour.

CASE EXAMPLES

Case: UX

This physician came to our attention when we were asked to examine him with a view to helping him to decide whether he should retire from practice. He was 58 years of age at the time of examination. The history was provided by his wife in his presence.

UX had been injured in a motor vehicle accident over ten years before. He was unconscious for eight days and spent three weeks in hospital. He was reported as suffering from cerebral oedema with uninhibited behaviour and diplopia. On discharge he showed no insight into his inappropriate behaviour. Apart from anosmia he suffered no physical disabilities. After a further three weeks he returned to work but was unable to cope, partly because of constant friction with his partners.

The patient's wife described him as a previously easy-going but hard-working doctor who had had a fine record as a medical student and had built his practice from scratch to a thriving concern with numerous junior partners. She noted numerous changes in her husband after the accident which had placed great strains on their marriage. He was now irascible and had outbursts on little provocation, especially after even a small amount of alcohol, so that they had lost many friends. His anosmia deprived him of the pleasures of the wine and food society of which he was an active member.

Some two years after the accident he finally left the multiple practice and after some months of idleness began a limited practice on his own several days a week. It was apparent that even here his wife served as a surrogate set of frontal lobes. He had ongoing memory problems and continued to lack full insight into the nature and extent of his deficits. He tended to forget people's names and arrangements concerning the practice, so that his wife had constantly to remind him. She felt that he had retained his medical knowledge and it is noteworthy that he had been a skilled practitioner for many years before the accident. However, he tended to either misinterpret information or failed to attend to what was said or written, so that he tended to make mistakes where new information was concerned. At other times he showed apparent understanding by responding appropriately with words, but this did not guarantee correct action and showed the 'curious dissociation between knowing and doing'. Despite all these problems the marriage remained a happy one and UX was popular with his relatively small number of patients. He continued in this way for ten years until the present.

At interview UX proffered little information. He was aware that his limitations placed a burden on his wife but he had been anxious to continue practising medicine as the sole remaining interest in his life. He was pleasantly co-operative but a trifle bewildered, with a partial realization that changes had to be made because of mistakes he had been making. He seemed prepared to accept our advice even if that meant retiring at a relatively early age. Independent medical examinations were proceeding at the same time as the neuropsychological assessments. UX was examined at the family's request by two neuropsychologists from different hospitals, parallel forms of tests being used where possible. Both sought to clarify the memory and adaptive behaviour disorders so apparent in the history. As the examinations were essentially the same and only a short time apart they are grouped together.

Wechsler Memory Scale, Form I

Information	6	Digits Total	14 (8,6)
Orientation	5	Visual Reproduction	12
Mental Control	9	Associate Learning	17 (6,2;6,2;6,4)
Logical Memory	13		
MQ 143			

Rey Auditory Verbal Learning Test

List A						List B	List A
Trial	1	2	3	4	5	Recall	Recall
First test	6	9	10	15	15	10	12
Second test	6	9	8	10	12	6	6

The first RAVLT examination showed that there was no significant deficit of acquisition of the type seen with temporal lobe damage, but the second performance was unexpectedly much poorer.

Naylor-Harwood Adult Intelligence Scale

Information	18	Letter Symbol	10
Comprehension	19	Picture Completion	13
Similarities	11	Block Design	10
Arithmetic	13	Picture Arrangement	12
Memory for Digits	12	Object Assembly	8
Vocabulary	16		
VIQ 131; PIQ 117; FSIQ 126			

If one takes the two or three highest scores as representing prior ability, then the remaining subtests, most of which have a loading on problem-solving and dealing with novel situations, show a significant lowering of these latter skills.

The quality of his difficulties on the Arithmetic subtest led to the administration

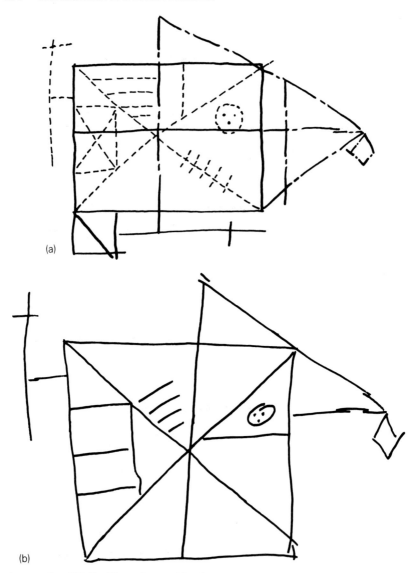

Fig. 5.3   Case UX. Rey Figure. Copy and Recall.

of a set of Complex Arithmetical problems (see Appendix). While straightforward arithmetical operations provided no difficulty, he had problems where the preliminary data was complex or where he had to take into account several different items of information simultaneously. In fact, he was only able to solve one such item.

On other NHAIS subtests he showed most of the features described in the first part of this chapter. One neuropsychologist commented:

'He showed poor attention to complex instructions, often getting details confused when carrying them out. He had difficulty analysing complex problems and systematically planning a solution. Instead, he tended to show a somewhat impulsive and unsystematic approach and his responses reflected his inability to take into account all aspects of the problem when attempting to solve it. He did not check his responses for errors and correct them, even when his errors were pointed out. He was also somewhat inflexible in his approach.

Verbal fluency appeared to be close to that anticipated:

Test 1	F−19	A−13	S−18
Test 2	F−16	A−13	S−14

Rey Figure. The complex figure was well copied but the reproduction from memory after only three minutes was greatly impoverished. (Fig. 5.3)

Austin Maze (Milner pathway). This test was discontinued after 31 trials. On trial one he made only 14 errors indicating that he had grasped the general nature of the problem, and was down to only four errors by the fifth trial. However, he continued to make errors and although he was fully able to tell the examiner where he was going wrong, he could not use this information to eradicate them on a subsequent trial. Note that to have accepted one errorless trial as the criterion of learning would have grossly underestimated the degree of this man's difficulty.

Errors on consecutive trials: 14 13 8 8 4 5 7 7 6 7 5 5 6 7 5 3 2 **0** 5 3 4 2 1 1 7 3 5 2 2 3 2 (discontinued)

It is noteworthy that this patient made only one error on the whole of the *Porteus Maze Test* which provides constant visual support for selecting the turns at choice points, whereas the Austin type of maze requires the pathway to be carried in abstracto.

Moving onto tests of conceptual behaviour, he had no difficulty on the *Colour-Form Sorting Test* but much difficulty with the *Wisconsin Card Sorting Test*. Here he attained the first two concepts with little difficulty but continued to perseverate on these when the correct concept was number and, despite constant disconfirmation of his incorrect choices, he took 38 trials finally to grasp this concept.

The finding of clear evidence of frontal lobe impairment seemed entirely consistent with the history as given by the patient's wife. Shortly after neuropsychological assessment an examining medical specialist sent a copy of the following report of a CT scan (Fig. 5.4):

The CT scan of this patient is truly remarkable and one wonders how he could possibly have functioned professionally all these years. There is extensive destruction of the frontal poles on each side with more widespread atrophy of the frontal lobes behind this. The destruction begins on the floor of the anterior fossa, i.e. the orbital cortex, and spreads right up to the superior frontal gyri. This indicates that he must have had severe contusion–laceration of the frontal lobes on each side at the time of his accident. This type of injury does not correlate accurately with the duration of unconsciousness and therefore it can sometimes be quite severe even when the patient has been unconscious for only a few days. This would appear to be the case in this particular instance. The findings correlate well with the neuropsychologic testing which, I understand, indicate frontal lobe disorder.

One can only speculate on how long this patient could have coped without the constant vigilance of his intelligent and devoted wife. The case presents an instance

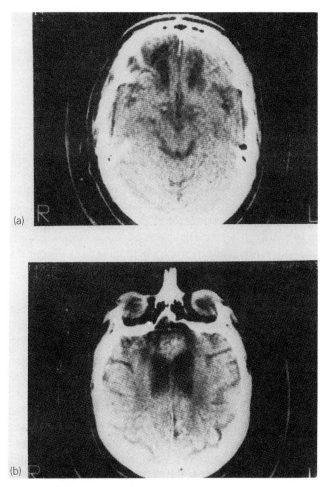

Fig. 5.4 Case UX. CT scan showing frontal atrophy

where there was both physical and psychometric recovery, the latter to 'average or above average levels', while there was significant lowering of adaptive ability and psychosocial deficit.

Case: VO

This woman was referred at the age of 26 by the psychological service of a government employment agency. The referring psychologist described a history of the client's continual failures to succeed for even the briefest time in a wide variety of occupations. This presented a paradox as the young woman was courteous, well spoken and had a verbal intelligence quotient of 135. There was a history of head injury twelve years before when VO fell from her horse. She was unconscious for three weeks but subsequently returned to school to complete year 11 successfully and passed some subjects in year 12. Her school results following her accident had been below those attained previously, but no details were available as VO came from a distant state.

Following secondary schooling her mother found it impossible to teach her housework and she also failed when enrolled in a residential course in domestic science. She then tried business school without success and after the death of her parents travelled to Europe with a friend. While there she had various live-in jobs looking after children. She herself commented that one mother had said that while she was with the household 'it was like having four children in the house instead of three'.

Two years before her referral she had been accepted for nursing training at our own hospital. She is recorded as being in the top third of the group at the end of her first six weeks of introductory theoretical teaching. She got into difficulty during her first few days on the wards and an appointment was made with the hospital psychologist, but she was dismissed as being totally unsuited (and unsuitable) for nursing before the appointment could be kept.

At interview VO was co-operative though a trifle verbose. She expressed interest in the tests and said that she was perplexed as to why she could not succeed at work. She described herself as making errors despite feeling confident that she knew what to do. Her description fitted that of the 'curious dissociation' but, as it was unclear whether she also had a memory difficulty, it was decided to clarify this early in the examination.

Wechsler Memory Scale, Form I

Information	6	Digits Total	12 (7,5)
Orientation	5	Visual Reproduction	14
Mental Control	7	Associate Learning	13.5 (5,1;6,1;6,3)
Logical Memory	11		
MQ 106			

Although this was quantitatively inferior to her reported VIQ there was no suggestion of any major amnesic syndrome.

Porteus Maze Test. M.A. 13 years. Though she had several failures there was nothing of note in the quality of her performance.

Austin Maze Test. This was introduced with the anticipation that the problem was one of adaptive behaviour. Errors on successive trials were 48–25–62–48–24–18–15–9–14–17–11–16–36 (discontinued).

No more striking illustration of her inability to learn from experience could be found. Despite repetition of the instructions not to retrace her steps she continued to do so. She showed through her verbal statements that she was aware of her errors ('I always go wrong here'). She was unable to modify her behaviour not only on successive trials, but even within the same trial, making repeated errors at the same choice point. She was mildly perplexed at her inability to learn but was quite happy to continue trying. Not once did she show any obvious frustration. As the source of her difficulty was obviously based on long-standing brain damage and as she was to return to the occupational psychologist, testing was discontinued at this point.

Further conversation after testing revealed that VO was aware of the reason for her dismissal as a trainee nurse. She described situations which she remembered clearly where she had correctly verbalized what she had to do but carried out a quite different action. These actions quite seriously threatened the safety of her patients and as the reasons were not understood by her superiors there was no option but to dismiss her.

We discussed the implications of her disorder with the occupational psychologist who arranged for her to be accepted as a routine clerical assistant under direct supervision in a government department. Here she remained for several years, more out of generosity than due to her competence. She still continued to make mistakes even in quite simple routine office procedures and was an obvious burden to her supervisors.

Over five years after her first examination she returned to seek help, as we had warned her that she might need such help if she were to marry and have children. She had married a man many years older than herself and was expecting her first child. She reported her difficulties at work and in daily living, stating that she was aware that she did not learn from experience and relied on her supportive husband to organize her life. We took the opportunity to repeat and extend the cognitive examination. Performance on the *Wechsler Memory Scale*, Form II was much as before:

Information	6	Digits Total	12 (6,6)
Orientation	5	Visual Reproduction	13
Mental Control	9	Associate Learning	16 (4,2;6,3;6,3)
Logical Memory	8.5		
MQ 112			

Naylor–Harwood Adult Intelligence Scale

Information	19	Letter Symbol	11
Comprehension	15	Picture Completion	11
Similarities	12	Block Design	9
Arithmetic	11	Picture Arrangement	8
Vocabulary	16	Object Assembly	2

The most notable failures were on the embedded items of the Block Design subtest. Placing a grid over the designs (as in Ch. 1) helped her to solve them with ease. She had considerable difficulty integrating the card series of Picture Arrangement into logical order, and found the Object Assembly task almost impossible.

Austin Maze Test. She showed the same pattern of lack of error utilization despite awareness of errors that she had shown years before, occasionally broke the rules, and was unable to inhibit impulsive errors. She was pleased when we terminated the test after the following errors on ten successive trials: 17−16−33−34−13−12−26−13−18−27.

Porteus Maze Test. Mental Age 14 years.

Verbal Fluency. F−10; A−16; S−10. Adjusted score at about the 85th centile with some examples of rule-breaking.

Rey Figure. The copy was carried out in a haphazard way with the result that her recall was extremely sparse (Fig. 5.5).

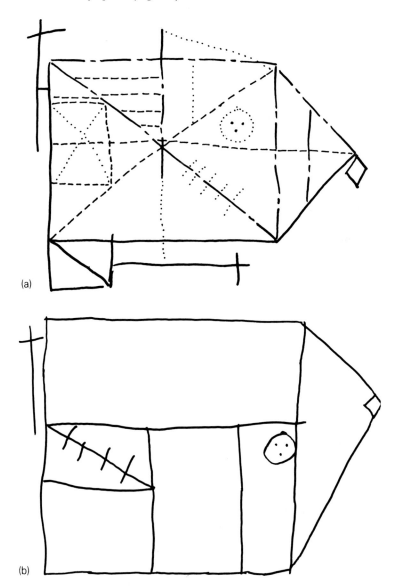

(a)

(b)

Fig. 5.5   Case VO. Rey Figure. Copy and Recall.

That her poor recall of the complex figure was largely determined by lack of organization is borne out by her almost perfect recall of the simpler Visual Reproduction designs.

RAVLT. This supported the impression gained from the WMS that her verbal memory was relatively well preserved though a frontal plateau was evident:

List						List B	List A	List A
Trial	1	2	3	4	5	Recall	Recall	Recognition
Correct	8	10	10	10	12	4	9	15

Colour–Form Sorting Test. This was executed normally.

Complex Arithmetical Problems. While her routine arithmetical operations were successful she was not able to solve any but the simpler problems.

In summary there had been no significant change in her constellation of signs and, indeed, none was to be expected. Her considerable insight was shown by her statement that she was a 'parasite because she used other people's brains'. This was very close to the mark but proved of no use in modifying her behaviour. Practical assistance was provided in arranging closer contact with helpful professionals to monitor her child-rearing practices and provide support for her husband. As one of the team of psychologists wrote, her husband 'was to be involved as much as possible so that a 'spare set of frontal lobes' could be called on in any novel situations regarding the baby.'

Case: QP

This young woman, a trainee teacher, had sustained a relatively minor head injury some eighteen months before referral at the end of the third year of a four year university degree. The medical details were unavailable but QP had finished her degree the next year graduating with honours and was enrolled in a postgraduate diploma at the time of examination. Not long after the head injury she began to experience 'blackouts' at infrequent intervals. Shortly before her referral for neuropsychological assessment a neurologist diagnosed temporal lobe epilepsy and the ensuing investigations revealed a severe hydrocephalus (Fig. 5.6).

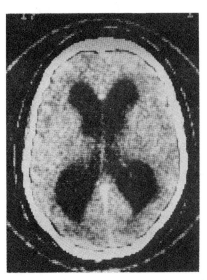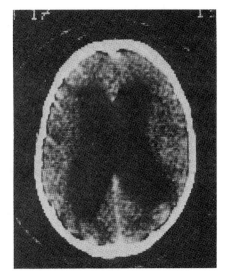

Fig. 5.6 Case QP. CT scan showing hydrocephalus.

The neurologist enquired: 'Could you give me any indication of her cerebral horsepower, whether there are temporal lobe signs and deficit and finally any evidence of recently acquired deficit. The problem is severe hydrocephalus. Is it stable or should we operate?'

Initial examination

At interview the patient and her father stated that they had felt there had been no intellectual decline since the accident. QP conversed freely in a relaxed manner.

It was felt that the neurologist's question might be approached by making certain assumptions. If there was a developing condition then it might best be reflected in the more subtle aspects of memory, learning and problem solving. In our experience the more adaptive and integrative a function is, the earlier it appears to be affected by a condition such as developing hydrocephalus which threatens the integrity of the brain. On the other hand measures biased towards crystallized intelligence might be quite insensitive and, in view of the fact that the university had recently carried out such an examination, it was felt that standard intellectual tasks would be inappropriate. Memory examination, even with the simple material of the WMS, immediately suggested that all was not well.

Wechsler Memory Scale, Form I

Information	6	Digits Total	11 (6,5)
Orientation	5	Visual Reproduction	10
Mental Control	6	Associate Learning	12 (4,0;6,2;6,2)
Logical Memory	8		
MQ 90			

This was thought to represent a considerable fall-off for a university graduate. QP showed marked proactive interference on the second prose passage and made numerous errors on serial addition. Two measures of learning and adaptive behaviour were then given.

Category Test. The patient clearly understood the nature of the task, making no errors on the training sets. However, the test was abandoned when she failed to reach even a chance level of responding on the first two major sets of items (30 errors out of the 40 items on Set III and 31 out of 40 on Set IV). She seemed totally unable to abstract information from the succeeding items to guide her behaviour. She also showed no insight into the poverty of her performance.

Austin Maze Test. Throughout her attempts QP made many infractions of the rules, seemed unable to inhibit the tendency to press buttons she clearly 'knew' were wrong and, in every way, acted like patients with serious frontal lobe damage. The error utilization problem was so evident that the test was abandoned: 32−14−22−14−11−17−15−19−9−9−8−9−6−6−6 (discontinued).

The answer to the neurologist's question was clear. The patient's intellectual powers were showing serious signs of waning. The patient was admitted to hospital where the neurosurgeon's opinion was that this was probably a case of congenital stenosis of the cerebral aqueduct and, after more serious causes of aqueductal obstruction were excluded, a ventriculo-atrial shunt was inserted. Following this the patient was discharged. The contribution of the head injury, if any, to the obstruction was never determined. A repeat scan showed that the ventricles had returned to a normal size and neuropsychological assessment was carried out three months later.

Post-operative examination

At this examination the patient volunteered that she could not understand how she had reported no fall-off in mental ability before her operation, as she now realized in retrospect that she had been obtunded at the time. Examination showed some obvious improvement but also residual difficulties.

Wechsler Memory Scale, Form II

Information	6	Digits Total	11 (6,5)
Orientation	5	Visual Reproduction	11
Mental Control	7	Associate Learning	18.5 (6,2;6,4;6,4)
Logical Memory	15		
MQ 116			

A vigilance reaction time test showed her to be performing normally for her age.

Porteus Maze Test. Mental Age 15 years.

Austin Maze Test. Successive errors: 25−18−10−9−7−15−4−5−8−5−6−5−6−5−6− − 1−1 (discontinued). The problem of error utilization was clearly present and the test was discontinued in order not to threaten the patient with too many failures.

Complex Arithmetical Problems. Question 1 produced an answer of 1360 1/5 planks, an answer so removed from the data that it should have provoked a recalculation, but QP appeared content. In Question 2, she failed to take into account the implications in the wording and wrote:

Van + Cargo = $16,000
Van = $700 less than cargo
Cargo is worth $15,300.

Questions 3 and 5 were answered correctly, requiring as they do, simple sequential operations. The other problems were failed. After several failed attempts on Question 6 she divided the total by 3 and credited this to person B adding 70 and subtracting 60 for A and B.

950 ÷ 3 = 316⅔   246 + 316 + 376 = 938 apples

It was thought that most of these problems would have been within her premorbid capacity.

Despite clear deficits it was obvious that some gains had been made and further cerebral impairment had been averted. Shortly after this QP obtained a position as a teacher in a country town, a post she held until her next referral three years later. She was coping well and enjoyed her teaching and had been free of epilepsy.

Third examination

Memory was examined with the *RAVLT*

List A						*List B*	*List A*
Trial	1	2	3	4	5	Recall	Recall
Correct	9	13	13	13	15	8	10

This was felt to represent a level comparable to her previous ability and she described no difficulties in daily life. She reported that her shunt had been replaced a year after its insertion. At the time she had felt mentally dull and had hastened to seek help.

Trail Making Test. She revealed her present alertness and mental flexibility. Part A–22 seconds; Part B–30 seconds.

This was confirmed by an excellent performance on the NHAIS Letter–Symbol subtest (scaled score 15). Pressure of time caused the examination to be abbreviated but she still showed problem solving difficulties on Block Design (SS,12) and Object Assembly (8). This latter performance was particularly poor, the score being bolstered by a good performance on the first item.

Rey Figure. Her copy contained one major omission and was begun by drawing around the periphery of the entire figure. The recall contained little of the original (Fig. 5.7).

VQ returned to her job. A year later she required replacement of her shunt after temporary decline in her conscious state; again, there was rapid postoperative improvement. When seen five years after the original shunting, repeated measures showed quality and levels of performance to be stable at the level of the previous examination.

This patient has been able to cope in a stable employment situation probably because of the restricted demands of the situation and the support of her colleagues. We advised against transferring her to another position which would place demands on her obviously fragile adaptive, problem solving abilities. She is also at considerable risk from complications of her shunt and it is felt that monitoring of her mental functions should be on a more regular basis since any further impairment will probably render her incapable of carrying on her occupation.

Case: QT

This young student librarian was injured in a motor vehicle accident in 1982. She was unconscious on arrival at hospital with decerebrate rigidity, right knee injury and extensive lacerations. CT scan was normal two days after admission. Her conscious state improved ten days after injury and she responded to some commands with a smile. A spastic left hemiparesis was now observable. At 17 days she was restless and disoriented, able to obey some commands and to open her eyes spontaneously, but she had no speech. On the 20th day she was conscious, alert and talking. Repeat CT scan showed minor dilatation of the ventricular system with a mild degree of communicating hydrocephalus. From this time her mental and physical condition

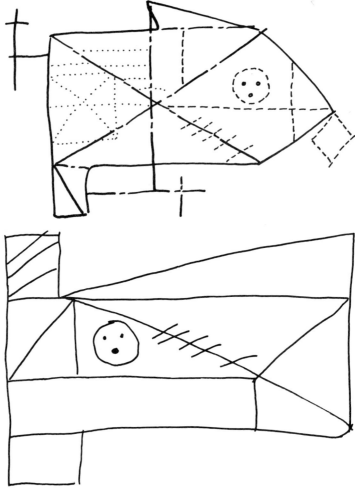

Fig. 5.7 Case QP. Rey Figure. Copy and Recall.

continued to improve. At nine weeks she was referred for assessment to monitor her cognitive improvement.

At interview QT reported a retrograde amnesia of about two and a half hours. She could remember virtually nothing of her first month in hospital and although she was aware that her memory had improved, she was still having difficulty remembering everyday events. The following tests were spread over three days in order to preserve the patient's full attention without tiring her.

Wechsler Memory Scale, Form I

Information	4	Digits Total	15 (8,7)
Orientation	5	Visual Reproduction	11
Mental Control	9	Associate Learning	15.5 (5,2;6,2;6,3)
Logical Memory	6		
MQ 100			

It was encouraging to note the returning ability to register new material at this early stage. After a second reading of passage B of Logical Memory she scored 13 on immediate recall and 8 after five minutes distraction.

Rey Figure. The copy had an orderly sequence with self corrected distortions, but little remained in the recall after an interpolated task lasting four minutes (Fig. 5.8).

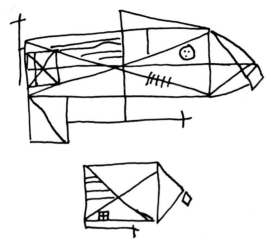

Fig. 5.8 Case QT. Rey Figure, Copy and Recall.

Verbal Fluency. F−9; A−5; S−9. Apart from a general poverty of responding there were no qualitative features of note.

Rey Auditory Verbal Learning Test

List A						List B	List A	List A
Trial	1	2	3	4	5		Recall	Recognition
	7	3	9	9	9	3	3	13

Again the recency of her injury and the fact that she was only a short time out of the period of PTA meant that no prediction should be made, though this performance was scarcely beyond her immediate memory span.

Trail Making Test. QT was slow but accurate. A−72 seconds, clearly impaired. B−115 seconds, moderate to marked slowing.

Complex Arithmetical Problems. She was unable to solve any.

Lhermitte and Signoret Tests. She made one errorless trial after only four attempts on the Spatial Arrangement task and succeeded on the Logical Arrangement in six. This also seemed to support an optimistic prognosis at this stage.

WAIS. Several subtests showed an obvious problem-solving difficulty on the complex Block Design items, and very great difficulty on Object Assembly.

Austin Maze. This showed a marked learning difficulty with no significant improvement from the third to the 17th trial when it was abandoned. Consecutive errors were: 22−10−8−14−17−12−10−8−7−6−6−6−8−4−5−4−7 (discontinued).

In summary, given the severity and recency of her injury, QT showed promising return to basic memory ability though she broke down as tasks became lengthy or complex. Old memories and skills seemed relatively intact. It was confidently expected that she would make more progress.

She was transferred to a rehabilitation hospital where she made further gains and there were no residual physical disabilities.

Reassessment seven months post-injury. At this time a comparison examination was requested as QT was keen to return to her studies. The assessment was made prior to her transfer to a centre with better facilities for cognitive retraining.

Wechsler Memory Scale, Form II

Information	not tested	Digits Total	14 (8,6)
Orientation	not tested	Visual Reproduction	14
Mental Control	9	Associate Learning	14 (3,1;5,2;6,4)
Logical Memory	13		

After ten minutes she recalled 8 points of the first Logical Memory passage, suggesting returning memory ability.

Rey Auditory Verbal Learning Test

List A						List B	List A	List A
Trial	1	2	3	4	5	Recall	Recall	Recognition
	5	8	10	11	10	6	7	12

This was thought to represent a significant degree of deficit for a person of her background, though further improvement was still thought possible.

Verbal Fluency. F−11; A−9; S−12. Again, this represented a performance well below expectation.

Rey Figure. The copy was complete though with distortions, but once again the recall was poor (Fig. 5.9).

Austin Maze. Consecutive errors: 12−4−6−4−5−2−1−0−3−1−1−1−0−1−1−0−0. This performance is slightly inferior to the control subjects in Milner's study (1965) and well below the expected performance of somebody of QT's estimated premorbid ability. Nevertheless, there did not seem to be a major problem.

Despite some obvious gains this patient had not yet made a full cognitive recovery. She was counselled to take the opportunity for further retraining before contemplating returning to her studies. The rehabilitation officers were conversant with the subtle but disruptive disorders described above and continued to monitor her ability to deal with complex material and to deal with novel situations of the type she would encounter in her occupational training. We felt that the prognosis should be guarded at this time since there was insufficient follow-up to know if progress was continuing or whether a plateau had been reached. If, in the ensuing year in

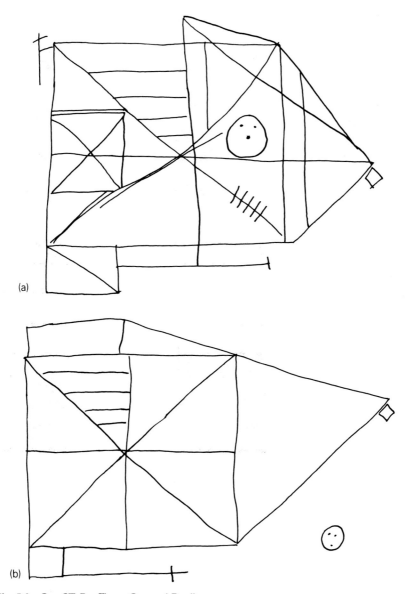

(a)

(b)

Fig. 5.9 Case QT. Rey Figure. Copy and Recall.

'advanced' rehabilitation little further improvement should take place, as we suspected, she may well need to be directed into an occupation of less complexity. Her case is a good example of a patient who may be described as recovered on superficial examination, but who may experience successive failures in the work force, with constant frustration and perplexity over the inability to cope. They often limp mentally from one job to another in a state of perplexity.

Case: VP

This 23-year-old nurse suffered an open compressed skull fracture with tearing of the dura and damage to the left frontal lobe when she was thrown onto the road as the touring bus in which she was travelling in Europe was involved in a collision. She was deeply unconscious when admitted to hospital. She showed her first pain reaction six weeks later and from that time there was steady improvement in her conscious state. At three months she was still disoriented and confused but able to converse with her father. She suffered from diplopia due to tearing of external ocular muscles. At four months she was repatriated to Australia. On admission to our hospital there was gross impairment of language, memory and frontal lobe function. Over the next three months she regained motor function and when first examined neuropsychologically she was continent and could walk with a stick. Speech therapy had been commenced and the state of her language functions was monitored because of the known left frontal damage though more widespread damage was probably present. Her articulation, object naming and repetition were good, as were simple reading and writing. She understood the significance of logico-grammatical constructions. However, independent meaningful expression was disturbed. Verbal reasoning was extremely concrete and she was unable to string together consecutive thoughts. There was a lack of spontaneous ideas and she frequently repeated herself. However, she had sufficient insight to be occasionally depressed by her language and memory difficulties.

Her first formal cognitive assessment at seven months showed marked difficulties in most areas.

Wechsler Memory Scale, Form I

Information	1	Digits Total	9 (5,4)
Orientation	5	Visual Reproduction	5
Mental Control	7	Associate Learning	6 (3,0;4,0;5,0)
Logical Memory	2		
MQ 61			

Despite the fact that she was perfectly well oriented she could not recall her birthdate. The test merely confirmed her clinically obvious memory difficulty. Despite this she cooperated with other tests before tiring.

NHAIS (scaled scores)

Information	7	Memory for Digits	7
Comprehension	7	Vocabulary	9
Similarities	7		

There was a childish character to many of her replies with disinhibition and attempts at simple jokes, e.g. What is an armadillo?—'An arm with a dillo on it.' Why do we brush our teeth?—'Keep them clean, white as normal. Keeps them happy. Oh, that was silly.' Other responses were of the simple concrete variety. Many of her responses on Vocabulary were perfectly acceptable definitions while others had some of the characteristics described in the earlier section of the chapter:

'elude': 'keep away from, some people are eluded, dislocated from the football team.' (Probably a response to exclude.)

'eminent': 'there in full force, such as this table, chair or wall.' (Possibly a response to evident.)

'exculpate': 'If I found a diamond I would dig it up.' (Probably clang association of excavate.)

Discussion as well as the excellence of her other responses clearly suggested that most words were in her lexicon. Her lack of selectivity, probably due to lack of inhibitory control, was seen on the *Verbal Fluency* test:

F. 'force, fool, fiddle, fink, find, fool, Friday, find, fool, find, fink, fool, Friday.'
A. 'add, a, alphabet, adjective, account, advance, answer, animal.'
S. 'skin, scoot, school, skin (I said skin), skittle, sun, son, sound, skin, skittle, son.'

On this first session she was introduced to the *Austin Maze* but this was discontinued as she could not be restrained from retracking and getting lost after several successful moves. Tried with the *Porteus Maze* she reached only a mental age of seven.

At nine months she was discharged to a rehabilitation hospital. The discharge summary said that 'her memory was now quite good although no further examination had been requested.

Second examination

At 21 months she was referred back to our hospital for cognitive re-evaluation. Considering the length of time in rehabilitation there were not thought to be any significant gains.

Wechsler Memory Scale, Form I

Information	3	Digits Total	10 (6,4)
Orientation	5	Visual Reproduction	6
Mental Control	7	Associate Learning	7.5 (5,0;5,0;5,0)
Logical Memory	4		

NHAIS (Scaled Scores)

Information	8	Letter Symbol	7
Comprehension	7	Block Design	10
Arithmetic	8	Object Assembly	8
Similarities	7		

Austin Maze. Discontinued after three trials. Errors 15–49–30.

Verbal Fluency. F–11; A–14; S–11 with numerous errors.

It seemed that her widespread deficits had undergone little or no resolution, the memory disorder being particularly profound. Over this long period frequent counselling was necessary and proved helpful on a day to day basis but produced no lasting gains. She was described as co-operative and mostly cheerful though strongly self depreciatory. She suffered one period of depression which remitted without treatment, and psychiatric help had not been needed since that time. Supportive counselling continued on a regular basis. She now lived at home and visited the centre daily. Her principal worry was that she had not been able to initiate social contact outside the centre and felt dependent and lonely.

Third examination (37 months)

Wechsler Memory Scale, Form I

Information	4	Digits Total	10 (6,4)
Orientation	5	Visual Reproduction	13
Mental Control	6	Associate Learning	14 (4,0;5,2;6,0)
Logical Memory	7.5		

There was a significant improvement in her nonverbal memory so that her memory disorder might at this stage be described as verbal specific. Her verbal fluency score was a little higher but contained the same kinds of errors. Porteus Maze mental age was 11½ years. She failed on all but the three simplest arithmetic problems of Luria (Christensen 1975).

Austin Maze Test. This was discontinued after ten trials. Errors: 20–16–28–17–10–14–10–12–10–12. She showed clear recognition of her errors at several choice points. On the first choice point, with only two possibilities, she made the wrong choice on most occasions, saying 'I always make that mistake' and at another choice point 'and that one.' She disobeyed the rules several times. It was thought that the error utilization difficulty was possibly compounded by her memory difficulty.

Despite the stable deficits her rehabilitation centre obtained two work trials for her, one at elementary nursing and one at simple clerical work. Not unexpectedly, both were unsuccessful. One doctor commented: 'She appears unable to achieve more than one-step tasks, anything more complicated requiring reasoning is beyond her.'

A year later the situation was unchanged though she had now moved to a centre where she continued an interest in art and craft classes. She was described as warm and friendly with only partial insight into her problems and doubts of her own worth. She lived at home with her father and moved around freely on public transport. Further attempts to employ her even on a voluntary basis had failed. To many lay observers she still appeared to be a 'normal' young woman. The eventual loss of her father will bring about a serious crisis in her life since she is still unable to manage the planning of her life's activities. We also have no clear idea of how the process of ageing will affect the steadily accumulating number of accident victims with such serious cognitive disorders and their impact on the person's total life adjustment.

REFERENCES

Adams J H 1975 The neuropathology of head injuries. In: Vinken P J, Bruyn G W (eds) Handbook of clinical neurology. North–Holland, Amsterdam, vol 23, ch 3, p 35–65
Artiola i Fortuny L, Briggs M, Newcombe F, Ratcliff G, Thomas C 1980 Measuring the duration of post traumatic amnesia. Journal of Neurology, Neurosurgery and Psychiatry 43: 377–379
Barbizet J 1970 Human Memory and its pathology. Freeman, San Francisco
Barbizet J, Lorilloux J, Fuchs D et al 1965 Le syndrome amnésique des traumatismes crâniens. Semaine des Hôpitaux de Paris 41: 1678-1687
Bender M B, Furlow L T, Teuber H L 1949 Alterations in behaviour after massive cerebral trauma (intraventricular foreign body) . Confinia Neurologica 9: 140–157
Benton A L 1968 Differential behavioral effects of frontal lobe disease. Neuropsychologia 6: 53–60
Bond M R 1975 Assessment of psychosocial outcome after severe head injury. In: Porter R, Fitzsimmons D W (eds) Outcome of severe damage to the central nervous system. Ciba Foundation Symposium 34 (new series) Elsevier, Amsterdam p 141–157
Bond M R, Brooks D N 1976 Understanding the process of recovery as a basis for the investigation of rehabilitation for the brain injured. Scandinavian Journal of Rehabilitation Medicine 8: 127–133
Broe A et al 1981 The nature and effects of brain damage following severe head injury in young subjects. In: Dinning TAR, Connelly T J (eds) Head injuries. Wiley, Brisbane, p 92–97
Brooks D N 1972 Memory and head injury. Journal of Nervous and Mental Disease 155: 350–355
Brooks D N 1974a Recognition memory after head injury: a signal detection analysis. Cortex 10: 224–230
Brooks D N 1974b Recognition memory and head injury. Journal of Neurology, Neurosurgery and Psychiatry 37: 794–801
Brooks D N 1975 Long and short term memory in head injured patients. Cortex 11: 329–340
Brooks D N 1976 Wechsler memory scale performance and its relationship to brain damage after severe closed head injury. Journal of Neurology, Neurosurgery and Psychiatry 39: 593–601
Brooks D N, Aughton M E, Bond M R, Jones P, Rizvi S 1980 Cognitive sequelae in relationship to early indices of severity of brain damage after severe blunt head injury. Journal of Neurology, Neurosurgery and Psychiatry 43: 529–534
Brooks D N, Aughton M E 1979 Psychological consequences of blunt head injury. International Rehabilitation Medicine 1: 166
Brooks N 1988 Personality change after severe head injury. Acta Neurochirurgica Supplementum 44: 59–64
Brooks N, Campsie L, Symington C, Beattie A, McKinlay W 1986 The five year outcome of severe blunt head injury: a relative's view. Journal of Neurology, Neurosurgery and Psychiatry 49: 764–770
Brooks N, Mckinlay W 1983 Personality and behavioural change after severe blunt head injury: A relative's view. Journal of Neurology, Neurosurgery and Psychiatry 46: 336–344
Brooks N, McKinlay W, Symington C, Beatie A, Campsie L 1987 Return to work within the first seven years of severe head injury. Brain Injury 1: 5–19
Brooks N, Symington C, Beattie A, Campsie L, Bryden J, McKinlay W, 1989 Alcohol and other predictors of cognitive recovery after severe head injury. Brain Injury 3: 235–246
Cattell R B 1943 The measurement of adult intelligence. Psychological Bulletin 40: 153–193
Christensen A L, 1975 Luria's neuropsychological investigation. Munksgaard, Copenhagen
Courville C B 1942 Coup-contrecoup mechanism of craniocerebral injuries: some observations. Archives of Surgery 54: 19–43
Courville C B 1945 Pathology of the nervous system, 2nd edn. Pacific Press, Mountain View, California
Courville C B 1955 Effects of alcohol on the nervous system of man. San Lucas Press, Los Angeles
Crosby E C, Humphrey T, Lauer E W 1962 Correlative anatomy of the nervous system. Macmillan, New York
Derouesné C 1973 Le syndrome 'pré-moteur'. Revue Neurologique 128. 353-363
Fahy T J, Irving M H, Millac P 1967 Severe head injuries: a 6 year follow up. Lancet 2: 475–479
Goldstein K, Scheerer M 1941 Abstract and concrete behaviour: an experimental study with special tests. Psychological Monographs 43: 1–151
Grant A D, Berg E A 1948, A behavioral analysis of degree of reinforcement and ease of shifting to new responses in a Weigl-type card sorting. Journal of Experimental Psychology 38: 404–411
Gronwall D 1976 Performance changes during recovery from closed head injury. Proceedings of the Australian Association of Neurologists 13: 143–147

Gronwall D, Sampson 1974 The Psychological Effects of Concussion. Auckland University/Oxford University Press, Auckland

Gronwall D, Wrightson P 1974 Delayed recovery in intellectual function after minor head injury. Lancet 2: 605–609

Gronwall D, Wrightson P 1975 The cumulative effect of concussion. Lancet 2: 995–997

Gurdjian E S 1975 Impact head injury. Thomas, Springfield, Illinois

Gurdjian E G, Lissner H R, Hodgson V R, Patrick L M 1966 Mechanisms of head injury. Clinical Neurosurgery 12: 112–128

Gurdjian E S, Webster J E, Arnkoff H 1943 Acute craniocerebral trauma. Surgery 13: 333–353

Gurdjian E S, Webster J E, Lissner H R 1955 Observations on the mechanism of brain concussion contusion and laceration. Surgery, Gynaecology and Obstetrics 101: 680–690

Hadley D M, Teasdale G M, Jenkins A et al 1988 Magnetic resonance imaging in acute head injury. Clinical Radiology 39: 131–139

Hannay H, Levin H S, Grossman R G 1979 Impaired recognition memory after head injury. Cortex 15: 209–283

Hebb D O 1942 The effect of early and late brain injury upon test scores and the nature of adult intelligence. Proceedings of the American Philosophical Society 85: 275–292

Hebb D O 1949 The organization of behavior. Wiley, New York

Heiden J S, Small R, Caton W, Weiss M H, Kurze T 1979 In: Popp A J et al (eds) Neural trauma. Raven Press, New York

Hillbom E, Jahro L 1969 Post-traumatic Korsakoff syndrome. In: Walker A E, Caveness W F, Critchely M (eds) The late effects of head injury. Thomas Springfield, Illinois p 98–109

Holburn A H S 1943 Mechanics of head injury. Lancet 2: 438–441

Hooper R S 1966 Head injuries: past present and future. Medical Journal of Australia 2: 45–54

Hooper R S 1969 Patterns of acute head injury. Edward Arnold, London

Jamieson K G 1971 A first notebook of head injury, 2nd edn. Butterworth, Sydney, p 31

Jennett B 1976 Prognosis after head injury. In: Vinken P L, Bruyn G W (eds) Handbook of clinical neurology. North-Holland, Amsterdam, vol 24, ch 34, p 669–681

Jennett B, Snoek J, Bond M R, Brooks N 1981 Disability after severe head injury: observations on the use of the Glasgow Outcome Scale. Journal of Neurology, Neurosurgery and Psychiatry 44: 285–293

Jennett B, Bond M 1975 Assessment of outcome after severe brain damage. Lancet 1: 480–484

Jennett B, Teasdale G, Braakman R, Minderhoud J, Knill-Jones R 1976 Predicting outcome in individual patients after severe head injury. Lancet 1: 1031–1034

Jennett W B 1969 Head injuries and the temporal lobe. In: Herrington R N (ed) Current problems in neuropsychiatry: Schizophrenia, epilepsy, the temporal lobe. British Journal of Psychiatry, Special Publication No 4: 40–41

Jennett W B 1981 Prediction of outcome. In: Dining T A R, Connelly T J (eds) Head injuries. Wiley, Brisbane p 119–131

Jones-Gotman M, Milner B 1977 Design fluency: the invention of nonsense drawing after focal cortical lesions. Neuropsychologia 15: 653–674

Kear-Colwell J J, Heller M 1980 The Wechsler Memory Scale and closed head injury. Journal of Clinical Psychology 36: 782–787

Kimble D P 1963 Physiological psychology. Addison-Wesley, Reading, Massachusetts

Kløve H, Cleeland C S 1972 The relationship of neuropsychological impairment to other indices of severity of head injury. Scandinavian Journal of Rehabilitation Medicine 4: 55–60

Konow A, Pribram K H 1970 Error recognition and utilization produced by injury to the frontal cortex in man. Neuropsychologia 8: 489–491

Lehtonen R 1973 Learning memory and intellectual performance in a chronic state of amnesic syndrome. In: Jahro L (ed) Korsakoff-like amnesic syndrome in penetrating brain injury. Acta Neurologica Scandanavica Supplementum 54: 107–133

Levin H S, Amparo E, Eisebberg H M et al 1987 Magnetic resonance imaging and computerized tomography in relation to the neurobehavioral sequelae of mild and moderate head injuries. Journal of Neurosurgery 66: 706–713

Levin H S, Amparo E G, Eisenberg H M et al 1989 Magnetic resonance imaging after closed head injury in children. Neurosurgery 24: 223–227

Levin H S, Benton A L, Grossman R G 1982 Neurobehavioral consequences of closed head injury. Oxford University Press, New York

Levin H S, Eisenberg H M 1979 Neuropsychological outcome of closed head injury in children and adolescents. Child's Brain 5: 281–292

Levin H S, Grafman J, Eisenberg H M (eds) 1987 Neurobehavioral recovery from head injury. Oxford University Press, New York

Levin H S, Grossman R G, Rose J E, Teasdale G 1979 Longterm neuropsychological outcome of closed head injury. Journal of Neurosurgery 50: 412–422

Levin H S, Grafman J, Eisenberg H M (eds) 1987 Neurobehavioral recovery from head injury. Oxford University Press, New York

Levin H S, O'Donnell V M, Grossman R G 1979 The Galveston Orientation and Amnesia Test: a practical scale to assess cognition after head injury. Journal of Nervous and Mental Disease 167: 675–684

Lewin W, Marshall T F, DeC Roberts A J 1979 Longterm outcome after severe head injury. British Medical Journal 2: 1533-1538

Lezak M D 1978a Subtle sequelae of brain damage: perplexity, distractibility and fatigue. American Journal of Physical Medicine 57: 9–15

Lezak M D 1978b Living with the characterologically altered brain injured patient. Journal of Clinical Psychiatry 39: 592–598

Lezak M D 1979a Recovery of memory and learning functions following traumatic brain injury. Cortex 15: 63–72

Lezak M D 1979b Personal communication

Lezak M D 1981 Assessing initiative, planning, and executive capabilities. Bulletin of the Postgraduate Committee in Medicine, University of Sydney, Supplement, 53–58

Lindenberg R, Freytag E 1957 Morphology of cortical contusions. Archives of Pathology 63: 23–42

Lindenberg R, Freytag E 1960 The mechanism of cerebral contusions: a pathologic-anatomic study. Archives of Pathology 69: 440–469

Lishman W A 1973 The psychiatric sequelae of head injury: a review. Psychological Medicine 3: 304–318

Luria A R 1969 Frontal lobe syndromes. In: Vinken P J, Bruyn G W (eds) Handbook of clinical neurology. North-Holland, Amsterdam, vol 2, ch 23

Luria A R 1973 The working brain. Allen Lane Penguin Press, London

Luria A R, Homskaya E D 1964 Disturbance in the regulative role of speech with frontal lobe lesions. In: Warren J M, Akert K (eds) The frontal granular cortex and behavior. McGraw Hill, New York, ch 17

Luria A R, Homskaya E D, Blinkov S M, Critchley M 1967 Impaired selectivity of mental processes in association with a lesion of the frontal lobe. Neuropsychologia 6: 97–104

Luria A R, Pribram K H, Homskaya E D 1964 An experimental analysis of the behavioural disturbance produced by a left frontal arachnoidal endothelioma (meningioma). Neuropsychologia 2: 257–280

Luria A R, Sokolov E N, Klimkovsky M 1967 Towards a neuro-dynamic analysis of memory disturbances with lesions of the left temporal lobe. Neuropsychologia 5: 1012

Luria A R, Tsvetkova L S 1964 The programming of constructive activity in local brain injuries. Neuropsychologia 2: 95–108

Luria A R, Tsvetkova L S 1967 Les troubles de la résolution des problèmes. Analyse neuropsychologique. Gauthier–Villars, Paris

McClelland R J 1988 Psychosocial sequelae of head injury: anatomy of a relationship. British Journal of Psychiatry 153: 141–146

McFie J, Thompson J A 1972 Picture Arrangement: a measure of frontal lobe friction? British Journal of Psychiatry 121: 547–552

Mandelberg I A, Brooks D N 1975 Cognitive recovery after severe head injury. 1: Serial testing on the Wechsler Adult Intelligence Scale. Journal of Neurology, Neurosurgery and Psychiatry 38: 1121–1126

Messerli P, Seron X, Tissot R 1979 Quelques aspects des troubles de la programmation dans le syndrome frontal. Archives Suisses de Neurologie, Neurochirurgie et de Psychiatrie 125: 23–35

Miller E 1979 The long-term consequences of head injury: a discussion of the evidence with special reference to the preparation of legal reports. British Journal of Social and Clinical Psychology 18: 87–98

Miller H, Stern G 1965 The long term prognosis of severe head injury. Lancet 1: 225-229

Milner B 1963 Effects of different brain lesions on card sorting. Archives of Neurology 9: 90–100

Milner B 1964 Some effects of frontal lobectomy in man. In: Warren J M, Akert K (eds) The frontal granular cortex and behaviour. McGraw–Hill, New York

Milner B 1965 Visually-guided maze learning in man: effects of bilateral hippocampal, bilateral frontal and unilateral cerebral lesions. Neuropsychologia 3: 317–338

Milner B 1971 Interhemispheric differences in the localisation of psychological processes in man. British Medical Bulletin 27: 272–277

Najenson T, Groswasser Z, Mendelson L, Hackett P 1980 Rehabilitative outcome of brain damaged patients after severe head injury. International Rehabilitation Medicine 2: 17–22

Newcombe F 1982 The psychological consequences of closed head injury: assessment and rehabilitation. Injury 14: 111–136

Newcombe F, Artiola i Fortuny L 1979 Problems and perspectives in the evaluation of psychological deficits after cerebral lesions. International Rehabilitation Medicine 1: 182

Oddy M, Humphrey M, Uttley D 1978a Stress upon relatives of head injury patients. British Journal of Psychiatry 133: 507–513

Oddy M, Humphrey M, Uttley D 1978b Subjective impairment of social recovery after closed head injury. Journal of Neurology, Neurosurgery and Psychiatry 41: 611–616

Oddy M, Humphrey M 1980 Social recovery during the year following severe head injury. Journal of Neurology, Neurosurgery and Psychiatry 43: 798–802

Ommaya A K, Gennarelli T A 1974 Cerebral concussion and traumatic unconsciousness. Brain 97: 633–654

Penfield W, Evans J 1935 The frontal lobe in man: a clinical study of maximum removals. Brain 58: 115–133

Perret E 1974 The left frontal lobe of man and the suppression of habitual responses in verbal categorical behaviour. Neuropsychologia 12: 323–330

Pimental P A, Kingsbury N A 1989 Neuropsychological aspects of right brain injury. Pro-ed, Austin, Texas

Porteus S D 1958 What do the Maze Tests measure? Australian Journal of Psychology 10: 245–256

Porteus S D 1959 Recent Maze Test studies. British Journal of Medical Psychology 32: 38–43

Porteus S D 1965 Porteus Maze Test: fifty years' application. Pacific, Palo Alto, California

Porteus S D, Kepner R DeM 1944 Mental changes after bilateral prefrontal lobotomy. Genetic Psychology Monographs 29: 4

Porteus S D, Peters H N 1947 Psychosurgery and test validity. Journal of Abnormal and Social Psychology 42: 473–475

Ramier A M, Hécaen H 1970 Rôle respectif des atteintes frontales et de la latéralisation lésionelle dans les déficits de la 'fluence verbale'. Revue Neurologique 123: 17–22

Rappaport M, Hall K M, Hopkins K, Belleza T, Cope D N 1982 Disability rating scale for severe head trauma: coma to community. Archives of Physical Medicine and Rehabilitation 63: 118–123

Reitan R M 1972 Verbal problem solving as related to cerebral damage. Perceptual and Motor Skills 34: 515–524

Rowbotham G F 1964 Acute injuries of the head, 4th edn. Churchill Livingstone, Edinburgh

Russell E W 1980 Fluid and crystallized intelligence: effects of diffuse brain damage on the WAIS. Perceptual and Motor Skills 51: 121–122

Russell W R 1932 Cerebral involvement in head injury. Brain 55: 549–603

Russell W R 1935 Amnesia following head injuries. Lancet 2: 762–763

Russell W R 1971 The traumatic amnesias. Oxford University Press, New York

Russell W R, Espir M L E 1961 Traumatic aphasia. A study of aphasia in war wounds of the brain. Oxford University Press, New York

Russell W R, Nathan P W 1946 Traumatic amnesia. Brain 69: 183–187

Russell W R, Smith A 1961 Post-traumatic amnesia in closed head injury. Archives of Neurology 5: 4–17

Rzechorzek A J 1978 A qualitative analysis of functional disturbances resulting from unilateral frontal lobe lesions in man. Unpublished Master of Arts thesis, University of Melbourne

Sampson H 1956 Pacing and performance on a serial addition task. Canadian Journal of Psychology 10: 219–225

Shores E A 1989 Comparison of the Westmead PTA Scale and Glasgow Coma Scale following extremely severe head injury. Journal of Neurology, Neurosurgery and Psychiatry 52: 126–127

Shores E A, Marosszeky J E, Sandanam J, Batchelor J 1986 Preliminary validation of a clinical scale for measuring the duration of post-traumatic amnesia. Medical Journal of Australia 144: 569–572

Strich S J 1969 The Pathology of brain damage due to blunt head injuries. In: Walker A E, Caveness W F, Critchley M (eds) The late effects of head injury. Thomas, Springfield, Illinois

Stroop J R 1935 Studies of interference in serial verbal reactions. Journal of Experimental Psychology 18: 643–662

Stuss D T 1987 Contribution of frontal lobe injury to cognitive impairment after closed head injury: methods of assessment and recent findings. In: Levin H S, Graftman J, Eisenberg H M (eds)

Neurobehavioral recovery from head injury. Oxford University Press, New York

Stuss D T, Benson D F 1986 The frontal lobes. Raven, New York

Tate R L, Lulham J M, Strettles B 1982 Severe head injury. Outcome, impact and adjustment. In: Brain impairment. Proceedings of the fifth annual brain impairment conference, Bulletin of the Postgraduate Committee in Medicine (supplement), University of Sydney.

Teasdale G, Jennett B 1974 Assessment of coma and impaired consciousness: a practical scale. Lancet 2: 81–84

Teuber H L 1964 The riddle of frontal lobe function in man. In: Warren J M, Akert K (eds) The frontal granular cortex and behavior. McGraw–Hill, New York, ch 20

Walsh K W 1960 Surgical modification of the personality. Unpublished Master's thesis, University of Melbourne

Walsh K W 1982 Neuropsychological aspects of rehabilitation following brain injury. In : Garrett J F (ed) International Exchange of Information in Rehabilitation 19: 36–40

Walsh K W 1987 Neuropsychology: a clinical approach, 2nd edn. Churchill Livingstone, Edinburgh

Warwick R, Williams P L (eds) 1973 Gray's anatomy, 35th edn. Longman, Edinburgh

Wechsler D 1944 The measurement of adult intelligence. Williams and Wilkins, Baltimore

Whitty C W M, Zangwill O L 1977 Amnesia: clinical psychological and medicolegal aspects, 2nd edn. Butterworths, London

Wilberger J E, Deeb Z, Rothfus W 1987 Magnetic resonance imaging in cases of severe head injury. Neurosurgery 20: 571–576

Wilson J T, Wiedmann K D, Hadley D M, Condon B, Teasdale G, Brooks D N 1988 Early and late magnetic resonance imaging and neuropsychological outcome. Journal of Neurology, Neurosurgery and Psychiatry 51: 391–396

Zangwill O 1978 Personal communication

6. Cerebrovascular disorders

The term cerebrovascular disorder can be taken to mean any disruption of brain function arising from some pathological process related to the blood vessels. Such disorders are among the most common in the practice of neurology and present an array of problems of bewildering complexity. In order for neuropsychology to progress in this area, a basic understanding of anatomy and pathology is needed, together with clinical experience with a wide range of disorders in various stages of evolution and resolution. It is not surprising then that neuropsychological studies of stroke are sparse. Even to understand the literature requires the grasp of a new terminology. For this reason key terms are defined in the glossary at the end of the review section of this chapter.

The vascular pathology may take many forms, e.g. lesions of the walls of the blood vessels themselves in the form of deposited material (atheroma) with or without ulceration, rupture of the vessel wall itself, narrowing (stenosis) or total occlusion of the lumen from thickening of the vessel wall or the presence of an obstructing clot (thrombus) or embolus, or changes in the characteristics of the blood itself.

Neuropsychological deficits are among the most common sequelae of cerebrovascular disease yet, despite the overwhelming importance shown by epidemiological studies (Wylie 1972, Kurtzke 1976), only one text (Benton 1970) has devoted itself solely to this important area. Despite the excellence of this latter work and the passing of two decades which have seen great progress in understanding the pathophysiology, little has been added to our systematized knowledge of the neuropsychological consequences. This is due in no small part to the complexity of the area coupled with the lack of neurological experience in the training of many neuropsychologists.

In no other area of brain impairment are neuropsychological deficits so likely to be overlooked or underestimated than in cerebrovascular disorders, where striking neurological conditions such as hemiplegia capture the attention of clinicians. yet a full appreciation of these disorders of higher function may play a vital role in determining the success or otherwise of management and rehabilitation. The situation is closely akin to that of the head injured patient where the psychosocial factors have been shown to be so decisive in determining outcome. Considering this, it is surprising that there are still so few studies relating neuropsychological indices to outcome of stroke.

207

PATHOLOGICAL CONDITIONS

The types of cerebrovascular disease are numerous but the majority of cases are due to ischaemia or haemorrhage. Cerebral ischaemia may be transient with symptoms which recover. Any prolonged ischaemia will lead to death of tissue, or infarction. The most common cause of infarction is thromboembolism and this accounts for two thirds of all cases of cerebrovascular disability. 15–25% of cases are due to intracerebral or subarachnoid haemorrhage, while the remaining 5–10% are due to less common causes.

CEREBRAL INFARCTION

The basic pathological process in infarction is atherosclerosis. This is not a uniform process but one which affects certain parts of the arterial system more than others. The deposition of material, mostly cholesterol, causes plaques which narrow the artery and thus restrict the flow. This may progress to complete occlusion of the affected vessel. Whether infarction occurs depends upon whether there is a collateral source of supply for the affected region (see below). However, in general, the size of an infarct depends to a large extent on the size of the vessel occluded. This may range from the minute to massive death of a large part of the hemisphere due to sudden occlusion of an internal carotid artery.

There are certain sites of predilection in the formation of atheromatous plaques, mostly where arteries branch or bifurcate. The most common sites are the origin of the internal carotid artery, the upper end of the vertebrals and the lower portion of the basilar, the stem of the middle cerebral, and the posterior cerebral, though other vessels are also commonly affected. The plaques may ulcerate and the debris which collects, e.g. platelets, fibrin and cholesterol, may detach in the form of emboli and travel further afield to block smaller vessels. The operation of endarterectomy has proved valuable in preventing this catastrophe. However, the most common cause of cerebral embolism arises from thrombi forming in the heart due to arrhythmias or myocardial infarction.

The symptoms and signs of infarction will reflect the loss of function in the territory of the affected vessels. In larger infarction there may be swelling which may affect the function of nearby regions. Using positron emission tomography Kuhl et al (1980) have shown disturbance of cerebral function at sites remote from an ischaemic area. This provides strong support for functional examinations, including neuropsychological assessment, which are not focussed solely on the obvious area of deficit as shown by CT scan.

Anatomy of the cerebral arteries

An understanding of the normal arterial anatomy, the normal arterial perfusion areas, and the more common anomalous arterial configurations is important in clinicopathological correlation of 'stroke' syndromes (McCormick & Schochet 1976).

The patterns of deficit associated with occlusion of the various major cerebral vessels are sufficiently consistent over a large series of cases to be abstracted in the form of classical syndromes. However, the features present in any single case may differ, often considerably, according to a number of factors. One of these sources of difference arises from the fact that the arrangement and distribution of vessels are subject to a degree of individual variation even without the presence of pathology. The pattern of distribution described in standard anatomical texts must be thought of as a modal one, not necessarily present in all cases. Detailed anatomy of the cerebrovascular supply can be found in Kaplan & Ford 1966, Salamon 1971, Krayenbuhl & Yasargil 1972. The knowledge gained from traditional neuroanatomy has been greatly expanded by more recent methods such as cerebral angiography and regional cerebral blood flow.

The effects on the brain of occlusion of a blood vessel will depend on a number of factors, the principal of which are:

1. the availability of collateral or anastomotic channels
2. rate of occlusion
3. blood pressure—insufficient pressure may reduce the effectiveness of the anastomotic circulation
4. the presence of anomalous circulation.

Collaterals, anastomoses and anomalies

These terms are often used interchangeably but have different meanings. Collaterals are vessels which serve a common end point, e.g. the two vertebral arteries run in parallel to supply the single basilar artery and thus either may serve effectively for the other in the case of narrowing (stenosis) or occlusion. 'Anastomoses, on the other hand, are interconnections of a network character in one or between two or more functionally separate systems allowing the possibility of draining blood from them.' (Zülch 1971). The arterial circle (circle of Willis) provides such a naturally occurring anastomosis joining the left and right carotid circulations with that of the vertebrobasilar supply. Anastomoses may also arise or enlarge in other situations in response to pathological conditions in parts of the circulation. The adequacy of such alternative supply routes will depend in large part on the rate of occlusion. A slowly occluding vessel will allow time for adequate anastomotic channels to open up so that complete occlusion of a vessel as major as the internal carotid artery may occur without observable clinical evidence, whereas the sudden occlusion of a smaller vessel may bring serious lasting neurological deficit. To such structural factors will be added dynamic factors such as blood pressure changes and blood viscosity.

Deviations from the modal distribution may occur in the absence of pathology. Such anomalies are described in the anatomical works cited. An extreme example is provided by Toole & Patel (1974, fig 1-4). Examples of these anomalies would be where the two anterior cerebral arteries arise from a common stem or where the posterior cerebral artery receives its supply from the anterior circulation (internal carotid artery) rather than the posterior circulation (basilar artery). The fact that many cases of undoubted cerebral infarction do not conform to any of the classical syndromes referable to specific arteries attests to the variability in distribution and the presence of anastomotic channels.

Major arteries of the brain and associated disorders

The brain is supplied by two major systems, the internal carotid and the vertebrobasilar. These have communication with each other at the base of the brain in the arterial circle. The paired internal carotid arteries divide into two major terminal branches on each side, the anterior and middle cerebral arteries, to be described later. The single basilar artery is formed by the two vertebral arteries. Its branches supply the brain stem and cerebellum before terminating in the left and right posterior arteries which supply posterior and inferior structures of the cerebrum.

The following outline is restricted to a description of the distribution of the three major arteries, the anterior, middle, and posterior cerebrals, together with a brief outline of the consequences of pathology affecting their territories of supply. In keeping with the aim of the text, emphasis is placed on disorders of higher function. More detailed neurological accounts may be found in Toole & Patel 1974, Adams & Victor 1977, Bannister 1978. A particularly detailed treatment is provided in volume 1 of the textbook on stroke edited by Barnett et al (1986).

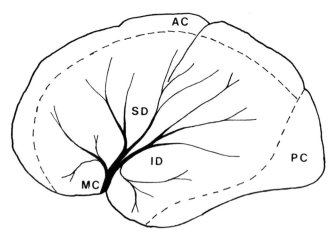

Fig. 6.1 Middle cerebral artery (MC): SD, superior division; ID, inferior division. AC, anterior cerebral artery territory; PC, posterior cerebral artery territory.

The anterior cerebral artery (Figs. 6.1, 6.3)

The anterior cerebral artery is joined a short distance from its origin to its paired artery of the other side by the anterior communicating artery, a vessel often only millimetres in length. Deep penetrating branches arise between the origin and the communication. There are several fine branches and one long penetrating branch (the medial striate artery or recurrent artery of Heubner). The fine branches supply anterior diencephalic nuclei, the anterior commissure and the genu of the corpus callosum. The long branch supplies the anterior part of the internal capsule and part of the putamen, pallidum and caudate nucleus.

Beyond the communicating artery cortical branches supply the anterior two-thirds or so of the medial aspect of the hemisphere as far as the parieto-occipital sulcus. Their territory also extends a little way over the superomedial border as well as the medial portion of the inferior surface of the frontal lobe. Another major branch, the pericallosal artery, supplies the anterior four-fifths of the corpus callosum.

As Adams & Victor comment: 'Well studied cases of infarction of the territory of this artery are not numerous; hence the syndromes are imperfectly known' (1977, p 1506). However, it is well established that occlusion of one anterior cerebral beyond the communicating vessel leads to contralateral paralysis of the foot and leg with relative sparing of the upper limb and complete sparing of the face.

However, three disorders of higher function associated with anterior cerebral artery pathology are of interest to neuropsychologists. These are adynamia, aphasia and amnesia. Less common disorders in the form of partial disconnection syndromes may arise in conjunction with damage to the anterior portion of the corpus callosum. Such disorders are quite likely to be overlooked unless appropriate methods of examination are undertaken (Beukelman et al 1980).

Adynamia. This condition was mentioned in the preceding chapter. In its extreme form it is termed akinetic mutism, a state first described by Cairns et al (1941) and subsequently reported with a variety of deeply placed brain lesions (Skultety 1968). The patient gives a clear impression of being alert and aware of his surroundings and yet remains inert and neither proffers any verbal utterance nor replies to questioning. It may even appear that the patient is being deliberately silent. The mutism is accompanied by a profound lack of general activity. The condition is particularly associated with destruction of midline structures, the deep parts of the frontal lobes, septal nuclei and cingulate gyrus. Perhaps the crucial lesion is one which disconnects the frontal cortex from the midbrain reticular formation (Segarra & Angelo 1970). It may be a prominent feature after haemorrhage from an aneurysm of the anterior communicating artery or its associated surgery, though it also occurs with occlusion of deep penetrating arteries at the upper end of the basilar artery. In this context, adynamia was a prominent feature in Case PN (below).

Akinetic mutism can be intractable or undergo full or partial resolution. The latter is often termed abulia, a condition differing largely in degree and characterized by a lack of spontaneity in word and deed, anergia and psychomotor retardation. The patient may be temporarily roused by external stimulation only to lapse back into the passive state when it is removed.

Aphasia. Critchley's exhaustive description of syndromes associated with the anterior cerebral artery (Critchley 1930) mentioned the occasional presence of aphasia without specifying the nature of the language disorder. More recent reports suggest that the disorder is closely akin to what Wernicke termed 'transcortical motor aphasia' (Rubens 1976, Damasio & Kassel 1978, Alexander & Schmitt 1979) though the two conditions are not necessarily identical. The condition may be related in part to damage to the supplementary motor area. Muteness appears at the onset, to be followed by great difficulty in speech initiation though repetition and comprehension of speech remain relatively intact. As described in the preceding section, verbal adynamia may be accompanied by a more general behavioural adynamia. Comprehension of written material is also said to be poor, especially for more complex linguistic structures.

Amnesia. The earliest report of amnesia following subarachnoid haemorrhage was possibly that of Flateau (1921). Subsequent investigators reported an incidence of around 2–3% after such haemorrhage (Tarachow 1939, Walton 1953). However, it was Norlén & Olivecrona (1953) who noted the specific association with anterior communicating artery aneurysms in two cases after surgery. Subsequently this association was confirmed by themselves and others (Lindqvist & Norlén 1966, Logue et al 1968, Sengupta et al 1975, Luria 1976). The amnesia, which bears a striking resemblance to the Korsakoff amnesic syndrome, appears in the immediate post-operative state in a proportion of cases which varies considerably from study to study. The acute state is marked by confusion, temporo-spatial disorientation and confabulation. Even in the acute state, immediate memory (as represented by digit span) is preserved. As the acute state clears the patient is noted to have a general amnesic syndrome. In the majority of cases this amnesia improves, though it may take months to do so. A small proportion of patients are left with a lasting, stable amnesia. There have been only a few cases in which a detailed specification of the amnesia has been attempted (Talland et al 1967, Brion et al 1968, Luria 1976).

Our own experience accords well with the recent description of the neuropsychological characteristics of two cases by Volpe & Hirst (1983) (see case ZQ below): (1) intact immediate memory; (2) non-specific anterograde amnesia marked by great susceptibility to proactive interference; and (3) differentially better recognition memory than spontaneous recall with patients showing some improvement with cued recall. Volpe & Hirst comment: 'The high recognition scores for our patients may be peculiar to this form of amnesia.'(op. cit. p 707).

These two cases are of importance since it was established by operative observation and CT scan that there was no evidence of obvious focal brain damage while arteriography had clearly established that both patients had arterial vasospasm.

The anatomical dependence of this form of amnesia is far from clear and there do not appear to be any cases where post-mortem histopathological changes have been correlated with prior neuropsychological status. Several features of the amnesia, however, stamp it as belonging to the thalamic rather than the hippocampal form of amnesic disorder.

The distinction between these two forms of the amnesic syndrome was put forward by Lhermitte & Signoret (1972) and supported by the studies of Mattis et al (1978) as well as clinical observations. A notable difference, if not the main one, relates to the 'familiarity' aspect of recognition memory. Simpson (1969) suggested that what he termed coincidence detection circuits may be related to the temporal lobes. These were conceptualized as the matching of present input with past experience. Thus, a mismatch might occur in two directions producing experiences of déjà vu or jamais vu. Such disorders of coincidence detection do not appear with lesions outside the temporal lobes. If such temporal circuits are preserved, as they should be in frontomamillo-thalamic lesions, then there is a possible explanation for the preservation of key aspects of recognition memory and the related benefit from cued recall of thalamic cases such as those described by Barbizet et al (1981) and later in this chapter, whereas cases with hippocampal lesions do not benefit in this way.

Recently Gade (1982) has reported a series of cases followed for two years. They have a striking similarity to case ZQ (below) in the form of a severe and stable amnesia although, like our case, some of the patients improved in their orientation over the period and some had better memory of personal affairs. Many lacked drive and initiative. Gade reviews the recent anatomical evidence which shows significant penetrating branches arising from or near the anterior communicating artery which supply midline structures. Evidence from this collaborative Danish study together with reappraisal of some previous studies argues strongly in favour of entrapment of these arteries at operation as the probable basis for the amnesic disorder. Conversely, operations sparing these vessels seem much freer of the amnesic complication.

The middle cerebral artery (Figs. 6.1, 6.3)

A short distance from its origin the middle cerebral artery divides into a superior and inferior division. Before doing so it gives rise to deep penetrating branches which supply parts of the globus pallidus, internal capsule and caudate nucleus. These vessels stop short of the thalamus. The superior division supplies the lateral orbitofrontal and dorsolateral prefrontal areas, the greater part of the premotor, motor and somatosensory cortex and the anterior parietal region. This zone includes anterior language areas (including Broca's area) in the dominant hemisphere. The inferior division supplies the temporal pole, anterior and posterior temporal regions down to the inferior temporal gyrus, together with the angular gyrus and posterior parietal region. Thus it embraces the posterior language areas (including Wernicke's area).

Symptomatology will depend on the side of occlusion. Total occlusion is followed by contralateral hemiplegia, hemisensory loss and hemianopia. Lesions on the dominant side also give rise to aphasia while non-dominant occlusions produce spatial disorders.

The superior division is more often occluded than the inferior. Superior occlusion also gives rise to a dense sensory and motor loss, and aphasia, which may be global in the early stages, but which becomes predominantly a non-fluent aphasia with improvement in comprehension. Since a good portion of the dorsolateral cortex may be included in the affected territory, there may be subtle yet disruptive intellectual disorders that may be masked by the non-fluent dysphasia. Collaboration between the neuropsychologist and the speech therapist may be productive in these cases.

The inferior division is less often occluded. Occlusion on the dominant side produces a fluent aphasia while that on the non-dominant side produces spatial disorders.

It should be noted that dominant lesions also produce spatial difficulties that may be overlooked because of the dysphasia. They appear to differ qualitatively as well as quantitatively from those of the non-dominant side. Finally, lesions of both arterial divisions may produce homonymous hemianopia.

The posterior cerebral artery (Figs. 6.2, 6.3)

The first part or stem of the artery runs around the midbrain to the medial aspect of the temporal lobe, then along the calcarine region of the occipital lobe to the occipital pole. In the early part of its course the posterior cerebral artery gives off penetrating arteries to the tegmentum of the midbrain, subthalamus, the medial posterior part of the thalamus, the mamillary bodies and hypothalamus. Further along, the artery gives off penetrating branches to both medial and lateral geniculate bodies and the posteroventral and superior lateral nuclei of the thalamus.

The superficial branches are the anterior and posterior temporal, hippocampal, calcarine and parieto-occipital arteries, each supplying the named territories (Fig. 6.2). The hippocampal branch may consist of a number of small, separate branches or a single branch which later gives rise to multiple branches (often likened to a candelabrum).

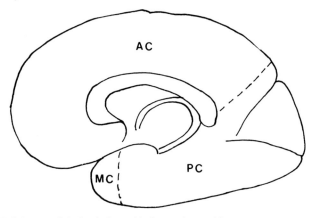

Fig. 6.2   Medial aspect of the hemisphere with three major arterial areas.

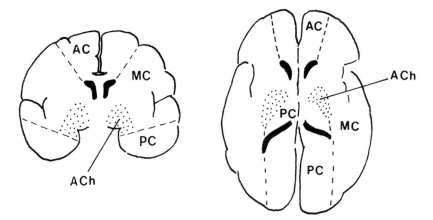

Fig. 6.3   Arterial supply of deep brain structures from the three major arteries and the anterior choroidal artery (A Ch), which is usually a branch of the internal cartoid artery.

Syndromes of the posterior cerebral artery may be classified as cortical and subcortical.

The subcortical disorders include severe sensory loss (the thalamic syndrome), paralysis of vertical gaze, extra-pyramidal movement disorders, stupor, homonymous hemianopia and occasionally, amnesia. The latter disorder is discussed under the lacunar state.

Cortical syndromes also produce homonymous hemianopia or upper quadrantanopia. Bilateral lesions produce cortical blindness. This is accompanied in the acute stages by confusion and by a general amnesic syndrome in the resolving phase. Some degree of memory difficulty may remain even after restitution of a fair degree of visual function. Cortical blindness accompanied by denial of the deficit is termed Anton's syndrome.

Pure alexia (alexia without agraphia, word blindness). This form of reading difficulty consists of failure to recognize words, without evidence of dysphasia in the form of speech and writing disorders seen with middle cerebral artery lesions. A right homonymous hemianopia is almost always present though the presence of this field defect serves as evidence for the location of the lesion and does not explain the reading difficulty, since patients with homonymous hemianopia from more anteriorly placed lesions do not have alexia.

The lesion is such that it disconnects the intact visual analysis in the non-dominant hemisphere from the language zones of the dominant hemisphere. Usually there is

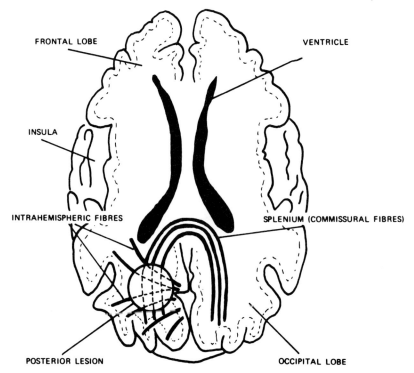

Fig. 6.4   Lesion producing alexia without agraphia (from Walsh 1987).

damage to part of the occipital lobe and fibres of the splenium of the corpus callosum (Fig. 6.4). More detail is provided in Walsh (1987) and other texts of neuropsychology.

Amnesia with posterior vascular lesions. Memory problems attributable to posterior cerebral arterial ischaemia may be of a transient or permanent nature. Occasionally, after several transient amnesic episodes, the patient may die of a massive vascular accident. Lasting disorders with the major features of the general amnesic syndrome have been described with bilateral infarction in the territories of the two posterior cerebral arteries. The patient of Victor et al (1961) who was followed for five years showed:

> . . . a profound defect in recent memory and inability to learn new facts and skills. His general intellectual functions remained at a 'bright normal' level, although certain mild and relatively inconspicuous abnormalities were disclosed by the tests designed to measure concentration, shifting of mental set, and abstract thinking. He also showed an incomplete retrograde amnesia, covering the two-year period prior to the onset of his illness. His memory for remote events was virtually unaffected.

Post-mortem examination of the brain showed old bilateral infarctions in the inferomedial portions of the temporal lobes. Since that time further studies have described the association of serious memory defect in life with post-mortem evidence of bilateral infarction in the territory of the posterior cerebral arteries (Boudin et al 1967, Boudin et al 1968, De Jong et al 1968, 1969).

Benson et al (1974) reported the acute onset of amnesia in ten patients, associated with unilateral or bilateral visual field defects clearly due to posterior cerebral artery territory infarction. In our experience there is always CT evidence of infarction in such cases.

A severe amnesia may be produced by infarction in the dominant hemisphere only (Geschwind & Fusillo 1966, Mohr et al 1971). It is possible that, because of the common use of largely verbal or verbally mediated tests of memory, these cases may appear to be instances of the general amnesic syndrome rather than, as we believe, cases of severe verbal-specific memory deficits. It is also possible that there may be bilateral but asymmetrical involvement of the posterior regions with pathological emphasis on the dominant side.

Whatever turns out to be the cause, severe memory impairment seems more related to the dominant than the non-dominant hemisphere in unilateral cases. The predominant mechanism of production of amnesia may be involvement of the inferomedial parts of the temporal lobes including the hippocampus. Amnesia produced by infarction of the paramedian arteries is outlined below (see under 'lacunar state').

Transient global amnesia (TGA). This term was coined by Fisher & Adams (1964) for a condition described earlier by Bender (1956) and Guyotat & Courjon (1956). It is most commonly seen in patients over 50 and is usually a single event lasting a variable time, but most commonly four to eight hours. The attack is characterized by confusion during which the patient has repetitive queries and shows a total inability to form any new memories. There is retrograde amnesia during the attack for events extending back for days, or in some cases even years, before the present but, as the confusion and anterograde amnesia clear, the retrograde amnesia shrinks to leave only amnesia for the period of the attack itself or slightly longer. There are usually no accompanying neurological signs and symptoms. On some occasions the episode or episodes appear to have been precipitated by special circumstances such as immersion in cold or hot water, sexual intercourse, or highly emotional experience. For reviews see Caplan et al (1981) and Fisher (1982).

Pathophysiology. Until recently the most common opinion was that the condition was due to temporary ischaemia in the territory of the posterior cerebral arteries, though Fisher (1982) strongly opposed this view and believed that the greater part of the evidence was consistent with cerebral seizure. This explanation is now most unlikely. Cole et al (1987) described a case with the onset of TGA while undergoing electroencephalography. The latter remained normal. Miller et al (1987) carried out EEG in 13 episodes of TGA in 13 patients, none of whom showed epileptiform activity in their records, and EEG examinations in nearly 100 patients after their attacks also failed to find support for an epileptic explanation. Similar negative results are provided by Jacome (1989).

It is possible that the clinical condition may, in fact, have a number of causes. Though it is unusual to find a cause, some cases with a proven vascular aetiology support the local ischaemia hypothesis (Ponsford & Donnan 1980). Such a case is described in detail below (Case KN). However, TGA appears to differ from classical attacks of transient ischaemia (TIAs) in that the latter but not the former are associated with occlusive vascular disease in the extracranial circulation (Feuer & Weinberger 1987).

Neuropsychological testing. With the growing interest in TGA, especially as a tool for the understanding of the neural basis of memory functions, there have been a number of reports of test findings both during and after the attacks. Two recent series totalling 11 cases have been particularly well documented (Kritchevsky et al 1987, Kritchevsky & Squire 1989, Hodges & Ward 1989). In essence the transient condition closely resembles the lasting general amnesic syndrome of central origin following bilateral damage to the medial temporal or medial diencephalic regions. For this reason the present author would prefer the term transient *general* amnesia for the condition. The test features are:

1. Preservation of immediate memory (not seen in the *global* amnesia of conditions such as Alzheimer's disease).
2. Anterograde amnesia for both verbal and nonverbal material, i.e. a general versus a specific amnesia. On occasions we have noted cases where nonverbal memory does not appear to be as severely affected as verbal memory. Okada et al (1987) describe two such cases whose nonverbal memory also recovered earlier.
3. Some retrograde amnesia. This may be patchy and in the series cited above was highly variable ranging from a day or two to several years. Following the attack this retrograde amnesia shrank rapidly though many were left with a hiatus of a day or two.
4. Other cognitive functions such as language, problem solving, and visuospatial functions are generally well preserved though Kritchevsky et al (1988) reported poor copying of a complex figure and possible difficulty with confrontation naming.

Perhaps more detailed testing will reveal other difficulties. Nevertheless, preservation of other functions stands in stark contrast to the amnesia.

Recovery. Most writers stress the rapid recovery of the faulty memory. In line with this Hodges and Ward (1989) found all of their subjects subjectively normal within 24 hours. However, all of them showed impairment of new learning for at least a week after the attack. This slow restoration is shown by Case KN (below) though it must be admitted that this is not a typical 'neurologically asymptomatic' case. Gallassi et al (1988), in follow-up of their cases, also report what they describe as a fragility of memory for some time after the event. It is possible that further studies utilizing neuropsychological tests will show this to be a common finding.

In recent times the strongest association emerging appears to be with migraine, and modern investigative techniques such as cerebral blood flow studies and positron emission tomography (PET) give some support to a primary neuronal mechanism as a basis. The question of aetiology remains open.

Finally, though there may be a superficial resemblance between TGA and an hysterical or dissociative amnesia (or fugue) there is little difficulty with differential diagnosis provided the episode has been witnessed and reported by a reliable observer.

Vertebrobasilar insufficiency (VBI)

Atherosclerosis in the posterior circulation, viz vertebral, basilar and posterior cerebral arteries, may cause transient attacks of brain stem vascular insufficiency, the most common symptoms being those of vestibular and cerebellar disturbance. Very little attention was paid to possible disorders of higher cerebral function. More recently it has been noted that patients showing symptoms of VBI are often forgetful, have poor concentration and occasionally have attacks of transient global amnesia (Rivera & Meyer 1976). Two small studies (Donnan et al 1978, Ponsford et al 1980) suggest that patients with evidence of chronic VBI may show evidence of a mild memory problem which has the characteristics of an axial amnesia.

Lacunar state (état lacunaire, Marie 1901)

This condition is almost invariably associated with hypertension and atherosclerosis. It takes its name from the cavities or lacunes resulting from absorption of softened material produced by infarcts which are caused by the occlusion of fine penetrating branches of the major brain arteries. The lesions are usually multiple, commonly four to six in number though they may be more numerous. They are usually small in size, 2-15 mm in diameter. Regions most affected are the diencephalon, deep cerebral white matter and brainstem (Fisher 1965, 1968, 1969). This latter author has described the extension of atherosclerosis in these cases from the large vessels, which are the usual site of atheroma, into the finer branches (Adams & Victor 1977). Symptoms will depend on the location and size of the lesions. In general, lacunes have been considered not to produce disorders of higher functions (language, intellect, memory and perception) but largely sensory and motor symptoms (Fisher & Curry 1965, Fisher 1978a,b), and symptoms often undergo apparently complete resolution.

One important exception, in the area of neuropsychological disorder, is the report of memory deficit with infarcts in the thalamus. While some of these infarcts are relatively larger than those traditionally considered under the title of 'lacunes', there is no doubt that quite small, strategically placed lacunes can produce major, lasting amnesic states (see Case PN below). The vascular anatomy of the thalamus has been provided by Percheron (1973, 1976), Lazorthes et al (1976) and others. Of particular interest is the observation that small, strategically placed lesions can disrupt the regions most frequently implicated in the production of the general amnesic syndrome. Castaigne et al (1981) have surveyed the general features of paramedian thalamic and midbrain infarcts. Percheron (1976) has described a not uncommon anatomical variant in the blood supply of these paramedian structures whereby the small vessels on either side of the midline arise from a common pedicle. Occlusion of this pedicle can thus produce bilateral infarction which is the sine qua non for the production of the general or axial amnesic syndrome. Cases of thalamic infarction in which memory disturbance has been a prominent feature have been reported in recent years (Mills & Swanson 1978, von Cramon & Zihl 1979, Schott et al 1980, Barbizet et al 1981) together with CT scan evidence of lesion location. Recent methods of locating the lesions accurately in three dimensions by the use of CT scan methods (Nguyen et al 1980) promises further refinement in studying brain-behaviour correlations.

Finally, recent studies (Speedie & Heilman 1982, 1983) seem to support the evidence which has been accumulating that unilateral thalamic lesions may produce material-specific memory losses according to the double dissociation paradigm—the latter being now well established for mesial temporal lesions, verbal-specific memory loss with dominant hemisphere damage and nonverbal memory loss with non-dominant damage.

Transient ischaemic attacks (TIAs)

This term refers to recurrent attacks of short-lived focal neurological deficit produced by temporary ischaemia. By accepted definition recovery should take place within 24 hours but is often complete within a much shorter time. Although the episodes take many forms they are often rather similar, even stereotyped, in the one individual. The patient experiences sudden loss of neurological function. This may be loss of power which often begins distally but may progress to affect the whole limb or an entire side. There may be sudden sensory loss, particularly loss of vision in one eye (amaurosis fugax, fleeting blindness) or loss of speech, memory or the functions referable to the cerebral hemisphere territories supplied by the internal carotid system. It is unusual for the brain and the eye to be affected simultaneously in one attack. Where the vertebrobasilar system is compromised there may be symptoms such as ataxia and vertigo signalling dysfunction in the cerebellum or brain stem. The attacks vary from infrequent (e.g. less than once per month) to very frequent (several times per day). During the attack the neurological signs will be indistinguishable from a developing infarct but examination between the episodes will be normal.

The term 'reversible ischaemic neurological deficit' has been used by some authors to indicate a neurological deficit of duration somewhat longer than 24 hours but which also shows apparently full clinical recovery (Sahs et al 1979). With the improvement in imaging techniques it appears that the majority of such cases are caused by small infarcts and the older term 'recovered stroke' is still preferred.

This brief description is clinical, and most authorities agree that many different factors may be involved in the attacks in different individuals though they have a very common association with atherosclerosis of the two main blood vessel systems which supply the cranial contents. It is often assumed that ischaemia has occurred without actual death of neurones, but this may not necessarily be the case and the apparent absence of findings may represent the insensitivity of functional measures as well as the relatively 'silent' location of the affected territory. Careful neuropsychological examination sometimes reveals that lasting decrease in higher function is present in some of these cases even where they appear to be neurologically intact between episodes. As in other situations, the decision as to whether 'asymptomatic' is synonymous with the preservation of the integrity of the brain will be a function of the sensitivity and appropriateness of the examinations used. Approximately a third of patients do go on to suffer obvious infarction. In keeping with the higher incidence of atherosclerosis in males than females and in hypertensive patients, some two-thirds of those suffering from TIAs are male or hypertensive or both. Another third will continue to have attacks without any apparent permanent disability, while the remainder will have attacks which cease spontaneously. It is impossible to predict the outcome and this suggests that the term 'TIA' may still be preferable to the terms incipient stroke or impending stroke which have sometimes been used.

Surgical treatment

Two major types of surgical procedure have been devised to prevent strokes and ischaemic attacks by reconstituting the arterial blood flow. The most common is the operation of endarterectomy which aims at correction of stenosis, removal of atheromatous plaques, and removal of organized thrombus and other obstructions compromising the circulation. It is sometimes necessary to remove totally a diseased segment of artery and replace it with a vein graft. The operations are carried out at the sites of predilection for atheroma formation, e.g. at the origin of the internal carotid artery. The indication for operation is usually the presence of transient ischaemic attacks in the territory distal to a radiologically demonstrated stenotic or ulcerated lesion. Neuropsychologists may be called upon to assess patients before and after surgery and there is by now a large number of reports of the results of such examinations.

Occlusive lesions not accessible from the neck may be approached surgically by some form of bypass operation, e.g. where a branch of the external carotid artery such as the superficial temporal artery is grafted via an opening in the skull to a portion of the middle cerebral artery, the so-called transcranial anastomosis. While the effectiveness of endarterectomy in preventing stroke and even in restoring function has become widely established the place of bypass operations is still under evaluation.

CEREBRAL HAEMORRHAGE

Bleeding within the cranial cavity may be due to a large number of causes (see Adams & Victor 1977, p 536). However, three conditions account for the majority of cases. In each condition the severity may vary from a small, almost symptomless bleed to a massive haemorrhage leading to sudden death:

1. Hypertensive intracerebral haemorrhage. This is the most common form of haemorrhage, with extravasation or bursting out of blood into the substance or parenchyma of the cerebral hemisphere. The bleeding destroys brain tissue and, if it continues, causes pressure effects on neighbouring tissue by compression or displacement. Large haemorrhages may so displace vital centres that they lead to death. Less serious pressure may disrupt the function of adjacent or nearby tissue without destroying it and this accounts for the partial, though often considerable, recovery of a function after the acute stages. While the onset of symptoms is rapid, hence the term 'stroke' the full development of the clinical picture may take an appreciable time, sometimes hours, depending on the rate of bleeding and its final cessation. When bleeding stops there is no recurrence from the same site, a situation unlike that of bleeding from aneurysms. While the bleeding may commence in the brain substance, it breaks into the ventricular system and thus into the cerebrospinal fluid in a high proportion of cases.

The accentuation of symptomatology with intracerebral haemorrhage tends to be on neurological rather than behavioural features since the cortex is often relatively spared. Sites of primary haemorrhage, in order of frequency, are the basal ganglia, thalamus, cerebellar hemispheres, pons and subcortical areas. Haemorrhages arise mainly from the penetrating branches of the middle cerebral, posterior cerebral and basilar arteries. The arteries undergo a pathological process which results in irregularity of the lumen and the formation of micro-aneurysms (Charcot-Bouchard aneurysms), which are the probable site of rupture. The subcortical haemorrhages arise from the penetrating branches of arteries on the surface of the brain that supply the deeper layers of the cortex and subjacent white matter. In these cases there is a mixture of cortical and subcortical signs.

2. Ruptured aneurysm. These thin-walled protrusions are most common on the vessels which form the arterial circle (circle of Willis) or their major branches. They are assumed to be developmental defects in the arterial walls and are prone to rupture. Over 90% are found on vessels of the internal carotid system, only a few being on the vertebrobasilar system. The most frequent sites of rupture are the anterior communicating region and the middle cerebral bifurcation, accounting for nearly half the cases. Sometimes the aneurysms are multiple.

In rupturing, blood may be spurted into the subarachnoid space or into the adjacent brain substance, producing an intracerebral haematoma. Bleeding into the cerebral substance is particularly prone to occur at the two most common locations mentioned. The territories of vessels in the areas often show infarction and this is possibly related to arterial vasospasm, since at autopsy the vessels may be patent.

The clinical symptoms and signs are those related to blood under pressure in the subarachnoid space—usually excruciating headache and collapse, followed in survivors by features of local disruption of function due to local pressure from extracerebral blood clot, intracerebral haemorrhage and infarction.

3.   Ruptured arteriovenous malformation (AVM). These developmental malformations vary from a small localized abnormality of a few millimetres to a large mass of vessels occupying considerable space, often in the form of a wedge extending from the cortex to the ventricle. The blood vessels forming the mass interposed between the feeding arteries and the draining veins are pathologically thin-walled and liable to rupture. Rupture of the larger malformations may produce intracerebral as well as subarachnoid bleeding. Like saccular aneurysms, AVMs have a tendency to recurrent bleeding. Hydrocephalus is a complication in some cases. Symptoms and signs will thus be extremely varied.

GLOSSARY

Abulia. A deficit or loss of the ability to make decisions.

Aneurysm. These are usually rounded outpouchings on the cerebral arteries; they occur most frequently at the branching of vessels and are common in certain sites such as the Circle of Willis.

Arteriovenous malformations. These are developmental abnormalities where abnormal communications exist between arteries and veins and may be large enough to form a space-occupying lesion. They may bleed into the substance of the brain or outside, and also rupture into the cerebral ventricles. Many of the constituent vessels are neither typical arteries nor venous channels.

Atherosclerosis. A complex pathological process in which deposits (or plaques) of cholesterol and other materials are laid down within the walls of arteries. The surface over affected areas may ulcerate and these ulcerated plaques may contain atheromatous debris, platelets etc.

Embolism. The sudden blocking of a vessel, most commonly an artery, by fragments of blood clot, atheromatous debris or less commonly by air or fat cells.

Infarct. An area of dead tissue, neurones, supporting cells and small blood vessels, produced by obstruction of an end artery due to thrombosis, embolism, or spasm.

Ischaemia (ischemia). Insufficient blood supply to a part, usually the result of pathology of the blood vessels supplying the part.

Plaque. A localized area of atherosclerosis. A focal accumulation of atheromatous material. (See atherosclerosis)

Stenosis. The narrowing of the space within a tube or the constriction of an orifice.

Stroke. 'The term "stroke" is generally applied to a sudden attack of ischemic or haemorrhagic disorder of the brain, often resulting in a focal neurological deficit, most often paralysis.' (Sahs et al 1979, p 5).

Thromboembolism. Embolism caused by the dislodgement of a thrombus (clot) or part thereof.

Thrombosis. Coagulation within a blood vessel during life.

CASE EXAMPLES

Transient ischaemic attacks

Case: RQ

This 68-year-old woman, who had worked formerly as a cook and then as a psychiatric nurse, presented with a three month history of transient left sided weakness and difficulty with speech. Subsequent questioning of the relatives elicited the fact that there was slurring of speech during the attacks, but their description also raised the possibility of true dysphasia rather than (or in addition to) dysarthria.

Seven years before, RQ had been admitted to hospital following episodes of dysarthria, stuttering and left sided weakness. An arteriogram at that time showed marked stenosis of the right internal carotid artery and mild stenosis at the origin of the left internal carotid. The right hemisphere was largely supplied via anastomoses from the external carotid, the vertebrobasilar system and cross-flow from the left middle cerebral artery. A right internal and external carotid endarterectomy was performed but this was not totally successful.

An arteriogram following the recent admission revealed that both internal carotid arteries were blocked at their origins, with intracranial flow being derived from a complex system of anastomoses. RQ was referred for assessment of her neuropsychological function.

She presented as an intelligent woman despite only basic education. She had always been an avid reader though she was no longer able to concentrate as before. There were no subjective complaints of memory or language difficulties. She had been a capable dressmaker but volunteered that she had to relinquish this hobby as she was no longer able to sew a straight line. An examination of her current intellectual status began with the *Wechsler Memory Scale,* Form I.

Information	5	Digits Total	10 (6,4)
Orientation	5	Visual Reproduction	5
Mental Control	6	Associate Learning	18 (6,1; 6,4; 6,4)
Memory Passages	11.5		
MQ 120			

The only notable finding was the poor Visual Reproduction score compared with the very good verbal learning. The adequacy of verbal learning for a woman of her age was also shown on the *RAVLT:*

List A			List B	List A
Trials	1 2 3 4 5		Recall	Recall
Correct	5 8 11 13 12		8	12

Rey Figure: This was given to extend testing of her visual memory. Her copy was piecemeal and incomplete and she had obvious difficulty in integrating the parts (Fig. 6.5,(a)). Her recall four minutes later reflected the originally disjointed attempt. She had to be encouraged to produce even the few fragments which she managed (Fig. 6.5,(b)). Such a performance seemed typical of degradation of right hemisphere function.

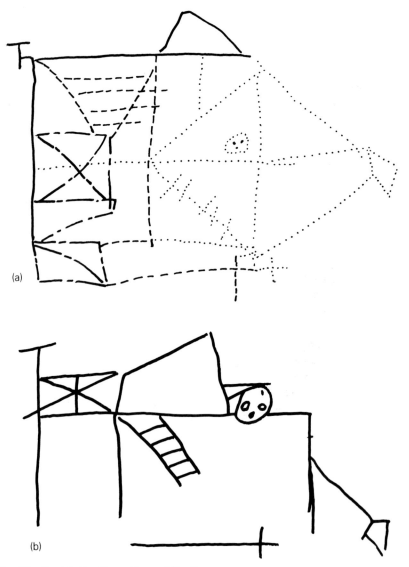

Fig. 6.5   Case RQ. Rey Figure, Copy and Recall.

Her efforts demonstrate both the spatial planning difficulty seen with purely frontal lesions as well as the poor orientation of parts to each other (spatial fragmentation) seen with posterior lesions. It would be difficult in such a case to tease out the relevant contribution, if such exists, of different parts of the brain, but it is noteworthy that her copying of simpler figures was much closer to normal, i.e. the difficulty became more pronounced as the material became complex thus requiring organization.

Associative Word Fluency. This was used as the interpolated task for the Rey Figure and produced a performance (F–10; A–9; S–11) which might be thought to be adequate for her background but was clearly inferior to other verbal performances mentioned below.

WAIS. Basic documentation of her intellectual abilities was completed with certain subtests of the WAIS (age scaled scores in brackets):

Information	16 (16)	Digit Symbol	9 (17)
Comprehension	17 (18)	Block Design	8 (19)
Similarities	16 (19)	Object Assembly	9 (11)

The excellence of many of her performances warns against making too simple an equation between education, occupation and expected cognitive test results. The difficulty she encountered on Block Design appeared to be largely of the frontal problem-solving variety. She had much difficulty with 'embedded' designs but succeeded where single block copying of separate sections of the design would suffice.

Embedded items	2 Fail	4 Pass	6 Fail	8,9,10 Fail
Non-embedded items	1 Pass	3 Pass	5 Pass	7 Pass

She resorted to a good deal of verbalization while struggling to complete the Object Assembly items.

In summary, RQ experienced difficulty with tasks involving visual memory, visuospatial organization, and construction. Such performances are in sharp contrast with very good performances on standard verbal tasks of intelligence and memory. Examination of language throughout her stay revealed no dysphasic elements. In spite of bilateral internal carotid artery occlusion the verbal capabilities probably dependent upon the left hemisphere seemed largely preserved while it was impossible to say whether the observed 'right hemisphere deficits' dated from the time of her right carotid endarterectomy of seven years ago or were, at least in part, of more recent origin.

The following CT scan report arrived after the neuropsychological report had been written. 'An irregular low density area overlies the right fronto-parietal region and, showing no contrast enhancement, probably represents an infarct of long standing duration involving the right middle cerebral artery territory.' The neuropsychological examination seemed consistent with the demonstrated lesion while revealing no evidence of deficits related to other parts of the brain. The adequacy with which anastomotic circulation can support cerebral function if the occlusion takes place slowly is amply illustrated in this case.

Several months later RQ underwent right sided transcranial anastomosis in the fronto-parietal region. Following this her attacks ceased in the six month period of her follow-up. She was able to carry on her home duties effectively apart from her sewing. As is often the case, her mild to moderate constructional apraxia has not intruded on her everyday activities.

Cerebral infarction

Case: VH

This 53-year-old man, who had been suffering from mild diabetes for the preceding four years, had awoken on the morning of his admission to hospital with paraesthesia of the left hand. Within the next hour he described a feeling of 'numbness' in his left arm and leg, and found that his left arm was 'clumsy' and that he was unable to stand. There was some double vision but no other symptoms. He had not experienced any episode of a similar nature before.

On examination he was not distressed and was able to move all limbs though there was clumsiness on attempted skilled movements with the left arm. He was unable to walk, tending to topple to the left, although power in his limbs appeared normal. A left convergent squint was present. Other signs elicited by the attendant neurologist were: (1) Cogan's sign (The patient is asked to deviate his eyes to one side after closing the lids and is then asked to open them. The sign is present if the eyes remain deviated as in this patient whose eyes remained turned to the left); (2) a difficulty in naming objects by touch when they were placed in the left hand (astereognosis); (3) pyramidal ataxia of the left arm; and (4) fine nystagmus to the left. There was no diabetic retinopathy and a CT scan three days after the event reported: 'an area of low density in the right temporal lobe probably represents an artefact.'

The signs and symptoms slowly improved and a neuropsychological assessment was sought after seven days to check for any residual deficit and, if possible, to assist with the localization of the pathological process, which was thought to be either a right hemisphere cortical or parathalamic event. A standard evaluation with the Wechsler Scales showed a relatively well preserved level of functioning on most tests.

Wechsler Memory Scale, Form I

Information	5	Digits Total	13 (8,5)
Orientation	5	Visual Reproduction	9
Mental Control	8	Associate Learning	16 (6,1; 6,2; 6,4)
Logical Memory	16.5		

Despite the fact that this performance yields a quotient at the ceiling of the scale (a quotient of 137), he managed only a simplified version of card B on Visual Reproduction, and expressed amazement when he was unable to recall anything of one of the designs on card C. It was felt that this might represent a mild degree of nonverbal memory impairment.

Rey Figure. His copy showed some distortion of spatial relations, and his recall was significantly impoverished (Fig. 6.6) after four minutes of interpolated activity in the form of the Associative Verbal Fluency test on which he returned a good performance.

WAIS (scaled scores)

Information	14	Digit-Symbol	9
Comprehension	16	Block Design	11
Digit Span	12	Picture Arrangement	10

Apart from an obvious slowness on the Digit–Symbol task it was felt that the score on Picture Arrangement might be slightly inflated since, although he placed the cards in the correct order on some items, he showed that he did not understand why they should be placed in this way. However, it was thought that the performance was insufficiently deviant to warrant much significance, though McFie (1975) has

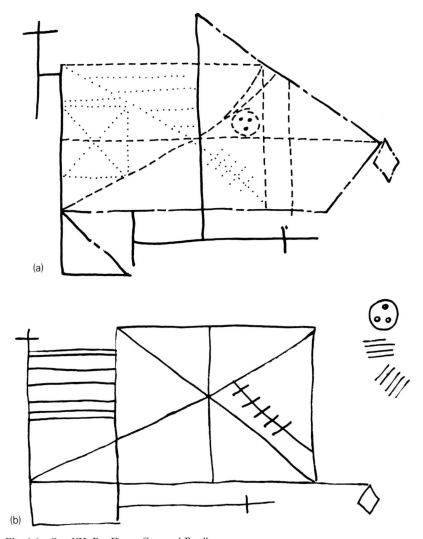

Fig. 6.6   Case VH. Rey Figure, Copy and Recall.

described poor performance on this task in patients with right hemisphere, particularly temporal, lesions.

Trail Making and *Colour-Form Sorting Tests*. VH gave an excellent performance on both tests.

In summary, it was felt that the testing showed only mild signs of depression of right hemisphere function, without any convincing localizing signs, though the opinion was given that there was minimal evidence of disturbance in the right temporal or temporo-parietal area.

VH was discharged a few days later with a probable diagnosis of infarction though it was felt that the presence of a tumour could not be excluded. There was still some clumsiness of the left arm and astereognosis but other signs had resolved.

Reviewed at three months the left astereognosis was still present. VH had returned to work but did not appear to be coping as well as before and had been given a less exacting job. There had been no further clinical event in the interim. Repeat CT scan showed two low density areas in the left external capsule consistent with old infarcts. Neuropsychological assessment revealed a marked improvement in the few areas on which he had previously performed poorly, e.g. his copy and recall of the Rey Figure were at the high level of his other performances. A year later his condition remained the same with residual mild astereognosis only.

Aneursymal amnesia

Case: ZQ

At the age of 56 this previously healthy man experienced sudden severe headache accompanied by photophobia and fever. On admission to a general hospital it was soon established that he had suffered a subarachnoid haemorrhage. Carotid arteriography revealed the presence of an aneurysm of the anterior communicating artery. This was surgically repaired 17 days later and after a further three weeks recuperation he was transferred to a rehabilitation hospital. At this stage he was still disoriented and confused and thought to be suffering from anterograde amnesia.

Neuropsychological assessment was requested to establish the presence, nature and degree of amnesia and a baseline evaluation of overall cognitive function preparatory to attempts at rehabilitation.

Neuropsychological assessment (three weeks post-operatively)

Wechsler Memory Scale, Form II

Information	3	Digits Total	11 (6,5)
Orientation	0	Visual Reproduction	7
Mental Control	7	Associate Learning	5 (2,0; 4,0; 4,0)
Memory Passages	4.5 (9,0)		
MQ 80			

This was thought to represent the hallmarks of the general amnesic syndrome, with preservation of immediate memory and inability to acquire new information. ZQ was stiff disoriented for both time and place and was easily provoked to confabulate.

NHAIS (scaled scores)

Information	12	Letter Symbol	5
Comprehension	9	Block Design	12
Similarities	12	Object Assembly	6
Memory for Digits	11		

Even in his somewhat confused state it was apparent that his intellectual abilities were relatively well preserved. The poor scores on two of the intelligence scale subtests seemed to be the result of slowness. Examination concluded with further tests of memory:

Luria's Ten Word List (Christensen 1975)

Trials	1	2	3	4	5
Correct	0	1	0	3	1

Rey Figure. Copy, Score 33, with poor sequential organization (Fig. 6.7). Recall, Score 8·5, with only a modicum of information (Fig. 6.8).

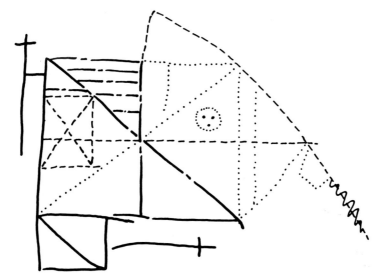

Fig. 6.7 Case ZQ. Rey Figure, Copy three weeks post-operative.

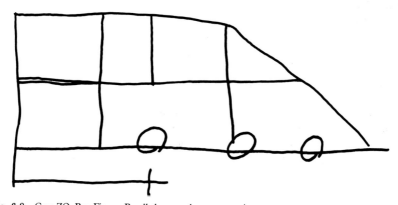

Fig. 6.8 Case ZQ. Rey Figure, Recall three weeks post-operative.

It was not thought that rehabilitation had anything specific to offer and the patient returned home to the care of his wife where he remained until reassessment 4½ months after operation. His wife reported considerable difficulty in his everyday management, occasioned by his total inability to retain any information for even a few minutes. This made it impossible for him to be independent even in the activities of daily living. He was still confabulating and it had become obvious that no significant improvement had taken place in the period between examinations. He was still partly oriented and his memory disorder was virtually unchanged. He obtained a better score for recall of prose passages but his recall of material was variable and always subject to rapid forgetting. Anything he retained was immediately lost if homogeneous material was interpolated between acquisition and recall. His scores on this occasion are given below in comparison with those obtained over a year later.

Scaled scores on WAIS and WMS at 4½ months (left column) and 17½ months (right column) were as follows:

WAIS

Information	12	12
Comprehension	9	11
Similarities	10	10
Arithmetic	13	—
Digit Span	12	9
Digit–Symbol	6	5
Block Design	10	11
Picture Arrangement	—	8
Object Assembly	6	11

WMS	Form II	Form I
Information	2	6
Orientation	3	5
Mental Control	9	9
Logical Memory	11	8
Digits Total	13 (7,6)	10 (6,4)
Visual Reproduction	9	8
Associate Learning	5 (3,0; 3,0; 4,0)	7 (3,0; 5,0; 6,0)

Other measures of memory remained as depressed as before.

Rey Figure. Recall Score 9 (Fig. 6.9).

ZQ remained robust and retained his ability to play golf but ceased his attempts because he was unable to keep track of his score. On this visit his wife reported that he was impotent, a feature we have seen in other cases.

At 17½ months the condition remained stable. He was still unable to retain any new information and continued to confabulate when pressed.

Rey Auditory Verbal Learning Test

Trials	1	2	3	4	5	Recall
Correct	4	4	7	3	5	1

Rey Figure. Recall Score 7 (Fig. 6.10)

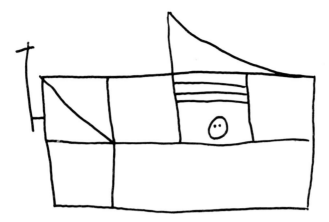

Fig. 6.9 Case ZQ. Rey Figure, Recall 4½ months post-operative.

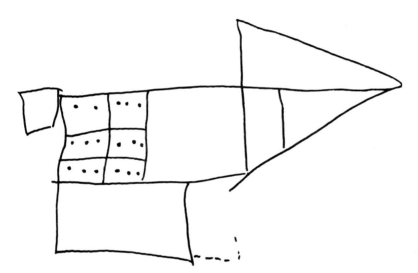

Fig. 6.10 Case ZQ. Rey Figure, Recall 17½ months post-operative.

Finally, ZQ was contacted nearly 4½ years after his vascular accident when he agreed to take part in an experimental study of amnesia. He had no idea of when he had been in hospital and thought that when he had been there it was for two days. He suggested that he filled in his time at home gardening and playing lawn bowls but his wife said that he never went into the garden. He was still unable to go to the store without a note as he forgot why he was going. The strain on the family was high and his wife likened the situation to having a child in the house again who was constantly in need of attention. Unfortunately, there was no expectation that this child would ever improve. There was no change in this final examination. This case is presented because it was singularly free of other major intellectual involvement.

Transient global amnesia

Case: KN

This 35-year-old foreman carpenter was eating his evening meal when he experienced an episode of vertigo lasting for a period of five minutes. There were no other associated neurological symptoms, and in particular no headache followed the event. Four days later he was present at a local meeting. Minutes before he was due to deliver a speech, he noted paraesthesia in the right side of his face, dysarthria and vertigo. He commenced his address, but was unable to complete it because of further exacerbation of these symptoms. After several minutes he developed a severe occipital headache associated with ataxia to the right. There was no diplopia or other visual disturbance.

He was admitted to hospital the next day for investigation. He was alert and well oriented with no observable memory difficulty. Cardiovascular examination was normal and there were no carotid or other vascular bruits.

Neurological examination showed nystagmus on gaze to the right and incoordination of the right arm and leg with ataxia to the right on standing. The remainder of the neurological examination, including examination of the optic fundi, was normal.

Over the next 48 hours these neurological signs resolved completely but three days after admission he developed a further episode of vertigo, nausea and vomiting. He was extremely pale and complained of incoordination of his right hand, and bilateral blurring of vision. He remained ambulant but his wife, who was visiting the hospital, reported that he could not recognize her and was indeed unaware of the reason for his admission to hospital. It was then noted that he also failed to recognize his attending physician.

Detailed neurological examination including neuropsychological assessment was undertaken two hours after the onset of this episode and repeated the following day, when the amnesic episode, which lasted approximately four hours, had resolved.

First Examination

During the episode KN was friendly and cooperative, but totally confused and disoriented, showing much agitation. He repeatedly asked where he was and what was happening to him. Several minutes after being given a cup of coffee he said 'Whose coffee is that?' He commented on the funny taste in his mouth and asked whether he had been vomiting (as he had shortly prior to the examination). He was unable to describe the events of the past few days, but gave details of his job and family without difficulty. He showed no confabulation and his reasoning powers were good.

He was given the verbal scale of the WAIS, the WMS, two of Luria's verbal learning tasks, and the Lhermitte and Signoret Spatial and Logical Arrangement Tasks. The aim was to discover the exact nature of his memory disorder. In addition to this, colour naming, reading, writing, drawing and word-finding abilities were assessed, since defects of these in isolation or combination are known to result from infarction in the region of the posterior cerebral artery (Benson et al 1974).

Wechsler Memory Scale, Form I

Information	4	Digits Total	10 (6,4)
Orientation	1	Visual Reproduction	4
Mental Control	5	Associate Learning	4.5 (3,0; 1,0; 5,1)
Memory Passages	4		
MQ 63			

KN did not know the date and thought that he was in a nearby veteran's hospital. He recalled nothing of the prose passages after half an hour. His performance on two subtests of the WAIS supported the clinical finding of preservation of a good deal of remote memory (Information 12; Similarities 12).

Luria's Ten Word List (Christensen 1975)

Trial	1	2	3	4	5	6	7	Recall after 3 min
Correct	4	5	3	7	2	4	2	0

He repeatedly asked 'Is this the same list?'

Verbal recall with homogeneous interference (Christensen 1975)
1. cat—house—forest: correctly repeated
2. night—needle—pie: correctly repeated
Recall 1. house—cat—needle
Recall 2. night—needle—pie

Lhermitte and Signoret tasks

Spatial Arrangement Test. KN was totally unable to learn this.
Logical Arrangement Test. After the second presentation KN understood that there was a conceptual arrangement, describing the downward pattern of symbols and the colour arrangement. By applying this 'information' he managed a significant reduction in errors, although he did have some difficulty holding both the colour and symbol patterns in his mind between presentations. His performance overall was far better than on the Spatial Arrangement Test.

Colour naming, reading and drawing were good, his writing was poor due to incoordination of his right hand, and he showed no language difficulties.

Second Examination
The following day KN was well oriented and his memory appeared to have returned to normal. He had no recollection of the period of, and shortly preceding, the amnesic episode. He showed some improvement on the tests of general knowledge and his performance on all memory tasks improved greatly. The tests were repeated together with some Performance subtests of the WAIS.

Wechsler Memory Scale, Form I

Information	6	Digits Total	11 (6,5)
Orientation	5	Visual Reproduction	9
Mental Control	8	Associate Learning	14 (6,1; 6,2; 6,2)
Memory Passages	13		
MQ 110			

There was good recall of the prose passages after half an hour.

Luria's Ten Word List

Trial	1	2	3	Recall after 3 min
Correct	6	8	10	8

Logical Arrangement Test. After the first trial he described the arrangement perfectly and recalled it after several minutes of intervening activity.

WAIS (scaled scores)

Information	13	Picture Completion	14
Similarities	16	Block Design	10
Digit Span	10	Object Assembly	11

Colour naming, reading, writing, drawing and word-finding were all good.

Further investigations included a CT scan, which revealed a right cerebellar infarct, and four vessel angiography which demonstrated a tight stenosis at the origin of the right vertebral artery. There was no evidence of a general vasculopathy.

One month later, right vertebral origin endarterectomy was undertaken. Operative findings were of a large atheromatous plaque at the origin, causing 'significant stenosis.' During the six month follow-up period no further clinical disturbance of hindbrain circulation had occurred. Further neuropsychological assessment was undertaken six weeks post-operatively. Parallel forms of all tests were used on this occasion to minimize practice effects:

Third examination (six weeks after endarterectomy)

Wechsler Memory Scale, Form II

Information	6	Digits Total	10 (5,5)
Orientation	5	Visual Reproduction	11
Mental Control	9	Associate Learning	20 (6,3; 6,4; 6,4)
Memory Passages	15		
MQ 132			

NHAIS (scaled scores)

Information	11	Picture Completion	15
Similarities	13	Block Design	15
Memory for Digits	9		

In summary, KN presented with clinical features of transient global amnesia in association with other signs of vascular disturbance of the posterior circulation.

There was sudden onset of confusion and disorientation, associated with a profound but isolated inability to register any new information, and some retrograde amnesia. Testing revealed the classical axial amnesic pattern. His immediate memory as tested by digit span was close to normal, as was his general knowledge and ability to handle concepts. He handled visual perceptual and constructive tasks at a high level and with ease. On the other hand, he exhibited a profound inability to retain any new material whether it was verbal or nonverbal or presented visually or auditorily. This suggested the likelihood of bilateral pathology.

The results of the Spatial and Logical Arrangement Tests of Lhermitte & Signoret were particularly interesting. KN's inability to learn the Spatial Arrangement contrasted with a vastly better performance on the Logical Arrangement Test. This suggests that his problem was not one of information processing (the logical or conceptual manipulation of material in order to store it efficiently), but rather a simple defect in the activation-consolidation process.

The pattern of neuropsychological findings conforms well with the post-encephalitic picture described by Lhermitte and Signoret, where the lesions are confined to the medial temporal areas on each side. This contrasts with the pattern seen with the Korsakoff form of the amnesic syndrome described in the same article. We have had a number of opportunities to confirm this dissociation with these two aetiologies using the same tests. KN also demonstrated the preservation of insight and the lack of confabulation, which are added clinical features of the post-encephalitic (medial temporal) variety.

It appeared that occipital lobe function was relatively spared. There was no visual field defect, nor any disturbance of colour naming, reading, drawing, or word-finding abilities. Such disturbances, in isolation or in combination, usually result from infarction in the splenial or calcarine branches of the posterior cerebral artery. The day following the transient global amnesic episode, KN's memory appeared to have largely returned to normal, except that he had no recollection of the period of, and shortly preceding, the amnesic episode. He showed some improvement on tests of general knowledge and verbal abstraction which suggested that there may have been some depression of cerebral function during the episode. On tests of visuospatial ability he had no apparent difficulty, although he performed slowly.

In conclusion, it appears clear that KN suffered an attack of transient global amnesia of vascular aetiology. Vertebrobasilar disturbance was clearly demonstrated by the clinical constellation of symptoms and signs, with angiographic and CT scan confirmation of right vertebral dysfunction. One likely sequence of events was an episode of vasospasm of the basilar artery, initiated by the passage of an embolus from its origin in the stenotic right vertebral artery to the right cerebellar hemisphere via the posterior inferior cerebellar artery. His extreme pallor also suggested a vasospastic element. Consequent bilateral reduction in blood flow through the posterior cerebral arteries may then have resulted in his amnesic state, since they supply the mesial temporal regions critical in memory processes.

This is one of very few cases where reasonably detailed neuropsychological data has been gathered both during and after the attack. It also illustrates one particular correctable cause for transient global amnesic attacks.

Thalamic amnesia

Case: PN

This 50-year-old successful businessman was seen shortly after admission. He was quiet and seemingly withdrawn although he responded accurately and appropriately to direct questioning. The history was confirmed by his wife. The principal feature of the history was the presence of a memory difficulty of relatively sudden onset extending back several weeks and remaining stable ever since. PN told of forgetting phone calls, people's names and conversations which he had over this time. He seemed mildly perplexed and anxious but not acutely troubled by his condition. His wife told of a similar episode of dysmnesia lasting two or three days on a previous occasion some five years before, followed by restoration of normal function. PN complained of bilateral frontal headaches, constant in nature lasting three to four hours and occurring in the late morning and early afternoon. He had also complained of headaches at the time of his previous episode of amnesic difficulty.

On examination his conscious state was normal, there was no loss of power or sensory disturbance, and physical examination was essentially normal apart from hyperactive reflexes and a blood pressure of 175/100. The day after admission clinical examination revealed a general amnesic syndrome. The Wechsler Memory Scale showed very poor new learning of both verbal and nonverbal material with excellent immediate memory and adequate orientation. As this patient was seen on a number of subsequent occasions the memory scale scores are summarized in tabular form:

Wechsler Memory Scale examinations

Test Form	Admission I	6 wks I	4 mths II	4yrs 10 mths I
Information	2	4	3	2
Orientation	4	5	5	4
Mental Control	5	8	8	8
Memory Passages	2.5	2	5	1.5
Digits Total	12	13	12	14
Visual reproduction	2	5	12*	5
Associate learning	7	7	4	3
MQ	70	83	90	72

With a single exception (*), which remains unexplained the scores remained stable over more than three years of follow-up. His complete inability to form new memories is shown very clearly in his numerous attempts on Paired Associate learning. While he was able to recall some of the easy associations, he failed completely to establish any new linkages:

Date	Form	Trial 1	Trial 2	Trial 3
Admission	I	4,0	4,0	6,0
6 weeks	I	4,0	5,0	5,0
4 months	II	4,0	2,0	2,0
9 months	I	1,0	2,0	3,0

A week after the first examination several subtests of the WAIS were administered:

Intelligence subtests

Date Test	Admission WAIS	6 weeks NHAIS	3 yrs 10 mths WAIS
Information	10	9	8
Comprehension	—	10	11
Similarities	10	12	—
Digit Span	11	13	14
Digit-Symbol	8	10	7
Picture Completion	12	—	—
Block Design	10	4	6
Object Assembly	(6)*	9	—

There was nothing in the quality of his responses to suggest any disturbance of intellect outside his memory and conative difficulties. This combination of deficits was responsible for his relatively poor score on the coding task (Digit-Symbol) and he gave up on the last item of Object Assembly*, having succeeded on the first three.

On subsequent occasions his poor scores seemed more associated with his anergia than any intellectual difficulty, e.g. he tended to give up on tests like Block Design though he was still able to do problems of some complexity if constantly stimulated.

The overall picture emerging at the early stage of his admission was of an 'axial' amnesia and both the psychologist and neurologist felt that alcohol was the most likely cause. However, both clinicians held reservations about the aetiology based on the presence of a verbal and behavioural adynamia and the apparently rapid onset of the dysmnesia and the history of an earlier transient amnesic episode. Longer contact with the patient revealed that while he was cooperative to direct questioning he proffered absolutely no conversation and he had to be directed to carry out the activities of daily living.

Speaking of cases of 'latent aphasia', Critchley (1972) commented:

Although the patient can keep pace with his interlocutor and betrays no obvious shrinkage of his vocabulary, he seems reluctant to embark on the seas of conversation. Inordinately protracted periods of silence are evident when the patient with ingravescent dysphasia is observed in the home, at the conference table or in the Board Room. He can and will reply to questions adequately enough. If sufficiently inspired, he can pose questions on his own initiative. In general, however, he appears unwilling to break silence with pertinent observations or even with small talk . . .

To the casual observer this lack of activity and spontaneity in our patient gave the impression of depression, but this was not borne out on direct questioning. Other investigations, including repeated electroencephalograms, all yielded negative results and the patient was discharged home to the care of his wife.

He was next seen six weeks after his first admission. Cognitive examination remained essentially as before, with the amnesic syndrome and adynamia completely unchanged. PN's wife recounted how he would remain abed, remain in a chair, remain unshaven unless directly bidden. This feature of her husband's disorder afforded her more concern than his inability to remember things. With a half formulated suspicion that his adynamia might be associated with frontal pathology despite earlier negative neurological findings, the psychologist added two tests, the Rey Figure and the Porteus Mazes, to the examination. He also suggested that on a subsequent occasion the tests of Lhermitte and Signoret (1972) might be applied to study the nature of the amnesic disorder, since the diagnosis of an alcohol based amnesic disorder was by now seriously in doubt.

Rey Figure. His copy was complete except for one small omission, but the recall at three minutes produced very little indeed (Fig. 6.11). The order of drawing was not recorded.

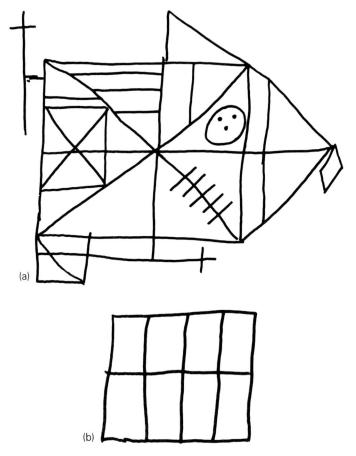

Fig. 6.11   Case PN. Rey Figure, Copy and Recall.

Porteus Maze Test. PN passed every problem in one trial with the exception of the Adult level, which was successfully completed in three. This added further support to earlier examinations that had revealed no associated intellectual difficulty.

At review at six months PN's clinical state remained exactly as before. Examination on this occasion was confined to the tests of Lhemitte and Signoret:

Test of Spatial Arrangement. PN was unable to learn the position of the nine cards despite 20 trials. This is one of the worst performances we have seen, even from subjects with Korsakoff psychosis. However, like the latter, he showed clear benefit from cued recall by placing all nine cards correctly after one hour's delay when given the whole pack of cards, whereas he had been able to place correctly only a few of the nine when asked to recall them with the empty board in front of him three minutes after twenty successive exposures of the complete set.

Test of Logical Arrangement. Our patient was successful on the fifth trial but his learning was unstable in that he made errors on three of the succeeding trials. This was a much better performance than alcoholic patients with this severity of amnesia but not as good as Lhermitte and Signoret's or our own post-encephalitic amnesic patients.

Test of Ordered Recall. Like post-encephalitic patients (and quite unlike alcoholic patients with amnesia) PN had no difficulty with this task, giving the correct order on the first trial. We have also confirmed this aspect of Lhermitte and Signoret's work, namely that alcoholic subjects have difficulty with this task and have noted that this difficulty may antedate clinically apparent amnesia.

Code Learning. PN had much difficulty with this task which is passed by post-encephalitic subjects with little trouble. He failed two, three and five item codes but passed the four item series. Once again the resemblance was more akin to the mamillo-thalamic subtype than the hippocampal.

In summary, the performance of PN on this group of tests did not accord closely enough with either the mamillo-thalamic or hippocampal variety to allow the case to be categorized in this way. The consulting neurosurgeon, in reviewing the investigations to that time, said: 'While... not fully convinced as to its alcoholic genesis, I would see this as a case of 'axial' amnesia in which reversible causes have been fully excluded. The sudden onset (and Mrs N. is an accurate, perceptive woman) suggests a cerebral vascular cause.'

Subsequent examinations at 9, 15, 21 and 23 months showed no alteration whatsoever in the two principal features of PN's disorder, i.e. the marked adynamia and amnesic syndrome. On several of these occasions attempts were made to study his maze learning ability but these were abandoned because of the lack of any learning whatsoever. On one occasion his arithmetical problem solving had some of the the characteristics described with frontal lesions. At 23 months, one of the neuropsychologists wrote: '. . . the more I see of him the more I am convinced that he has a lesion affecting the deep mesial frontal connections with the reticular system and I am inclined to agree that he has a vascular cause for his amnesic syndrome.'

The latter psychologist also commented that the picture looked 'very much like that seen after anterior communicating artery aneurysm surgery, namely adynamia, amnesia and impotence.' The latter symptom had been mentioned for the first time in a recent interview with PN's wife, who confirmed that it had been present throughout the duration of the disorder. It is noteworthy that despite the clinically apparent adynamia, the patient at this stage produced a very superior performance on a simple reaction-time vigilance task in which he was asked to press a key as quickly as possible to a light stimulus occurring at random interstimulus intervals varying from 0.5 to 1.5 seconds. It was thought that this finding strengthened the clinical impression that the adynamia was of the 'frontal' variety. While the patient could not activate his behaviour from within he could readily be roused from without. PN continued in this state until admitted to hospital with an inferior myocardial infarction 30 months after the onset of amnesia. His wife reported that his adynamia was still so profound that he failed to call for help despite obvious physical distress from his heart attack and it was only after a number of hours of vomiting that she summoned the doctor and he was admitted to the Intensive Care Unit. His condition responded to therapy but he required treatment for cardiac failure over the next year until he was admitted with a second cardiac infarction. Examination also revealed a right hemiplegia with dysarthria and dysphasia. He died a week later following a further extension of his myocardial infarct and pulmonary oedema. Post-mortem examination confirmed the presence of recent and old myocardial infarctions together with extensive atheromatous changes throughout the body. The brain was examined after fixation:

Macroscopic examination. Weight 1240 gms. The brain showed mild general atrophy. The large vessels were thin walled, but showed atheromatous plaques, widely scattered. Atheroma was extensive along the basilar artery and scattered in each vertebral artery. Atheroma was also scattered along the first part of the posterior cerebral artery. Anteriorly, atheroma was extensive in each internal carotid artery, but only scattered along the middle cerebral artery on each side. The mamilllary bodies were normal.

Sections of the brain stem and cerebellum did not show any definite pathological changes. Multiple coronal sections through the hemispheres showed irregular small lacunes scattered through the head of the caudate nucleus in the left hemisphere. Lacunes were also present in the putamen of each hemisphere and a small area of destruction was present in the anterior part of each thalamus (Fig. 6.12).

In the right hemisphere there was a large linear area of necrosis extending through the lenticular nucleus up to the lateral ventricle. The mamillary bodies appeared normal. Ammon's horn of the hippocampal region in each hemisphere appeared normal, but posteriorly in the left hippocampus there was a small ischaemic lacune.

Microscopic examination. Mamillary bodies appeared normal. In the basal nuclei of each hemisphere the small vessels showed hyaline thickening of the walls. There was much perivascular demyelination. The areas of old ischaemic necrosis showed much surrounding gliosis in the thalamus on each side. The median and anterior nuclear areas showed old ischaemic necrosis in patches. In the large vessels atheromatous plaques had severely constricted the lumen.

Conclusion The changes in the anterior and median nuclear areas would be consistent with severe disruption of the mamillo-thalamic tract and anterior thalamic nucleus. The small patch of ischaemic necrosis in the left hippocampus showed surrounding gliosi.

Summary

This case shows features of thalamic infarction described in the theoretical section above. While it might be taken as support for the mamillo-thalamic theory of amnesia, a review of the pathological sections shows dear evidence of dilatation of the third

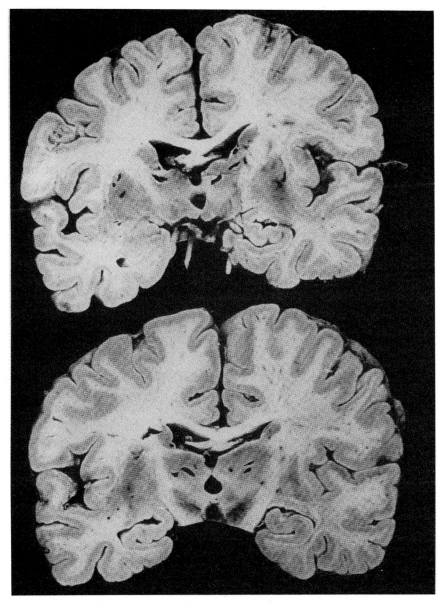

Fig. 6.12   Case PN. Coronal sections of the hemispheres showing lacunes deep in the brain substance.

ventricle indicating possible wasting of the dorsomedial nucleus or other structures as possible contributing or even vital factors.

Attention is once again drawn to the similarity of the clinical picture to that seen after anterior communicating artery aneurysms.

Non-invasive monitoring

Case: VP

This 64-year-old woman was referred by the vascular surgery department with the following history. Five years before, she began suffering symptoms of cerebrovascular ischaemia including dizziness and loss of balance. A right carotid endarterectomy was successfully performed in February of that year.

She remained well until four years later when she began suffering symptoms similar to her earlier episodes. These included loss of consciousness after standing up, episodes of blurred vision, spasmodic numbness in the right forearm, and several episodes of faintness when lifting her arms above the neck or when turning her head. She was admitted to hospital at which time bruits were noted over both left and right carotid arteries. A bilateral carotid arteriogram revealed: (1) a stenosis 1 cm from the origin of the right carotid artery; (2) a severe stenosis 1 cm beyond the origin of the left internal carotid artery; and (3) stenosis present at the origin of both vertebral arteries.

A left carotid endarterectomy was performed at which atheroma was removed from the common, external and internal carotid arteries. Three months later a repeat endarterectomy was carried out on the right side. The right common carotid artery was found to be completely occluded with severe atheroma and recent thrombus. The operation, which included almost the entire length of the artery, was performed with satisfactory results.

The vascular surgeons were concerned about VP's tendency to redevelop atheroma. They noted that she had been mentally quite dull before each of her two operations and had shown clear improvement post-operatively. It was felt that a regular neuropsychological check on her mental status would provide a preferable alternative to repeated carotid arteriography, with its attendant risks, in detecting any recurrence of circulatory compromise. A report of any sign of mental deterioration would lead automatically to neurovascular review. Testing sessions were carried out as follows:

A. One day before the repeat right endarterectomy.
B. One month after operation.
C. First annual testing session.
D. Second annual testing session.

Alternate forms of the *WMS* gave the following results:

A	B	C	D
Form I	Form II	Form I	Form II
MQ 118	MQ 120	MQ 137	MQ 124

Though some practice effect may be included in these scores there were neither quantitative nor qualitative features suggestive of deteriorating performance, Given the patient's age and educational background these were thought to be well up to expected level. Her recall for novel stories equated for length with the Wechsler material gave similar results.

The *Trail Making Test* was also given on each occasion:

	A	B	C	D
Part A	31s	22s	28s	31s
Part B	107s	77s	85s	82s

Although no parallel forms were available the improvement seen after the last operation seems to have been maintained.

Among other tests, several given at one year and two years post-operatively also supported the absence of any intellectual decline:

Associative Word Fluency. At one year F—8; A—9; S—9 Corrected score 38 (55%). At two years F—8; A—7; S—10 Corrected score 37 (58%)

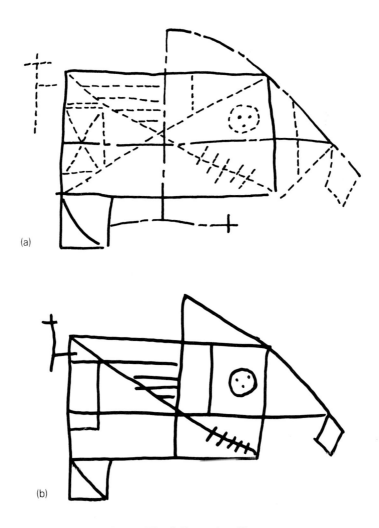

(a)

(b)

Fig. 6.13   Case VP. Rey Figure, Copy and Recall. **Formerly g.14.**

Verbal Learning. At one year VP produced an errorless recall on a ten word list on the third trial. After two years, examination with the *RAVLT* argued strongly for preservation of verbal learning:

Trials	1 2 3 4	List B	Recall A
Correct	7 12 13 15	7	12

Finally the copy and recall of the *Rey Figure* one year after operation can be compared with those of the roughly comparable Taylor figure in 1979. Little or no change is again apparent (Fig. 6.13).

The serial examinations strongly support the clinical impression that this patient became mentally more alert after her bilateral endarterectomy operations and maintained that improvement in the ensuing two years.

Though the serial assessment procedures were less than systematic the case illustrates the usefulness of neuropsychological assessment as a non-invasive and safer alternative to repeated angiography in monitoring the progress of patients after neurovascular surgery. This use of serial examinations points to the need for multiple equivalent forms of tests to cope with such factors as practice effects.

Intracerebral haemorrhage

Case: TD

Two days before admission to the neurology service, this 46-year-old photographer had complained of persistent, severe headache and pain behind the right eye since lifting a heavy load. Shortly after this, his wife noted that he was constantly veering to the left while driving, and that he had an asymmetry of his face which she described as the right side of his face being raised and the right lid lowered.

At interview the patient was drowsy but easily roused. He replied appropriately to questions but no further symptoms were elicited. In particular, he denied the presence of any motor, sensory or speech disturbance over the preceding two days. He was correctly oriented for time, place and person. He had suffered no major illnesses but knew that he had been hypertensive and had received treatment for this for a short period. He had been told on a recent visit to his doctor that his blood pressure was elevated but no antihypertensive treatment was recommended.

On examination he was markedly hypertensive and showed a clear seventh cranial nerve upper motor neurone weakness and slight weakness of the left arm and leg. A clinical diagnosis of right internal capsular haemorrhage was made and treatment for hypertension was instigated. CT scan confirmed the clinical diagnosis, a haemorrhage in the right lentiform nucleus being clearly demonstrated. EEG revealed widespread abnormalities over the right side, most marked in the right temporal region.

By the fifth day after the event, power had begun to return well to both the arm and the leg, and the patient's conscious state had returned to its normal alertness. There were no disorders of higher mental function noted in the clinical neurological examination but a neuropsychological assessment was sought to check for the presence or absence of such disorders in a more thorough and systematic way. The logic of this type of request becomes apparent in the discussion at the end of the case.

First examination (five days after episode)

Wechsler Memory Scale, Form I

Information	6	Digits Total	13 (7,6)
Orientation	5	Visual Reproduction	4
Mental Control	8	Associate Learning	18 (4,3; 6,3; 6,4)
Memory Passages	9		

MQ 112

The only obvious deficit was his pronounced difficulty with Visual Reproduction (Fig. 6.14). When he had completed drawing his recall of Card B, TD commented: 'That's not it at all.' Questioned about this he said: 'It should have been squares within a square.'

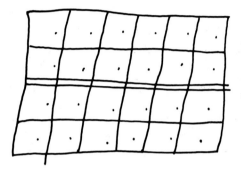

Fig. 6.14   Case TD. Attempted reproduction of Card B, Visual Reproduction, *WMS.*

His drawing was then covered and he was given another opportunity but produced almost a facsimile of his first attempt. On Card C he commented that he just could not recall anything of the second design. In view of the known right hemisphere pathology it was deemed advisable to explore visual memory further before extending the examination into other areas.

Benton Visual Retention Test. His score of 7 correct with 5 errors for administration A raised the question of impairment, if one assumes him to be in the bright normal to superior range of intelligence.

Rey Figure. His copy was produced very slowly and contained a major inaccuracy (Fig. 6.15(a)). After interpolating the Verbal Fluency test (4 minutes), TD produced his depicted recall (Fig. 6.15(b)), stating that he was having difficulty recalling the figure, and commenting: 'It looked like an old building with extensions to it. There were criss-crosses'. There seemed little doubt that he was having a real difficulty with this visuo-spatial class of material.

His verbal memory appeared intact and his Verbal Fluency performance had been at his expected level.

Further confirmation of his intact verbal skills was given by his performance on a short exploratory form of the WAIS which also demonstrated markedly poor performance on the three subtests from the Performance side of the scale.

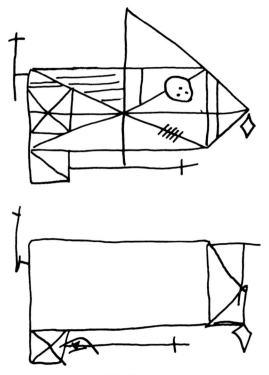

Fig. 6.15   Case TD. Rey Figure, Copy and Recall.

WAIS (scaled scores)

Information	12	Digit–Symbol	7
Similarities	12	Block Design	5
Digit Span	12	Object Assembly	5

It looked as though the 'depression' of right hemisphere function might extend beyond a specific memory deficit. The low score on Digit-Symbol substitution seemed largely, if not solely, due to psychomotor retardation. TD had shown a general slowing in the first two or three days after his vascular event but this was no longer clinically apparent at the time of his examination.

Qualitative observations from the two constructional tasks revealed a constructional dyspraxia which came as a surprise to the patient. TD had difficulty on the embedded items 2,4,6 and 8 as described in Chapter 1. He solved items 1,3 and 5 in 24,10 and 36 seconds respectively, and produced design 7 rapidly, though he at first omitted each of the white faces at the cardinal points of the compass, i.e. he produced the design without the background. When told to use all the blocks available he correctly filled in the missing portions.

Not only did he have difficulty with the embedded designs, but his unsuccessful efforts at construction were marked by approximately 45° rotations (Fig. 6.16). This phenomenon of rotation of the design by brain damaged individuals has been noted frequently in the literature since the 1950s.

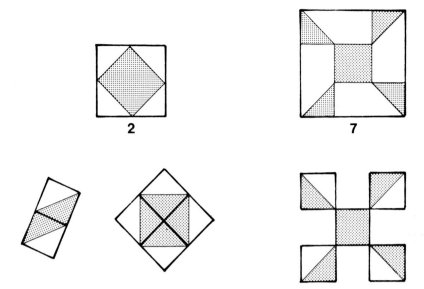

Fig. 6.16   Case TD. Block Design attempts.

The Object Assembly subtests provided further difficulties of a constructional nature. He was able to recognize with ease which object each set of pieces would make, i.e. his difficulty did not lie in an inability to create the perceptual *Gestalten*. However, despite this, he was able to complete only the first of the four assemblies in the allotted time. 'Testing the limits' by extending the time did not significantly improve his performance.

In answer to the referral question it was stated that there was strong evidence of considerable residual disruption of right hemisphere function as evidenced by the visual memory and visuo-constructive difficulties.

Second examination (five weeks after episode)

Wechsler Memory Scale, Form II. The patient reached the ceiling MQ of 143 on this parallel form. This included a maximum score for Visual Reproduction. Two parallel subtests from the NHAIS showed that there had also been significant improvement in his visuo-constructive ability. Block Design scaled score of 8 was below his anticipated ability but the depressed score on this occasion was largely the product of slowed performance. He was able to complete several of the problems with additional time and his efforts were not marked by the rotations seen previously. On Object Assembly his scaled score of 11 was probably approaching his optimum.

Other tests, which included the Benton Three-Dimensional Praxis task (Benton and Fogel 1962) and the tests of Spatial and Logical Arrangement, were performed perfectly.

With these signs of improvement the patient was allowed to return to work. Treatment of his hypertension continued on an outpatient basis.

Third examination (five months after episode)

This examination showed no apparent residual difficulties. The Taylor Complex

Figure (Appendix, under Rey Figure) was both copied and recalled well. Clearing of the psychomotor retardation was reflected in the scaled score of 12 on the WAIS Digit–Symbol subtest as well as a vigilance reaction time test in the laboratory. The patient was pleased with his progress and was now able to cope with all aspects of his work to his own and his employer's satisfaction.

Comment. This type of referral reflects the interaction between departments of neurology and neuropsychology (or between individuals). Both departments had become aware of the risk of advising return to work in such cases solely on the criteria of return of full motor functions and absence of major subjective complaints by the patient. In the preceding few years we had seen a number of similar cases who had made apparently full recovery as evidenced by resolution of paresis and other obvious neurological features who, nevertheless, found themselves unable to cope with their work for a considerable period. Some of these returned to the hospital and a number unfortunately acquired labels such as 'functional overlay' or 'exaggerated psychological reaction'. On neuropsychological examination a sizeable proportion, like the present case, revealed an obvious but latent cause for their inability to cope, in the form of constructional apraxia, problem solving difficulty or other clearly defined higher function disorder. Many of these, like TD, did resolve satisfactorily with further time, and hence it is our custom to check patients on discharge for such residual deficits. The neurological examination is not complete until such evidence is in.

REFERENCES

Adams R D, Victor M 1977 Principles of Neurology. McGraw-Hill, New York
Alexander M P, Schmitt M 1979 The aphasic syndrome of anterior cerebral artery distribution infarction. Archives of Neurology 37: 97–100
Bannister R 1978 Brain's clinical neurology, 5th edn. Oxford University Press, Oxford
Barbizet J, Degos J D, Lourn F, Nguyen J P, Mas J L 1981 Amnésie par lésion ischemique bithalamique. Revue Neurologique 137: 415–424
Barnett J M, Stein M S, Mohr J P, Yatsu F M (eds) 1986 Stroke: pathophysiology, diagnosis and management. Churchill Livingstone, Edinburgh, vol 1
Bender M B 1956 Syndrome of isolated episode of confusion with amnesia. Journal of the Hillside Hospital 5: 212–215
Benson D F, Marsden C D, Meadows J C 1974 The amnesic syndrome of posterior cerebral artery occlusion. Acta Neurologica Scandanavica 50: 133–145
Benton A L 1970 (ed) Behavioral change in cerebrovascular disease. Harper and Row, New York
Benton A L, Fogel M L 1962 Three dimensional praxis. Archives of Neurology 7: 347–354
Beukelman D R, Flowers C R, Swanson P D 1980 Cerebral disconnection associated with anterior communicating artery aneurysm: implication for evaluation of symptoms. Archives of Physical Medicine and Rehabilitation 61: 18–23
Boudin G, Barbizet J, Derouesné C, Van Amerongen P 1967 Cécité corticale et problème des amnésies occipitales'. Revue Neurologique 116: 89–97
Boudin G, Brion S, Pepin B, Barbizet J 1968 Syndrome de Korsakoff d'étiologie artériopathique. Revue Neurologique 119: 341–348
Brion S, Derome P, Guiot G, Teitgen Mme 1968 Syndrome de Korsakoff par anévrisme de l'artère communicante antérieure: le problème des syndromes de Korsakoff par hémorragie méningée. Revue Neurologique 118: 293–299
Cairns H, Oldfield R C, Pennybacker J B, Whitteridge D 1941 Akinetic mutism with an epidermoid cyst of the 3rd ventricle. Brain 64:273

Caplan L, Chedru F, Lhermitte F, Mayman C 1981 Transient global amnesia and migraine. Neurology
    31: 1167–1170
Castaigne P, Lhermitte F, Buge A, Escourolle R, Hauw J J, Lyon-Caen O 1981 Paramedian thalamic
    and midbrain infarct: clinical and neuropathological study. Annals of Neurology 10: 127–148
Christensen A L 1975 Luria's neuropsychological investigation. Munksgaard, Copenhagen
Cole A J, Gloor P, Kaplan R 1987 Transient global amnesia: the electroencephalogram at onset. Annals
    of Neurology 22: 771–772
Critchley M 1930 The anterior cerebral artery and its syndromes. Brain 53: 120–165
Critchley M 1972 Communication: recognition of its minimal impairments. In: Critchley M, O'Leary J
    L, Jennett B (eds) Scientific foundations of neurology. Heinemann, London, ch 4, p 223
Damasio A R, Kassel N F 1978 Transcortical motor aphasia in relation to lesions of the supplementary
    motor area. Presentation to 30th annual meeting, American Academy of Neurology, Los Angeles,
    California
De Jong R N, Itabashi H H, Olson J R 1968 'Pure' memory loss with hippocampal lesions: a case
    report. Transactions of the American Neurological Association 93: 31–34
De Jong R N, Itabashi H H, Olson J R 1969 Memory loss due to hippocampal lesions: report of a
    case. Archives of Neurology 20: 339–348
Donnan G A, Walsh K W, Bladin P F 1978 Memory disorder in vertebrobasilar disease. Journal of
    Clinical and Experimental Neurology 15: 215–220
Feuer D, Weinberger J 1987 Extracranial carotid artery in patients with transient global amnesia:
    evaluation by real-time B-mode ultrasonography with duplex Doppler flow. Stroke 18: 951–953
Fisher C M 1965 Lacunes: small deep cerebral infarcts. Neurology 15: 774–784
Fisher C 1968 Dementia in cerebral vascular disease. In : Toole J F, Sickert R G, Whisnant J P (eds)
    Cerebral vascular disease. Sixth Princeton conference, Grune and Stratton, New York
Fisher C M 1969 Arterial lesions underlying lacunes. Acta Neuropathologica 12: 1–15
Fisher C in 1978a Ataxic hemiparesis: a pathologic study. Archives of Neurology 35: 126–128
Fisher C M 1978b Thalamic pure sensory stroke: a pathologic study. Neurology 28: 1141–1148
Fisher C M 1982 Transient global amnesia: precipitating activities and other observations. Neurology
    39: 605–608
Fisher C M, Adams R D 1964 Transient global amnesia. Acta Neurologica Scandanavica 40
    (supplement 9) 1–83
Fisher C M, Curry H B 1975 Pure motor hemiplegia of vascular origin. Archives of Neurology 13:
    30–44
Flateau E 1921 Sur les hémorragies méningées idiopathiques. Gazette des hôpitaux 94: 1077–1081
Gade A 1982 Amnesia after operations on aneurysms of the anterior communicating artery. Surgical
    Neurology 18: 46–49
Gallassi R, Stracciari A, Morreale A, Lorusso S, Ciucci G 1988 Transient global amnesia follow-up: a
    neuropsychological investigation. Italian Journal of Neurological Science supplement 9: 33–34
Geschwind N, Fusillo M 1966 Color naming defects in association with alexia. Archives of Neurology
    15: 137–146
Guyotat J Courjon J 1956 Les ictus amnésiques. Journal de médecine de Lyon. 37: 697–701
Hodges J R, Ward C D 1989 Observations during transient global amnesia. A behavioural and
    neuropsychological study of five cases. Brain 112: 595–620
Jacome D E 1989 EEG features in transient global amnesia. Clinical Electroencephalography 20:
    183–192
Kaplan H A, Ford D H 1966 The brain vascular system. Elsevier, Amsterdam
Krayenbuhl H, Yasargil M G 1972 Radiological anatomy and topography of the cerebral arteries. In:
    Vinken P J, Bruyn G W (eds) Vascular diseases of the nervous system. North-Holland, Amsterdam,
    vol 2, ch 4, p 65–101
Kritchevsky M, Squire L R 1989 Transient global amnesia: evidence for extensive, temporally graded
    retrograde amnesia. Neurology 39: 213–218
Kritchevsky M, Squire L R, Zouzounis J A 1988 Transient global amnesia: characterization of
    anterograde and retrograde amnesia. Neurology 38: 213–219
Kuhl D E, Phelps M E, Kowell A P, Metter E J, Selin C, Winter J 1980 Effects of stroke on local
    cerebral metabolism and perfusion: mapping by emission computed tomography of 18FDG and
    13NH3. Annals of Neurology 8: 47– 60
Kurtzke J F 1976 An introduction to the epidemiology of cerebrovascular disease. In : Scheinberg P
    (ed) Cerebrovascular disease. Tenth Princeton conference. Raven Press, New York p 239–254
Lazorthes G, Gouaze A, Salamon G 1976 Vascularisation et circulation de l'encéphale. Masson, Paris

Lhermitte F, Signoret J L 1972 Analyse neuropsychologique et différenciation des syndromes amnésiques. Revue Neurologique 126: 161–178

Lindqvist G, Norlén G 1966 Korsakoff's syndrome after operation on ruptured aneurysm of the anterior communicating artery. Acta Psychiatrica Scandanavica 42: 24–34.

Logue V, Durward M, Pratt T R C et al 1986 The quality of survival after rupture of an anterior cerebral aneurysm. British Journal of Psychiatry 114: 137–160

Luria A R 1976 The neuropsychology of memory. Winston, Washington

McCormick W F, Schochet S S 1976 Atlas of cerebrovascular disease. Saunders, Philadelphia

McFie J 1975 Assessment of organic intellectual impairment. Academic Press. New York

Marie P 1901 Des foyers lacunaires de désintégration et de différents autres états cavitaires du cerveau. Revue de Médecine 21: 281–298

Mattis S, Kovner R, Goldmeier E 1978 Different patterns of amnestic syndromes. Brain and Language 6: 176–191

Miller J H, Yanagihara T, Petersen R C, Klass D W 1987 Transient global amnesia and epilepsy. Electroencephalographic distinction. Archives of Neurology 44: 629–633

Mills R P, Swanson D P 1978 Vertical oculomotor apraxia and memory loss. Annals of Neurology 4: 149–153

Mohr J O, Leicester J, Stoddard L T, Sidman M 1971 Right hemianopia with memory and color deficits in circumscribed left posterior cerebral artery territory infarction. Neurology 21: 1104–1113

Nguyen J P, Effenterre R, Fohanno D, Robert G, Sichez J P, Gardeur D 1980 Méthode pratique de repérage spatial préopératoire des petites néoformations intra-crâniennes à partir des données de la tomodensitométrie. Neurochirurgie 26: 333–339

Norlén G, Olivecrona H 1953 The treatment of aneurysms of the circle of Willis. Journal of Neurosurgery 10: 404–415

Okada F, Ito N, Tsukamoto R 1987 Two cases of transient partial amnesia in the course of transient global amnesia. Journal of Clinical Psychiatry 48: 449–450

Percheron G 1973 The anatomy of the arterial study of the human thalamus and its use for the interpretation of the thalamic vascular pathology. Journal of Neurology 20: 1–13

Percheron G 1976 Les artères du thalamus humain. Artères et territoires thalamiques paramédians de l'artère basilaire communicante. Revue Neurologique 132: 309–324

Ponsford J L, Donnan G A 1980 Transient global amnesia: a hippocampal phenomenon? Journal of Neurology, Neurosurgery and Psychiatry 43: 285–287

Ponsford J L, Donnan G A, Walsh K W 1980 Disorders of memory in vertebrobasilar disease. Journal of Clinical Neuropsychology 2: 267–276

Rivera V M, Meyer J S 1976 Dementia and cerebrovascular disease. In : Meyer J S (ed) Modern concepts of cerebrovascular disease. Eighth International Conference, Salzburg. Thieme, Stuttgart

Rubens A B 1976 Transcortical motor aphasia. In : Whitaker H, Whitaker H A (eds) Studies in neurolinguistics. Academic Press, New York, vol 1

Sahs A L, Hartman E C, Aronson S M 1979 Stroke: causes, prevention, treatment and rehabilitation. Castle House, London

Salamon G 1971 Atlas of the arteries of the human brain. Sandoz, Paris

Schott B, Mauguière F, Laurent B, Serclerat O, Fischer C 1980 L'amnésie thalamique. Revue Neurologique 136: 117–130

Segarra J, Angelo J 1970 Anatomical determinants of behavior change. In: Benton A L (ed) Behavioral change in cerebrovascular disease. Harper and Row, New York, p 3–14

Sengupta R P, Chiu J S P, Brierly H 1975 Quality of survival following direct surgery for anterior communicating artery aneurysms. Journal of Neurosurgery 43: 58–64

Simpson J A 1969 The clinical neurology of temporal lobe disorders. In: Herrington R N (ed) Current problems in neuropsychiatry: schizophrenia, epilepsy and the temporal lobe. British Journal of Psychiatry, special publication 4: 42–48

Skultety F M 1968 Clinical and experimental aspects of akinetic mutism. Archives of Neurology 19:1

Speedie L J, Heilman K M 1982 Amnestic disturbance following infarction of the left dorsomedial nucleus of the thalamus. Neuropsychologia 20: 597–604

Speedie L J, Heilman K M 1983 Anterograde memory deficits for visuospatial material after infarction of the right thalamus. Archives of Neurology 40: 183–186

Talland G A, Sweet W H, Ballantine H T 1967 Amnesic syndrome with anterior communicating artery aneurysm. Journal of Nervous and Mental Disease 145: 179–192

Tarachow S 1939 The Korsakoff psychosis in spontaneous subarachnoid haemorrhage. Report of three cases. American Journal of Psychiatry 95: 887–899

Toole J F, Patel A N 1974 Cerebrovascular disorders. McGraw-Hill, New York

Victor M, Angevine J B, Mancall E L, Fisher C M 1961 Memory loss with lesions of hippocampal formation. Archives of Neurology 5: 244–263

Volpe B T, Hirst W 1983 Amnesia following the rupture and repair of an anterior communicating artery aneurysm. Journal of Neurology, Neurosurgery and Psychiatry 46: 704–709

von Cramon D, Zihl J 1979 Roving eye movements with bilateral symmetrical lesions of the thalamus. Journal of Neurology 221: 105–112

Walsh K W 1987 Neuropsychology: a clinical approach, 2nd edn. Churchill Livingstone, Edinburgh

Walton J N 1953 The Korsakow syndrome in spontaneous subarachnoid haemorrhage. Journal of Mental Science 99: 521–530

Wylie C M 1972 Epidemiology of cerebrovascular disease. In: Vinken P J, Bruyn G W (eds) Handbook of clinical neurology: vascular diseases of the nervous system. Elsevier North-Holland, New York, vol 11, p 183–207

Zülch K J 1971 Some basic patterns of the collateral circulation. In: Zülch K J (ed) Cerebral circulation and stroke. Springer-Verlag, New York, 106–122

7. Epilogue: roles for the neuropsychologist

In a brief introductory book there are obvious limitations. The present primer can in no way stand on its own as a textbook of clinical neuropsychology. Nor is it suggested that the method outlined is the only way to proceed, but one which has proved itself both useful in training and capable of further development. The main purpose is to serve as an adjunct to clinical development in neuropsychology while the trainee is acquiring experience, hopefully under skilled supervision. In the colourful words of one neurologist 'clinical neuropsychology is a body contact sport', i.e. it is learned principally through practice and only practice will acquaint the developing clinician with the nature of disorders in various stages of evolution and resolution that will form the frame of reference against which later decisions will be made. Since the major emphasis in the present work has been on evaluation it will be helpful to underline some major points in this area before commenting on other roles for the neuropsychologist. These other roles all, however, flow from an appreciation of the individual case as revealed by insightful assessment.

THE EVALUATIVE ROLE

This is the basic role upon which all others depend. Without such evaluation there is no firm foundation, for example, for sensible rehabilitation.

The present method rests heavily on knowledge of psychoanatomical relations and this knowledge is continuing to grow in detail and specificity. The basic tenet is that psychological functions depend on the integrity of what may be termed distributed anatomical systems. These are akin to what Luria, in his numerous works, referred to as 'functional systems', and are made up of collections of nerve cells in the cerebral cortex (often in several geographically dispersed areas) together with cells in subcortical locations in many instances, all of these being joined together by sundry bundles of connecting nerve fibres to form what in common parlance might be called a set of integrated circuits. Damage at key points in a system subserving the multiple aspects of a complex psychological process, such as memory or language, will confer qualitatively different features on the compromise of the process. Cortical damage will produce different deficits from the so-called disconnection effects or syndromes produced by lesions which isolate cell collections from one another while leaving the cells themselves largely or wholly intact. Thus one should make a distinction between regional *localization* of function and regional *specialization*. While damage to local cortical regions will regularly produce disruption of a particular function or process this is only one point in the system which can cause disturbance. Moreover, it has become apparent that disruption at different points in a system confer particular features on functional change, and it will be important to detect these for the better understanding of the patient.

Clinical neuropsychology is no longer an exercise in localizing lesions. The major tenet is that signs of disruption of regional brain systems should lead the investigator not only to a further, detailed examination of the disordered function in the light of current neuropsychological knowledge, but also to the functioning of neighbouring or functionally related systems that may bring to light *unsuspected disorders* which may have been silent to neurological and other examinations. If clinical neuropsychology is to be useful it must add to the data base on which clinical decisions about management and rehabilitation are made.

The method is essentially that of differential diagnosis or approximation to known syndromes or patterns of disorder. *It is essential that the relations between observed facts and reported conclusions should make neuropsycholgical sense.* The method rests on knowledge of four main areas : (1) the accumulated facts of human neuropsychology; (2) knowledge of the structure of psychological functions derived from the developing science of cognitive neuropsychology; (3) an acquaintance with the general principles and details of relevant neurosciences, especially neuroanatomy, clinical neurology and neuropathology; and (4) psychological test theory and practice.

With regard to the latter, as in all professions, the practitioner will utilize certain tools over and over again. However, there will be questions or hypotheses that will require special tools which will produce pathognomonic data. *Test selection should be germane to the questions being asked or the hypotheses being tested* so that the 'compleat' neuropsychologist will gradually develop quite a large armamentarium from which to choose. While developing this, beginning neuropsychologists will find an encyclopaedic source of test data and wisdom in Lezak (1983). To this and other textual sources they should add a personal store of further qualitative observations. Such test familiarity is necessary for the rapid and economic evaluation associated with the branching decision-making process which is the basis of clinic evaluation on a scientific basis.

The fallacious inference

In Chapter 2 an example was given of how faulty logic may lead to unwarranted inferences. The *right hemisphere hypothesis* suggested that because chronic alcoholics perform poorly on tests usually considered sensitive to right hemisphere pathology, alcohol has a greater effect on the right hemisphere than the left. Miller (1983) cites two other similar examples in the literature one very similar to the right hemisphere hypothesis, namely that since normal elderly subjects did less well on tests sensitive to right hemisphere pathology, the right hemisphere ages more rapidly than the left.

This paralogical thinking is exploded by Miller:

If damage to structure X is known to produce a decline in performance on test T it is tempting to argue that any new subject or group of subjects, having relatively poor performance on T must have a lesion at X. In fact the logical status of this argument is the same as arguing that because a horse meets the test of being a large animal with four legs that any newly encountered large animal with four legs must be a horse. The newly encountered specimen could of course be a cow or hippopotamus and still meet the same test. Similarly new subjects who do badly on T *may do so for reasons other than having a lesion at X.* (Miller 1983) [my italic]

The last sentence explicitly recognizes the principle of multiple determination of test outcomes discussed in Chapter 1 and exemplified throughout. If, then, we are to continue to operate with tests of complex factorial composition, how may we strengthen the confidence of our predictions? At least two methods are available, namely sharing of variance and experimental investigation.

Sharing of variance

What at first may appear to be a broad pattern of failures may, on closer examination, turn out to be the reflection of a common disorder which contributes to failure in seemingly disparate tests. The magnitude of failure on separate tests will reflect the degree to which the disturbed function is represented in their composition. It is for this reason that emphasis has been placed on the importance of the quality of responses as well as their level, since the former will give valuable clues as to which factor or factors has led to the poor performance. In attempting to explain these factors it is wise to remember that the law of parsimony has never been repealed.

Experimental investigation

Hypotheses to be tested may be presented quite specifically by the referring source, as in the temporal lobe case described in the next section. More often their derivation is left to the neuropsychologist, based on the medical knowledge provided about the case or derived from the patient at interview. Often this may be insufficient and a certain amount of exploratory examination may be needed in order to clarify which areas should receive most attention. In such a situation experimental tests may well arise from the former process, i.e. observing shared variance.

To test emerging hypotheses it is advisable to use tests which are as factorially simple as possible. As these are few in number at the present time, the neuropsychologist may have to show considerable ingenuity in devising tests appropriate to the individual case. Fortunately, once devised they will serve on future occasions since the number of questions being asked will be relatively small, some occurring with considerable frequency, e.g. those related to the presence and nature of organically based memory disturbance.

In this stepwise method it is well to leave time out for rumination so that several short sessions will often prove more productive than one lengthy examination.

THE EDUCATIONAL ROLE

Neuropsychologists often stand in a central position in the multidisciplinary team concerned with the brain impaired patient. In the development of a team approach they will sometimes need to take on an educational role. Not all those wishing to avail themselves of the services of neuropsychology will know how to proceed, particularly at the outset. This will usually be reflected in requests which are far too general, e.g. after providing the briefest of clinical histories the request may simply state 'For neuropsychological assessment please'. As the referral agencies become more aware of the use of neuropsychological evaluation, the questions will become more specific and the background information provided about the patient will help greatly in shaping the nature and scope of the evaluation.

The following case from Walsh (1978) is rephrased to show a good working relationship between neurologist and neuropsychologist. The question posed was: 'Does this patient have an amnesia to which she is not entitled?'. Though not expressly stated the neuropsychologist is being asked to refer to the patient's hospital file, perusal of which revealed the following: A 56-year-old housewife (IN) had a history of sudden episodes of detachment from reality, staring eyes, and lack of awareness of her surroundings, each episode lasting about two minutes. The episodes had commenced shortly after a head injury 15 years before when she was struck on the right temple. EEG recordings had consistently shown the presence of a left temporal focus with no abnormal activity on the right side. All attempts to control the attacks with drug therapy had failed and the patient was proposed as a candidate for left unilateral temporal lobectomy. It was at this stage that the referral question was put.

The question thus placed in its context assumes that the neuropsychologist is familiar with the literature related to the question. The neurologist will not be surprised if the patient shows a differentially weaker verbal than nonverbal memory performance in line with the proven double dissociation shown with lateralized temporal lesions between verbal and nonverbal material. This would be a deficit to which the patient would be 'entitled' by virtue of a left medial temporal lobe dysfunction. However, a 'non-entitled' deficit of nonverbal memory would signal a possible dysfunction in the right temporal lobe. This dysfunction might also be silent to neurological examination since, in the case of an atrophic lesion, the area might be electrically silent, i.e. a normal EEG on the right side would not exclude pathology.

The import of finding a neuropsychological deficit would have the utmost significance, since surgical ablation of the electrically active focus in the left temporal lobe would be added to the atrophic damage in the previously unsuspected right side. Functionally, this would be equivalent to bilateral medial temporal damage, a condition which produces a general, profound, and lasting amnesic syndrome. Hence the finding of *an amnesia to which the patient was not entitled* would be the clearest possible contraindication to surgery.

In this case the neuropsychological examination did show a minor difficulty with one aspect of new verbal learning, though verbal short-term memory, memory for prose material and verbal intelligence measures were at an appropriate level. However, the patient clearly had much more difficulty with nonverbal memory (Fig. 7.1) together with evidence of constructional apraxia possibly due to more widespread disruption of function in the right hemisphere. It seemed that the proposed surgery ran the risk of producing a general amnesic syndrome. At this stage the patient died suddenly and at autopsy the site of the left sided irritative focus was essentially of normal appearance, while the electrically silent side was atrophic in the hippocampal region.

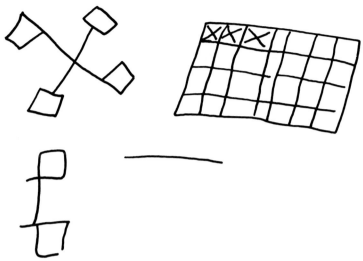

Fig. 7.1 Case IN. Visual Reproduction, Wechsler Memory Scale.

This is one of numerous examples where collaboration between neurologist and neuropsychologist can be very fruitful. In one sense the neuropsychological examination is the upper end of the neurological examination and one which has warranted specialization because of the rapid expansion of knowledge of brain–behaviour relations over recent decades. *No neurological examination of cerebral function is complete until the neuropsychological evidence is in.*

Such fruitful collaborations are not restricted to medical referrals but will develop with other psychologists, therapists and lawyers who are concerned with the patient's problems. The interaction can be furthered through written reports, verbal discussions, and didactic presentations such as workshops. Reports must be written with the specific reader in mind and not in 'psychologese'. The effectiveness of the communication will be shown by the increasing sophistication of the questions coming from the same source.

Verbal discussion, though not always feasible, is the most flexible and effective means of improving communication. These discussions often aid in clarifying the understanding of both parties and are sometimes better carried out before the definitive report is written.

Finally, didactic presentations help to bridge the gap between professionals by providing a shared basis of knowledge and terminology. They are at their best when they are regular, frequent, and brief.

THE REHABILITATIVE ROLE

The past few years have seen a great expansion of the involvement of neuropsychologists in rehabilitation. This is reflected in the origin of specialist journals of which the following form a sample : Cognitive Rehabilitation (1983), Journal of Head Trauma Rehabilitation (1986), Brain Injury, (1987) and Clinical Rehabilitation (1987). This has been accompanied by a large number of texts and handbooks. While a review is beyond the scope of the present work a few general comments are apposite.

Firstly, *accurate, detailed and insightful assessment of function is the basis of all good rehabilitation.* This makes it difficult to separate the rehabilitative from the evaluative role. Some of the points made earlier should be reinforced in the rehabilitation setting.

Summarizing measures

An early mistake made by psychologists was to place reliance on composite or summarizing scores, such as the IQ score, derived from a variety of subtests measuring a plethora of functions. The result was often to conceal quite specific and important deficits in the process of describing a lowering of 'intelligence'. This could be likened to summarizing scores from all four limbs to derive an index of 'motor power'. A 90% power score does not convey the information that the patient has three limbs with normal power together with a left arm paresis. Moreover, a composite score can be made up in endless individual ways. What is needed is a description which communicates both the level of function in separate areas together with the *nature* of any dysfunctions.

As already demonstrated in several cases, composite scores might be quite misleading as the basis for selection for rehabilitation. Physicians in rehabilitation found quite promptly that high levels on intelligence tests often failed to demonstrate quite serious impediments to rehabilitation such as the subtle, pervasive, and constantly frustrating frontal lobe deficits, so that cases with a 'high IQ' often did very poorly. It was as though these patients possessed 'intelligence' which they could not utilize effectively. On the other hand there were those with scores considerably below their estimated premorbid level who did tolerably well because preserved planning, executive and motivational factors allowed them to use their remaining assets to the full.

Individualized treatment

It is not uncommon for even experienced psychologists to advocate certain treatments without due consideration for what might be important differences in individual cases, e.g. to advise particular manoeuvres in the rehabilitation of memory disorders. To speak of amnesic patients or even of *the* amnesic syndrome as something unitary is to act as if there were no fundamental neuropsychological differences to be made between amnesic syndromes. Even for the very characteristic amnesia due to central brain lesions, important differences exist according to the location of the lesion. The patient with medial temporal lesions as the basis of the disorder benefits from logical structure in the material while the alcoholic Korsakoff patient with mamillo-thalamic (and other) lesions does not. On the other hand cued recall benefits the Korsakoff patient but not those with medial temporal lesions. This makes it highly probable that the rehabilitative procedures which will aid one patient will not necessarily aid the other. For this reason it is always mandatory to ascertain the nature of the disorder in the individual case.

Finally, although the emphasis throughout this text has been mainly on cognitive processes, the impact of these on the individual will depend on interaction with emotional and psychosocial factors that often determine the outcome. It is assumed that if they are not already skilled clinical psychologists, workers in this area will have a good working relationship with such professionals until they gain expertise.

Prognostic and outcome studies

At present there are very few studies which provide information about the factors which might predict the outcome of what is usually a lengthy, time consuming, labour intensive and expensive process. A vital question is when (if ever) to desist and this is best done through serial examination. Discovery of a stable state of deficit should suggest a reappraisal of aims based on preserved assets.

There are some deficits which will make prognosis guarded at the outset, e.g. patients with unilateral spatial neglect and left hemiplegia tend to show a lesser degree of improvement in independence and social adjustment than a corresponding group with right hemiplegia. Whether this is a function of the nature of the neuropsychological deficit or the location of the lesion is unclear but more studies of this kind are clearly needed. They will also need to include accurate knowledge of the relative effects of natural or spontaneous recovery versus intervention.

One of the many problems is to devise methods which evaluate progress from the patient's point of view. What may be only a small objective gain may have great significance for the patient. It is also likely that new psychological measures of function will need to be designed. Many currently used tests probably do not approximate closely enough to the processes involved in performance in occupations and professions. There is also a reciprocal need for functional task analysis in different work settings so that appropriate matching can be made between the patient's residual capabilities and the needs of the task. Neuropsychologists in rehabilitation settings should actively collaborate with colleagues in occupational and industrial psychology.

THE MEDICO-LEGAL ROLE

Neuropsychologists are finding themselves increasingly concerned with assessment in legal suits, particularly those relating to personal injury involving alleged damage to the brain. The situation will vary from country to country but certain common trends appear to be emerging, so a few comments are apposite.

Who is an expert?

The most obvious comment is that clinical neuropsychology is beginning to be recognized as an area of psychology in which expertise might be expected of its practitioners. This means that expert witnesses will need to demonstrate to courts and similar bodies that (1) they are conversant with the growing body of knowledge in clinical neuropsychology; (2) they have specific knowledge of the particular areas under consideration; (3) they have had supervised training in the speciality; and (4) they have clinical experience of a number of individual cases exhibiting the deficits which are the focus of the present claim.

It is becoming increasingly common for psychologists to be questioned closely on all these aspects, and what appears to be widely accepted, in this field as elsewhere, is a clearly reasoned argument where current observations are meaningfully related to the established corpus of knowledge. As the speciality continues and professional training becomes more readily available, evidence of specialist qualifications will no doubt become desirable if not obligatory. Kolpan (1989) reminds us that once qualified by the court as an expert the individual may then give 'opinion testimony' in the field in question but not in others. The purpose of this testimony is to aid the court in understanding complex information, and opinion will be expressed in terms of probability, i.e. 'more likely than not'. Kolpan (1986) has also reported an example, from a United States court, where a psychologist's evidence did not fulfil the requirements for admissibility since the different possibilities were given without conveying the relative weight which should be allotted to each.

As written submissions are often necessary before court proceedings, psychologists should be particularly careful not to present loosely written and argued statements which will lead them into unnecessary cross-examination. Readers are referred to papers such as that of Miller (1979).

One of the finest trainings for this exercise is to participate in detailed case presentations with colleagues adopting a critical attitude to every aspect of the presentation. We have found that having to justify publicly the basis of statements and inferences made in case reports rapidly improved both the understanding and the quality of the written reports of our graduates in training, and prepared them for the often rigorous business of cross-examination. All neuropsychologists who practise in English-speaking countries where common law prevails should prepare themselves by consulting a text such as that of Freckelton (1987) which presents the rules of evidence and deals extensively with problems of expert testimony. Information of the legal requirements regarding expert testimony should also assist in moulding reports to fit the medico-legal situation.

Faults in conducting the examination

One major weakness lies in failure to clarify the history where necessary: '... extra time spent on the history is likely to be more profitable than extra time spent on the examination.' Hampton et al (1975, p 489). Despite examination by various experts there are times when the history of events close to the time of injury remains unclear. Every effort should be made to clarify this but if no further information can be obtained the report should make it clear that the statements are made against the background as presented to the neuropsychologist. It is also helpful to have information about the rate and degree of improvement with the passage of time.

Traumatic injuries, even of great severity, are usually followed by improvement that may not reach a plateau for a year or even longer. Deficits which do not improve or which get worse with time must be suspected of having a non-neurological element. Those deficits which are not apparent until some time after the event are probably not neurological in origin. This is not to say that they are necessarily examples of malingering but that at least they are not based in neural incapacity, though they may be incapacitating and often have just as poor a prognosis. At this juncture the matter is better handed on to colleagues in clinical psychology or psychiatry for added consultation.

A second fault stems from the use of a fixed examination format without allowance for special features of the case. Relevant comments have already been made in Chapter 1 but most of these are particularly germane to medico-legal arguments. The use of a battery approach may mean that the examiner will be unprepared (or under-prepared) for questions from opposing counsel which may prove crucial. While a standard situation provides many advantages it may constrain the opportunity for observation of behaviour relevant to some questions. The neuropsychological examination should be planned according to the history and the previous findings of other specialists.

Observations should if possible be made on behaviour outside the immediately structured test situation. The present author refers to this as 'coffee break' testing. Often when the tests are pushed aside for a 'break' the patient may visibly relax and perform quite differently when observed informally in this non-test situation. The discrepancy may be quite great, e.g. a patient who has just failed on certain parts of a commonly used protocol such as the Boston Diagnostic Aphasia Examination may evince no difficulty whatever when the same linguistic constructions are used in conversation that takes place in the rest period and, on returning to the tests, begins to fail again.

It is also not uncommon for patients to indicate that they are having trouble understanding test instructions which, in most psychometric instruments, are spelled out with the greatest clarity by the tests' designers—psychometric tests should be unambiguous, having to cope with a wide range of intellectual levels. Once again these patients do not have comparable difficulties in understanding even complex grammatical or syntactical information introduced into normal conversation.

One must be prepared to have ready material appropriate to the particular case or to introduce them in a second session. The hypotheses for such informal testing may arise during the preliminary assessment but many will occur to the examiner after the first perusal of the relevant documents.

Faults in reporting the examination

The following list examines ten faults in the neuropsychological reporting of medico-legal cases:

1. Failure to report precise details (such as scores) upon which deductions are made. This includes use of terms such as 'average score', 'superior', 'abnormally low'. As there is much statistical psychometric data in common use this weakens the

arguments which might, in fact, be quite valid. It is wise on most occasions to append a summary sheet with all pertinent quantitative data so that the reader can see the basis on which claims are being made, i.e. the strength of this side of the argument. This obviates misunderstanding, particularly on the part of other psychologists.

2. Description of the individual's performance in terms of the test's reference population without sufficient attempt (often none) to place the person's expected level of performance. There are a number of ways of providing an approximate level, e.g. best estimates from 'hold' tests, or Lezak's notion of basing the estimate on the 'best' things the person does, which in turn finds support in the high general correlation between most of any intact individual's performances. Specific tests such as the National Adult Reading Test (Nelson & O'Connell 1978, Lezak 1983) are of great value where background detail is lacking, particularly with adult subjects. Other useful information may come from occupational history and education though caution must be exercised in generalizing. There are a number of individuals who have been under-achievers at school and who have moved into occupations with little demand on cognitive skills who, nevertheless, prove to be of high intelligence when examined.

3. Succumbing to face validity. This entails failure to take into account the numerous possible reasons for failure. The examiner may be unaware of some of the reasons, psychological as well as neurological, which cause failure on the particular test. Naive examiners will write as the though a failure on a test automatically means a deficit in the function said by the test originator to be measured by that test. Such reports are often accompanied by thinly disguised extracts from the particular manual and this procedure may be repeated with other tests.

As discussed earlier, much of this difficulty arises from the failure to note and utilize qualitative features of the person's responses as well as the direct scoring or the failure to use anything but standardized psychometric tests.

An interesting reverse argument sometimes encountered in court is based on the fact that an individual may pass on a test for one examiner but fail on a like-named test for another. Legal representatives may then argue that this represents variability of performance, i.e. that the person is competent at one time and not another. The strong inference is that the deficit is not a permanent one. In such a case it is even more important to show that the difference between the two performances depends not on fluctuation of the patient's cognitive abilities but on the fact that one test contains a factor which defeats the patient while the other does not. To support such a view the neuropsychologist must be able to demonstrate that the person fails whenever the function or ability in question is necessary for correct performance. A well trained examiner will have tested this hypothesis as a matter of course.

4. Moving outside the field of training and expertise. One of the principal strengths of a neuropsychological report is the way in which it integrates the neurological data with the behavioural and cognitive changes. Some less experienced psychologists like to comment about neurological matters and this should be resisted unless the issue is one where the writer or speaker can demonstrate proven competence. In fact, cases have already occurred where it has been ruled that psychologists not specifically trained in such matters will not be accepted as expert witnesses with regard to

comparisons between established brain changes and alterations in personality and cognition. In any case, presenting a weak or dubious set of statements is only likely to invite the listeners to 'throw out the baby with the bath water', i.e. in bringing to light some of the expert's weaknesses it may raise further doubt about the person's expertise in general and this may greatly weaken the impression on judge and/or jury of the strength of the psychologist's valid and cogent arguments in other areas of the case. In the courtroom it is bound to provide much material for cross-examination, usually with drastic consequences.

Example: Mr Z was injured in a collision between his motorcycle and a car. He was not unconscious, or only for the briefest time, and there were no neurological abnormalities. He suffered lasting personality changes and received psychiatric treatment. A lengthy period after the injury he began to complain of difficulty in seeing on his right-hand side. He told a psychologist that he had developed techniques to cope with his difficulty, e.g. walking on the extreme right of the pavement, and going around to the other side of the lathe at work to compensate for difficulties on that side. He even said that he had learned to ride his motorcycle side-saddle! (This must have been quite a sight but was uncorroborated.) The visual difficulty was not mentioned in most of the numerous medical reports and it seems likely that the patient did not allude to it.

A visual examination was carried out by an eye specialist three years and three months after the injury. The only finding was some restriction of vision in the right upper quadrant of the right eye while the left visual field was normal. Despite this the following are quotes from the psychologist's report:

'Your client also displayed deficits in that subtest measuring visual memory (Visual Reproduction of the WMS) and of note in this area is his obvious right visual field defect (temporal hemianopia). This may be indicative of a lesion in the occipital lobe area of the brain. This deficit may account for Mr Z's poor result on the Benton Visual Retention Test, where there are indications that his inability to perceive objects in his right visual field led to many errors, and while there may also be a memory defect it is difficult to differentiate clearly the relative effect of organic lesions relating to visual areas from those of other areas of the brain on this test...'

Later, in summary, the psychologist says, 'Mr Z has a right visual field defect indicating damage to the visual pathway, probably in the occipital lobe area. He is, simply, unable to see objects that appear to the right of his body.'

Such pseudoscientific claptrap shows a profound ignorance of the nature of visual field defects in general as well as lack of experience of what might be expected if the person did in fact have such a lesion. Clinically, people with defects of this magnitude are often unaware that they exist, the visual field loss being discovered on routine examination of vision. Movement of the eyes compensates fully and the author knows of no other case where such a small defect has had everyday consequences of the type described.

It is noteworthy that Mr Z had done the BVRT quite well for another psychologist some months before and when tested a year or so later he performed normally on tests specifically designed to bring out any right lateral visual defect should such have been present.

5. Using excessive detail without adequate summaries. In most cases there are only a few deficits in any individual and these should be reported as clearly as possible. Where confirmatory evidence arises from a number of tests these can be briefly summarized while indicating that the added information is available for presentation; scores can be given in the appendix.

6. The cross-sectional approach. Some reports of examination, often long after the event, fail to take cognizance of resolution, progression and change, or lack of it, over time. One of the crucial issues is that of prognosis, and this is always better viewed against the temporal aspects of the case in relation to known outcome in similar cases.

7. Weakness in relating the difficulties to other cases in one's own experience and the literature. Sometimes individuals write as though they have experience which they do not possess. In such cases it is quite permissible to mount an argument based on intimate knowledge of the literature but it would be wise to make evident that this is the basis of the argument. The less experienced practitioner would also be wise to be prepared to say that he does not know from personal experience when posed certain questions, rather than get in deeper and lose whatever credibility he had in the first place. If the matter under consideration is a contentious one in which the writer knows that experts hold divergent views, this must be made clear.

Behaviour inconsistent with the known or assumed lesions should be treated in adequate detail. Witnesses, expert or otherwise, should be prepared to state that there are things about a case which they do not understand rather than attempt to fit every single fact into their scheme of explanation.

8. Failing to note discrepancies, e.g. between (a) test and non-test behaviour; (b) everyday competence and test behaviour. This may be difficult since examining psychologists may not be provided with the relevant information and, in fact, much in the way of background information which could be used for corroboration may be kept from them. Except in cases where lawyers are suspicious of malingering or exaggeration little or no information about the 'natural' behaviour may be available, and the client and relatives may be quite defensive and resentful of attempts to elicit what is going on from day to day or may deliberately exaggerate or attempt to deceive.

9. Failure to note internal inconsistencies, the *sin of summation*. Since many psychometric instruments are graded internally from the simple to the more difficult items, it should make no sense simply to sum them. If this is done, it merely provides a false idea of the level of preservation or degradation of the psychological function or process under examination. A common finding is for an individual to fail on relatively simple items of a test or set of items while passing on some of the more difficult ones. One accident litigant failed on both the eight and nine year levels of the Porteus Maze Test but passed the Adult level on the first trial with consummate ease. It makes no neurological or neuropsychological sense to ascribe such failures to neural incapacity when a subject can perform well on even a modest number of difficult items while failing the less demanding. One should always assume that the difficult subsumes the easy.

10. Finally, many reports fail to fulfil the principal function of communication since they are couched in technical language or jargon which leaves the reader in doubt as to their meaning. A report to be read by the legal or medical professions or

for the average layman should be written with those particular readers in mind. Although the technical basis of the opinions may be difficult to translate into common usage, the general arguments and conclusions should not. Technical terms likely to be unknown to the reader should be explained at the appropriate place in the report. Furthermore, care should be taken to return to the basic concepts for each new case.

Cross-examination

The most common forms of attack fall into two categories. The first depends on lessening the degree of perceived expertise by showing lack of familiarity with the literature and restricted experience with the type of problem under consideration, and need not concern us in these brief notes. The second form is directly relevant to our exposition throughout and consists of counsel attempting to break down the statements or the psychologist's report point by point in a war of attrition. The strongest defence against this is to continue to stress the major position, namely that there are recognizable syndromes and that significance arises out of a constellation of symptoms and signs considered in the context of the history and not in the features taken separately. Thus the absence of one or more features does not invalidate the argument and it is important that the expert be allowed to present this position. It is closely akin to arguments that are familiar to courts and commonly accepted as valid. Consider, for example, a charge of receiving stolen goods. Counsel may argue item by item that the object in question is of very common occurrence and therefore it would be reasonable to claim that the item could well belong to the individual being charged. Opposing counsel will often argue successfully that the fact that all of the stolen items were found assembled together at the same place, at the same time, and in the possession of the accused immediately after their removal, greatly strengthens the probability that they are the items in question. If, at the same time, an object with a unique characteristic (such as a serial number) is also found with them, the case becomes almost unanswerable. Similarly the neuropsychologist is arguing that a certain concatenation of circumstances in the presence of a particular pattern of disturbance renders a particular conclusion highly probable. If there are pathognomonic signs in the examination the argument is even more strongly supported.

To conclude, much valuable time will be spared for all if care is taken to prepare the report in a competent manner, one which anticipates the questions which opposing counsel might put. This frequently results in the case being settled without the need for going to court.

CASE EXAMPLES

Many of the points covered above are exemplified in the following case extracts. The method can be applied to a variety of situations.

Whiplash

In medico-legal circles this term often takes on a pejorative character which can be difficult to counter. As the following two cases illustrate, each should be taken on its merits. Both involved a rear end collision while the plaintiff was at the wheel of his stationary car and both men claimed damages for deficits which included neuropsychological impairments. In both cases the impact was severe enough to damage the driver's seat and both were wearing seat belt restraints. Neither lost consciousness except momentarily and neither appeared to have struck his head.

Case: SG

This 45-year-old man was visiting a distant city in 1983 and was seated in the stationary car, which he had hired, at the kerbside studying a road map when the car was struck from behind on the driver's side by a car travelling at high speed. The driver's seat was fitted with a head rest, a point of significance in what follows. The report of a neurologist who examined the patient 12 days after the impact is worth reporting in some detail since it provides cogent evidence for a particular medico-legal stance. Unfortunately, one seldom has such a careful report made at a time close to the event.

> ... His wife, who was sitting beside him, recovered first from the impact and noticed that her husband was lying on his back within the car and that, on opening his eyes, he was attempting to speak, but could not do so clearly for about 30 seconds. He said something like 'it is not even our car' and was aware of the crash. Neither of them seemed to have hit their head. He was able to sit up and get out of the car by himself, but kept repeating a question about the other driver—'What was her excuse for the crash?' On being given an answer he would then, within a minute or so, repeat the question. When approached by an ambulance man he was able to give his name and address and that he was 'OK'. During the police interview he seemed vague on what happened and indicated that the car was slowing down at the time of the impact, disagreeing with his wife about the fact that the car was stationary. When their son's girlfriend arrived, he recognized her and addressed her by name. However, on being taken to—Hospital, he kept on asking his wife a series of questions which she estimated he repeated 'twenty times'. His speech was clear, but he was complaining of neck pain. He did not know the date and was not aware that they were in—(not his home town). This memory problem was pointed out to the examining doctor—and his tendency to repeated questioning existed for another six hours, until he became orientated and aware of his surroundings. He was kept in hospital overnight. He was aware of a severe headache and aching all over. On leaving hospital, the headache has improved, although he feels a pain at the base of his skull on any sudden movement or jarring when walking. He has had some tenderness to palpation and neck stiffness on the right side which was still present. He felt transiently dizzy on any sudden standing up or movement, but this did not sound like true vertigo. During the time after the accident, up until the day previous to my consultation ... he was still having problems with memory and continually asked about arrangements for that and the next day which he was unable to retain. He felt that his tongue was 'heavy and numb' with some numbness on the left side of the tongue, as if he 'had had a dental anaesthetic'. If he spoke at normal speed he would tend to mumble (this was also noted by his wife). He thought that his memory and speech had almost returned to normal at the time of my consultation.
>
> There is no relevant past history. He had not had any previous injury and was not taking any medication. He described himself as a 'fitness fanatic' who does not smoke and has a small alcohol intake.

A thorough neurological examination was reported as normal with only the following exceptions: 'when he protruded his tongue it did protrude slightly to the left, there was a suggestion of mild impairment of rapid repetitive movements and fasciculation of the tongue bilaterally ... [There was] only slight tenderness on palpation of cervical muscles.'

The remainder of the neurologist's letter is worth recording in full:

He was alert and appropriate during the interview. He recognized the day correctly, but was unsure whether it was 26th or 27th January. He could repeat seven numbers forward and four numbers backwards correctly. With the hundred minus sevens test, when he got down to seventy-two he paused and enquired whether he was taking six away. Subsequently he resumed and was correct in his subtraction. He was unable to repeat a Babcock sentence entirely word perfect after four attempts (missing one word). His general knowledge and awareness of recent world events seemed intact. He still felt that there was some lack of facility in his memory.

I think that this is a most unusual situation as he appears not to have had a head injury. The description of his amnesia is very similar to episodes of 'transient global amnesia' although there was a persisting problem with short-term memory to some degree for a further period of six or seven days. His case is like that described in an article entitled 'whiplash amnesia' (Fisher 1982) ... I thought it was of great interest to pursue further investigation and did obtain a skull x-ray ... There was definite C5/6 disc space narrowing and degeneration with osteophytic encroachment on the intervertebral foramina at the C5/6 level. An EEG examination was normal. Brain stem auditory evoked responses showed what seems to be a significant delay between wave two and three on the right hand side, suggestive of a ponto-medullary junction problem (although this is a preliminary report).

It seems most likely that he has suffered an episode of vertebro-basilar ischaemia, perhaps due to involvement of vertebral arteries at the level of the C5/6 degeneration with osteophytic encroachment on the arteries caused by the flexion/extension movement; or that a traction on the vertebral arteries had caused spasm and ischaemia of the thalamus and medial temporal lobes bilaterally. The problem with respect to his tongue is difficult as the tongue only slightly deviates to the left and the impairment and possible fasciculation of the tongue is difficult to interpret. There has been some brain stem ischaemia as indicated by the brain stem auditory evoked responses or there could have been some traction effect on the twelfth cranial nerves at the base of the skull.

I think it is likely that he will make a full recovery, but it is of great interest to speculate on the nature of the memory problem and there is some worry as to whether there has been some vertebral injury (and vertebral arteriography may be indicated) ...

Neuropsychological assessment

On his return home SG was referred for neuropsychological evaluation of his memory functions. The first examination was done three weeks after his injury. At this time the patient was conscious of his memory being below par, especially as his job involved keeping track of rapidly changing information concerning parts and machine models and he travelled interstate and overseas keeping up with developments. For the first time he became dependent on frequent note taking to support his memory in day to day affairs. Before the examination he produced two photographs of the car taken shortly after the accident. One of these showed the rear end of the vehicle while the other showed the seat broken from its moorings with the back of the seat now parallel to the floor and the head rest bent at right angles to that. This left a strong possibility that his head had been forced into extreme flexion.

WMS. Form I (three weeks after accident)

Information	5	Digits Total	12 (8,4)
Orientation	5	Visual Reproduction	14
Mental Control	9	Associate Learning	10 (4,1; 5,1;5,1)
Memory Passages	8		

MQ 112

We have found, in subjects whose intellect would be classified as bright normal or better, that this scale often shows differences in the direction of the Memory Quotient being significantly above the Intelligence Quotient. Subsequent examination with the WAIS-R gave this man a Verbal IQ of 127 and a Performance IQ of 126. Many of our patients with scores in this range reach the ceiling of the Memory Scale, an MQ of 147. Thus, to argue that there cannot be anything seriously amiss with a memory quotient around 110, for example, is grossly to underestimate the situation.

The following features were consistent with an impoverished memory performance and inconsistent with other possible bases for his complaints such as neurosis or enactment: (1) perfect scores on the first three subtests measuring orientation and routine mental operations, together with a maximum score for visual memory of a simple nature involving immediate recall, and an excellent score of digits forward, contrasting with (2) comparatively poor performance on recall of logical prose material (Memory Passages) and great difficulty with acquisition of the novel (difficult) pairs of the Paired Associate learning task with relatively little difficulty in acquiring the easy pairs which are based on well learned associations. This is a pattern frequently seen with organic amnesic syndromes so that the 'above average' Memory Quotient on its own can be quite misleading.

On the more lengthy *Rey Auditory Verbal Learning Test* he also encountered difficulty in learning the total list, a task he felt would have been easy for him before his injury.

List A						*List A*	*List B*	*List A*
Trials	1	2	3	4	5	Recall	Recall	Recognition
Correct	6	9	10	11	11	6	4	15

Again we felt that this had the characteristics of a moderate amnesic disorder with a learning curve peaking well below expectation based on his background as well as the test norms, followed by a considerable fall-off in recall after the presentation of the interfering list B but a perfect recognition memory score for the re-presentation of the first list. This pattern is exactly what we have experienced in our amnesic populations with confirmed pathology and is certainly not the configuration seen in neurotic or enacting individuals.

In this case the examination would have been improved by the introduction of measures of forgetting, since some of our patients with this degree of acquisition difficulty have also shown a very rapid rate of forgetting for the material that they have rather laboriously acquired. This rapid forgetting seems to correlate more with the patient's complaints than the acquisition capability, which might lead the inexperienced to think that the problem was not serious.

Symbol-Digit Modalities Test (Smith, 1973). A score of 54 was about 'average' but well below expectation for this man. It seemed from questioning that very little incidental learning was taking place. He found that he had to keep on checking each symbol on each occasion. He said he always set a high standard for himself and was acutely aware that before his injury he would have been much more efficient.

We explained to the patient that we considered that his problem was a real one and that it might be some time before his memory returned to its previous level. We counselled him to try to be patient and he was advised that if he was still left with any residual difficulty that there were therapists who might help with cognitive retraining though we stressed that this might not be necessary. In these cases it is sometimes hard to tread the middle ground between saying that everything will be all right (when clearly this may not be so), and alarming the person unnecessarily, since many organically based amnesia difficulties, particularly after trauma, appear to improve significantly with time.

SG remained concerned over the ensuing weeks and wrote several letters outlining very clearly how he had much more difficulty than formerly in learning and retaining things in relation to his job. At this juncture there was a tendency for the lawyers representing the insurance company to write him off as yet another neurotic 'whiplash' subject or someone who was trying to achieve gain by simulation or exaggeration.

Re-examination (15 weeks after accident)

WMS Form 1

Information	5	Digits Total	15 (8,7)
Orientation	5	Visual Reproduction	13
Mental Control	6	Associate Learning	9.5 (5,0;6,0;6,1)
Memory Passages	5		
MQ 104			

RAVLT

List A						List B	List A	List A
Trials	1	2	3	4	5	Recall	Recall	Recognition
Correct	8	8	11	12	12	—	9	15

This pattern and level of performance seemed very close to that produced three months before and corresponded with the patient's feeling that whatever recovery there might have been had now stopped. The lower score on Mental Control was caused by the subject getting lost on serial addition and the better score on the post-learning recall of the 15 word list is probably accounted for by the fact that no interfering list was given by the particular psychologist on this occasion. Nevertheless, it seemed that the condition had stabilized and he was referred for cognitive rehabilitation.

We learned subsequently that, although he may have been helped, he found it less taxing to take a lower level position with another firm where the demands on his memory were not so great. We also learned that he was considered conscientious in his former work, so much so that when he fell behind after his accident he took annual leave but returned to his office to clear up the backlog. This scarcely seems the behavior of a non-organic disorder.

In arguing the medico-legal case we supported the neurologist's original hypothesis and we felt that this man had been left with what was referred to in Chapter 6, in the section on transient global amnesia, as a 'fragility of memory'. The neurological and neuropsychological examinations seemed to be congruent with the events as described by the patient and his wife and at no time did a neuropsychological examination of other areas of cognitive function produce evidence of other difficulty. In the ensuing period before settlement of his claim other very similar cases appeared in the literature (Hofstad & Gjerde 1985, Matias-Guiu et al 1985).

Note: Fisher's original case had also involved a rear end collision to a stationary car with the patient wearing a seat belt. The 67-year-old woman sustained no direct head injury and did not lose consciousness. She showed features often described with transient global amnesia such as repetitive questioning. Her memory returned to normal after 72 hours.

Case: OH

This 45-year-old salesman was waiting to make a turn when he noticed in the rear vision mirror a car bearing down on him at high speed. He had time to brace himself and remembers attempting to accelerate to lessen the impact when his car was struck. As in the previous case, the force was sufficient to break the bolts holding his seat to the floor. He was uncertain whether he lost consciousness but thought that if he did it could only have been for a few seconds. He felt dizzy but got out of the car and shortly after helped the police to move his car out of the traffic. His wife came and took him to hospital where a crack fracture in one of his cervical vertebrae was diagnosed and he was given a cervical collar which he said he wore for four months.

Seven and a half months after the accident OH was examined by a psychologist. The latter was aware that a claim was being made against the other driver. The disabilities claimed included neck injury and loss of consciousness resulting in 'a very short concentration span, poor new learning ability and poor memory' together with 'sleeplessness, tension, loss of libido and impotence'.

The psychologist administered tests mainly in the areas of concentration, memory, and learning. The results were said to show poor new learning, very short concentration span, poor memory and depression. The psychologist was inclined to think that the memory difficulty was the result of decreased concentration and attention, and went on to hypothesize that there may have been a basis in brain impairment possibly affecting the midbrain reticular activating system. This theory was communicated to the patient. The psychologist in his report cited the work of Taylor (1967) on experimental studies of head injury in animals and agreed with Taylor's conclusion that the post-traumatic syndrome did not have a basis in neurosis but in demonstrated changes in the midbrain and white matter. The psychologist gave as his opinion that the man's depression and anxiety were secondary to the brain impairment.

A psychiatrist who was seeing OH at the time discussed this examination with the psychologist and wrote: 'we mutually feel that the anxiety is playing a role in his difficulties in learning new material and therefore contributing to his short-term memory deficit', but did not refer to brain impairment.

A year after the trauma an orthopaedic surgeon said that the neck injury required no further treatment and that the patient was well enough to return to work. He thought that many of the patient's complaints were 'non-organic'. These included difficulty with concentration and inability to cope with stress.

At 21 months a second psychiatrist felt that the concentration difficulty could be explained by anxiety as well as a neuropsychological condition. OH had been back at work for some months doing his usual work apparently in an adequate manner.

Finally, at 3 years and 8 months, with the court case to settle his claim in the offing, the insurer sought an up-to-date neuropsychological opinion.

Neurosychological assessment

At interview OH was, at least superficially, co-operative with the examiner and conversed readily. He said he was tired of the number of specialists to whom he had been sent over his claim but said this in an almost bantering tone without rancour. He repeated his main complaints of difficulty with his concentration and memory, reporting that he had been back to the original psychologist quite recently. He was told that some of these tests would probably be repeated as we wished to check his areas of difficulty.

Digit span and digit learning. Two lots of four digits were failed, as were five-digit series, despite the fact that he seemed at ease. Rather than appearing to have difficulty he gave the impression of saying any numbers at all so that even with such short series there was no similarity between his responses and the stimuli given. He was then asked to do his best to learn a set of four numbers which would be repeated over and over until he passed them. After eight trials he was still failing and on the last occasion, as on many preceding it, he gave four numbers not one of which was in the given series. Even at this early stage in the examination it seemed to suggest behaviour 'sicker than the sickest' as outlined for role enactment in Chapter 4.

Associate Learning (WMS II)

Trial	1	2	3
Knife–Sharp	Dig	Sharp	Sharp
Lead–Pencil*	Heavy	'No'	'No'
Jury–Eagle	Store	'No'	Crown
Country–France*	—	'No'	'No'
In–Out	Out	Out	'No'
Murder–Crime*	'No'	'No'	'No'
Necktie–Cracker	Shirt	Shirt	Shirt
Lock–Door	'No'	Jewellery	'No'
Dig–Guilty	—	Crime	'No'

Not only did he fail to learn any new pair of words but he failed to respond to well tried associations which are often achieved by patients with dementia. This set of responses is all the more surprising in a person who could converse sensibly in between the tests and told the examiner that for a time before coming to Australia he had worked as a journalist in London (note items marked *). There was no evidence from his behaviour here or on any other test that he had a concentration difficulty; he merely replied in a mildly amused manner and when questioned refused to elaborate on any response.

Fifteen Item Test of Rey. Once again he failed in a most unusual way, producing the following:

II   A   B   O   I

3

Smiling blandly, he said that was all he could recall.

Knox Cube Test. Only one item passed.

Verbal Fluency

F	A	S
Friend	Apple	Sugar
Fire	(sighs Ohhh)	Soap
Furniture*	'can't think'	Swing
Father		'no more'**

  *'All I can think of'
  ** Patient firm about not continuing

At this juncture the examiner said that they would move away from the areas of memory and concentration to sample his other mental abilities. Several subtests of an Australian intelligence scale were used as another means of looking at his attitude to testing in a broader framework. On each task, after the first few items, he made comments to draw attention to the fact that he was having trouble with the item even where these could be passed by a young child. He alternated this type of behaviour with frequent assertions that he did not know the answer almost before he had time to think about the matter at hand. When told that he could take more time he several times cut the examiner short by saying that it would be useless for him to continuing trying. His responses on general information reinforced earlier impressions that he was enacting or deliberately faking:

Q: Which is the largest Australian state?
A: Victoria. (In fact the smallest mainland state by far.)
Q: What is a peninsula?
A: Wouldn't have a clue.
Q: Who was Robinson Crusoe?
A: Wouldn't have a clue.
Q: Where did the Vikings come from?
A: Britain.

Q: What is meteorology?
A: To do with the fishing.
Q: Where is Durban?
A: *North* Africa.
Q: When is the shortest day of the year?
A: March.
Q: What is a barometer?
A: Reading. A weather reading ... degrees isn't it?
Q: What is an armadillo?
A: An army tank.
Q: What is the capital of Canada?
A: New Brunswick.
Q: Who wrote Alice in Wonderland?
A: Wouldn't have a clue.

On many tasks he adopted the posture, with eyes closed, of someone apparently trying very hard to concentrate. He made extravagant exclamations over the simplest problems and this continued over the two hour examination. When asked to copy an open cross drawn for him he made one arm much longer than the other three. When this deviation was brought to his attention and it was requested that he try again, his response was to make the deviant arm even more divergent from the original.

Unlike patients with neurological disorders he failed on everything he construed as a formal test of ability irrespective of its nature. The whole tenor of his performance was grossly out of keeping with his ability to function in a job with a commercial sales firm over the preceding two years, to converse normally, and to carry on his life without assistance. One cannot do better than paraphrase the statement of a surgeon who had seen this man for another claim related to a supposed back injury. 'He presents with a bizarre conglomeration of non-organic features and inconsistencies and the only question that arises is whether his condition is determined substantially on a psychological or on a voluntary basis'.

In his report—after discussing the absence of any evidence of brain injury at the time of the accident, such as unconsciousness or post-traumatic amnesia, and the singular lack of improvement (which is known to occur even in the most severe brain injuries)—the neuropsychologist gave as his opinion that the man was enacting the role, as he saw it, of a person with acquired deficit and stressed that the pattern of uniform failure on all types of test material, together with numerous qualitative features of his behaviour, was totally unlike that seen either with patients with cognitive impairment on a neurological basis or with psychiatric patients suffering from anxiety and/or depression. He added that some of the responses were such that he felt at least part of the motivation must be conscious but that there was no way in which a neuropsychologist could produce evidence to this effect. However, he repeated that the picture was *not* that of poor performance based on neural incapacity.

This last statement is a major contribution in such cases. To say that a condition is organically based when the case comes to judgment, usually after a considerable time, is to say that there will be no further improvement. On the other hand, to say that the condition is not organically determined is to leave open the possibility that there could be improvement, either spontaneously or following some intervention, although the author's experience with these cases is that the prognosis for such improvement is poor and financial compensation seldom affects the outcome. However, there are occasional dramatic improvements presumably in those whose motivations are largely conscious.

In summary, here are two individuals who were involved in almost identical accidents who present marked divergence in their complaints and whose test behaviour and scores differed widely. In the first case there is reasonable evidence of a logical relation between the conditions of the event, the medical evidence and the neuropsychological evaluation with no evidence of exaggeration, enactment, or malingering. In the second case there is no medical evidence to support such a striking set of failures on cognitive examination and the test performance is incongruent with the occupational adequacy of the person concerned.

Carbon monoxide poisoning

The third case is of a different nature but involves the same kind of argument.

Case: QN

This 44-year-old woman was referred by a neurologist who felt that she might have sustained generalized brain damage resulting from the following harrowing series of events which had occurred 16 months before. At that time, together with her husband and son, she had recently migrated from Europe, arriving in winter. The family moved into a new apartment, a fact which is of significance.

Several weeks later they all began to feel unwell in a non-specific way with what they felt might be influenza-like symptoms. After a week of lethargy, headache and vomiting they rang the local doctor on a Sunday and he left a prescription for them.

Later the same day the son collapsed and when the father tried to help he collapsed also. QN rang the doctor who summoned an ambulance. She retains only a vague recollection of this period. After spending the night under observation in hospital they all improved somewhat but no firm diagnosis was made and the next day they were sent home where they all rested in bed. Later the same day QN collapsed and was incontinent. Her husband called the doctor who said there was little he could do and said he would call in the morning.

When the doctor did come the next morning he found the husband dead and both QN and her son unconscious. He got them to hospital where both recovered slowly. This time a firm diagnosis was made, namely carbon monoxide poisoning.

Investigation of the apartment later revealed a faulty heater. Moreover, the so-called ventilators were false, i.e. they did not lead anywhere. Only a small part of this information was available to the neuropsychologist at the time of the first evaluation. A recent neurological examination had been normal.

Neuropsychological examination

The patient appeared mildly depressed as she recounted the sad circumstances and said she had moved from the distant city with her son to get away from painful associations. She was co-operative and volunteered no subjective complaints suggestive of cognitive difficulties. Knowing the common occurrence of amnesic difficulties after carbon monoxide poisoning, it was decided at the first session to explore memory and learning as well as to sample general intellectual functions.

On the Wechsler Memory Scale (see table below) it was reassuring to note that she was well able to perform adequately, particularly on the Paired Associate learning test which is so sensitive in amnesic disorders and especially that associated with carbon monoxide poisoning. The preservation of her ability to learn new material was supported by a good performance on the RAVLT where she recalled 14 of the list of fifteen words after the interpolated list, a very good performance indeed, especially as one might have expected her to be a little below par because of her depression:

List A						List B	List A
Trials	1	2	3	4	5	Recall	Recall
Correct	7	9	12	13	13	6	14

Her copy of the Rey Complex Figure was adequate (score 31) though her recall was poorer (score 10.5).

On the sampled subtests of the intelligence scale, while her age scaled scores were depressed on two subtests, there were no qualitative features suggestive of organic impairment and it was noted that she did better than expected on the two visuoconstructive tasks of Block Design and Object Assembly. This argued, together with preserved new learning ability, for an absence of any significant degree of brain impairment. This opinion was given to the neurologist with an offer of additional exploration after further treatment for her depression.

It should be pointed out that at this stage there was no suggestion of any medico-legal claim. This is significant since an examination for medico-legal purposes often needs to have a good deal more detail in the way of test data to sustain an argument in court, especially in cross-examination, than an opinion which would satisfy a medical colleague. The knowledge of a claim did not reach the neuropsychologist until a further three years had elapsed (some four years and three months after the trauma) when it was learned that she was claiming damages from the local doctor, the hospital, the heating appliance company and the builder. A psychologist had supported her claim for brain impairment based on an examination at this late stage. Another psychologist had carried out an examination at 28 months. The case was complex involving as it did the loss of her husband together with the emotional and financial consequences, as well as possible damage to herself from the poisoning. At this juncture the lawyers asked for an opinion from the neuropsychologist based on his early examination. His report made the following major points: (1) as reported earlier there had been no evidence of any memory or new learning difficulty and this would be an unusual finding in cases with cerebral impairment from carbon monoxide poisoning; (2) while there were two relatively poor performances on the intelligence scale (Digit Span and Digit-Symbol) he felt that these could be explained readily by her depression; (3) there were no qualitative features suggesting brain impairment; (4) in noting that the third psychologist had pointed to a relatively poorer verbal than performance quotient as supporting damage to the brain, he commented that in his experience of conditions causing general brain impairment the Verbal–Performance difference was invariably in the other direction i.e. with Performance IQ lower than Verbal. Moreover, he pointed out that the second psychologist had noted a similar discrepancy but had then elicited from the patient the history of a lifelong difficulty with reading and writing and on formal testing had found her functionally illiterate. Far from being an acquired deficit the difference had always been present; (5) the neuropsychologist also commented that the level of the patient's memory quotient had declined from around normal at 16 months to very poor at 51 months, and stressed that the usual finding for patients with amnesia, uncomplicated by major cognitive deficit, was for improvement rather than decline to take place, the memory sometimes returning to normal or at least reaching a stable plateau below the premorbid level (see Walsh 1987, Case QT, p 354-356). There did not appear to be any cases of long term decline described in the literature.

Wechsler Memory Scale examinations

Test Form	16 months I	28 months I	51 months II
Information	5	3	2
Orientation	5	5	2
Mental Control	6	3	0
Memory passages	8.5	5.5	5.5
Digits Total	9 (5,4)	7 (4,3)	7 (4,3)
Visual reproduction	8	13	6
Associate learning	13 (4,0;5,2;6,3)	8	9.5 (4,0;6,1;5,1)
MQ	96	84	67

WAIS examinations

	16 months	28 months	51 months
Verbal Scale			
Information	9	—	6
Comprehension	12	10	14
Arithmetic	—	8	7
Similarities	14	12	12
Digit Span	8	5	4
Vocabulary	—	9	12
Performance Scale			
Digit-Symbol	8	8	4
Picture Completion	—	15	16
Block Design	13	15	11
Picture Arrangement	—	11	10
Object Assembly	14	—	11
VIQ	(102)	92	97
PIQ	(101)	113	114

He concluded that there was no significant neuropsychological evidence to support a diagnosis of brain impairment from his own examination and this point was later accepted in the overall appraisal of the claim which involved numerous other factors as mentioned.

Conclusion

It has become clear that clinical neuropsychology already covers a wide range of areas, and neuropsychologists are finding professional roles in all situations where a knowledge of brain-behaviour relationships can prove useful. No doubt these expanding roles will prompt the development of a comprehensive compendium of practice. The present text is a small step in that direction.

We may close with a quote from Stuss (1987): 'What you test is what you get; i.e., what you test is based on a number of factors, including knowledge of neuropathology and neuroanatomy, and valid and reliable experimental procedures.'

REFERENCES

Bell D S 1981 Assessment of outcome. In: Dinning T A R, Connelly (eds) Head injuries : an integrated approach. Wiley, Brisbane, p 132–139
Broe G A, Lulham J M, Tate R L, Walsh C A, Ross G A 1981 The concept of head injury rehabilitation. Bulletin of the Postgraduate Committee, University of Sydney, Supplement, p 59–68
Fisher C M 1982 Whiplash amnesia. Neurology 32: 667–668
Freckelton I R 1987 The trial of the expert : a study of expert evidence and forensic experts. Oxford University Press, Melbourne
Hampton J R, Harrison M J G, Mitchell J R A, Pritchard J S, Seymour C 1975 Relative contributions of history taking, physical examination, and laboratory investigation to diagnosis and management of medical out-patients. British Medical Journal 2: 486–489
Hofstad H, Gjerde I O 1985 Transient global amnesia after whiplash injury. Journal of Neurology, Neurosurgery and Psychiatry 48: 956–957
Jennett W B 1981 Prediction of outcome. In : Dinning T A R, Connelly T J (eds) Head injuries : an integrated approach. Wiley, Brisbane, p 119–131
Kolpan K I 1986 Medicolegal issues. Journal of Head Trauma Rehabilitation 1: 79–80
Kolpan K I 1989 Expert courtroom testimony. Journal of Head Trauma Rehabilitation 4: 95–96
Lezak M D 1983 Neuropsychological assessment, 2nd edn. Oxford University Press, New York
Matias-Guiu J, Beunaventura I, Codina A 1985 Whiplash amnesia. Neurology 35: 1259
Meier M J, Benton A, Diller L (eds) 1987 Neuropsychological Rehabilitation. Guildford Press, New York
Miller E 1979 The long-term consequences of head injury: a discussion of the evidence with special reference to the preparation of legal reports. British Journal of Social and Clinical Psychology 18: 87–98
Miller E 1983 A note on the interpretation of test data derived from neuropsychological tests. Cortex 19: 131–132
Nelson H E, O'Connell A 1978 Dementia: the estimation of premorbid intelligence levels using the new adult reading test. Cortex 14: 234–244
Smith A 1973 Symbol Digit Modalities Test. Western Psychological Services, Los Angeles
Stuss D T 1987 Contribution of frontal lobe injury to cognitive impairment after closed head injury: methods of assessment and recent findings. In : Levin H S, Gratman J, Eisenberg H M (eds) Neurobehavioural recovery from head injury. Oxford University Press, New York
Taylor A R 1967 Post-concussional sequelae. British Medical Journal 3: 67–71
Uzzell B, Gross Y (eds) 1986 Clinical neuropsychology of intervention. Martinus–Nijhoff Press, Hingham, Maryland
Walsh K W 1978 Neuropsychology: a clinical approach. Churchill Livingstone, Edinburgh
Walsh K W 1987 Neuropsychology: a clinical approach, 2nd edn. Churchill Livingstone, Edinburgh

Appendix

The following are brief outlines of the tests commonly referred to in the text. More details may be found in the relevant manuals and in Lezak's exhaustive compendium of test wisdom (Lezak 1983).

Austin Maze Test

This is a direct descendant of the 'stepping-stone maze' of Barker (1931). The author has used sundry versions since 1950 but with the publication of a paper by Milner (1965) a ten by ten matrix of buttons was used so that the problem pathway used by Milner could be introduced into our work for future comparison with this important study. The pathway proved such an excellent way of examining complex learning in our neurological patients that we have retained it as our standard problem since.

The standard maze with the Milner pathway is shown in Figure A.1.

Instructions. The patient's attention is first drawn to the distinctive buttons at the start (S) and finish (F) of the pathway. The following instructions are then given to the subject:

Each of these buttons gives either a green light or red light when pressed (demonstration with one button on pathway and one off the pathway). There is one continuous pathway of 'green' buttons from Start to Finish. Your task is to first find this pathway by moving one step at a time across the board and then to see how much of it you can learn by going across a number of times.

There are several rules in this game. (1) You may move only in the following ways (demonstrating) left, right, forward, backward. You are not permitted to move diagonally (demonstrate), only left, right, forward, backward. (2) Remember, only one step at a time. From each button there are four possible choices. If you choose the next green one you are free to go on. If you choose a button which gives red, go back one step to your last correct choice and try another one.

We will use the first trial to make sure that you know what you have to do. Of course, at first you will have to proceed by trial and error since you have no idea of how the path moves from S to F.'

The instructions may be varied according to the sophistication of the subject. (It is helpful to wire a small section of the board in the top left of the matrix with red and green lights to use during the instructions).

If the subject begins retracking along a number of previously correct choices the trial should be interrupted and further instructions given.

279

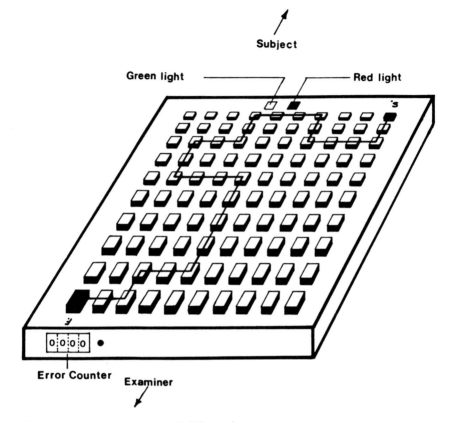

Fig. A.1 Austin Maze Apparatus with Milner pathway.

Sometimes a subject will neglect to move in one direction while repeating errors at the same choice point. This happens frequently where the pathway makes the first turn backward (i.e. towards the subject). The four possible moves should again be shown to the subject on a part of maze well away from the pathway. No further help is given.

Observations

Quantitative. The Milner pathway provides a serial learning task of some complexity which can be mastered by the majority of subjects of 'normal intelligence' (WAIS IQ 90–110) in from 10 to 15 trials. Normative data is not yet available though detailed studies are now beginning to emerge (Gates et al 1983). More intelligent subjects master the pathway in less than ten trials.

Probably the most valuable use of the maze is in the study of patients' error utilization. A deficit in the patient's ability to utilize information from one piece of behaviour to modify the next, e.g. eliminating errors as learning trials proceed, can form one of the most serious, and often insurmountable, obstacles to full rehabilitation. Examples are given in the preceding text but a few general points are worth making here.

Even quite dull subjects are able to learn material of the complexity of the Milner pathway though, of course, they take more trials than brighter subjects. After reducing their errors to zero, a small number of repetitions will allow them to retain the programme of behaviour often for very long periods. On the other hand, even very intelligent subjects with lateral frontal lobe damage may have extreme difficulty in totally eradicating errors to produce a stable, error-free performance. The maze thus provides an opportunity to observe the patient's performance in a learning situation with a task which approximates the complexity of many everyday life situations.

Qualitative. Note should be made of the following features:

1. Deviations from instructions after the first trial, e.g. jumping two or more steps at a time, or moving diagonally.
2. Retracking despite a further explanation that this will only lead back to the start.
3. Repetitions of the same error at one choice point on the same trial.
4. 'Running-on' errors. Some subjects, after reducing their errors to a small number, will continue on in a straight line one step beyond the correct choice in a row or column, but will always make the next correct choice (turn in the path) only to add one more, incorrect, step to the next series of correct responses. This sometimes represents a state of affairs where the subject knows that the extra step is incorrect but needs the confirmation of this fact by the red light before proceeding. Subjects may even verbalize the fact that they know it is going to be incorrect but are unable to inhibit the response. This, too, is seen almost exclusively with frontal lobe damage, and such errors may sometimes be eliminated by admonishing the subject to stop and think or by reminding him that only one or two trials remain. The difficulty appears to be related to Luria's notion of a disorder of the verbal regulation of behaviour (Luria, 1973 and elsewhere).

Other versions of the maze apparatus using microprocessor technology allow a range of problems to be presented and have facilities for the storage and print-out of errors suitable for experimental study of negative transfer, proactive interference and similar phenomena. The more sophisticated versions are being used for the study of the error utilization problem, mentioned in Chapter 5, which is seen as a major component of the frontal lobe syndrome, one which may have important implications for rehabilitation.

Colour-Form Sorting Test (Goldstein & Scheerer 1941).

The subject is shown 12 coloured shapes, four colours (red, blue, green and yellow) in each of three shapes (circle, triangle and square) and asked to sort them out into groups which go together. A perfect performance would be where the subject is able to verbalize and arrange the pieces according to the two concepts of shape and colour. Difficulties in sorting or shifting are examined in a qualitative way. Subjects with anterior lesions have more difficulty than those with posterior lesions and the most severely affected are those with left sided lesions.

Complex arithmetical problems

1. How many whole planks 5 feet long can be cut from 18 planks, each 29 ft 6 inches long?

2. A van and its cargo are worth $16,000. The van is worth $700 less than the cargo. How much is the cargo worth?

3. Tom had a bicycle which was worth $50. He sold it for that sum and afterwards bought it back again for $30. He afterwards sold it for $65. What was his gain from first to last?

4. If a ship can steam 16 miles an hour against a stream which runs at the rate of 2½ miles per hour, how far could the ship steam in 4 hours with the stream?

5. Jones caught 70 fish, Brown caught 8 more than twice as many as Jones, and Smith caught 3 times as many as Jones. How many did they catch altogether?

6. A, B and C had 950 apples between them. A had 60 more than B and B had 70 more than C. How many had C?

7. A man and a boy had a race for 4000 yards. The man ran at the rate of 330 yards a minute and the boy at the rate of 220 yards a minute. The boy had a start of 1500 yards and won. How many minutes did he win by?

Knox Cube Test

This was a component of the Arthur Point Scale (Arthur 1947) and has been incorporated in the Queensland Test (McElwain & Kearney 1970) since it can be used without verbal instructions, thus being useful in situations of reduced communication due to language barriers. It is also useful as a memory test in neurological patients for similar reasons.

The examiner taps, in sequences of varying composition and length, four small cubes attached to a board and the subject is asked to imitate this. The test correlates well with WAIS Digit Span.

Lhermitte and Signoret Tests

The three tests outlined here were first described by the authors in 1972. In this article they found differences in performance between the 'mamillo-thalamic' and 'hippocampal' versions of the general amnesic syndrome. The clinical use of these tests soon demonstrated to us their value in dissecting cases of non-specific amnesia and we have continued to use them. Our experience supports the French workers' distinction of two patterns of response according to different anatomical locations. However, we consider that the exceedingly poor performance of the alcoholic (mamillo-thalamic) group on the Logical Memory Task and the Code Learning Task is due to the associated lesions in the anterior parts of the cerebrum which cause considerable difficulty with conceptual manipulations, as outlined in Chapter 2.

Tasks 1 and 2 use a wooden or cardboard frame (200 x 200 mm) divided into nine equal areas, together with two sets of nine stimulus cards (Figures A.2, A.3) some 60 x 60 mm each.

1. Spatial Memory Task (Fig A.2).

Instructions. 'I want to see if you can learn the position of pictures in a frame. Each picture has its own location in one of the nine squares. I am going to show them to you one at a time. Try to remember where each one goes. After I have shown you the nine pictures I will show them to you again and see if you can remember where each one goes ... This one goes here [placing the card on its spot for 5 seconds and then removing it]. The next one goes here [placed in position and then removed].

Continue until all nine have been shown in random order (e.g. 6−1−8−5−7−2−9−3−4).

CHAIR	DRUM	KITTEN
SPOON	CHILD	TREE
BANANA	SAFETY PIN	YACHT

Fig. A.2 Lhermitte and Signoret Spatial Arrangement Task.

'Now you have seen them all, try to remember where this one goes.' Cards are now presented in a new random order, one at a time above the centre of the empty frame. At each response the examiner replies either 'Yes, that goes *there*' (placing the card on its spot for five seconds and then removing it), or 'No, that one goes *here*', (placing it on the correct spot for five seconds). Using this correction method the trials proceed until the subject can place all nine correctly on one trial or has reached a less stringent criterion depending on the examiner's purpose. Discontinue at ten trials. Subjects of normal intelligence will almost invariably reach a perfect score in six trials or less. Patients with general amnesic syndromes will seldom reach a perfect score, even after as many as 20 trials. The nature of the errors described by Lhermitte and Signoret should be noted.

(Note: we have employed simple line drawings of readily identifiable objects in place of the photographs used in the original study.)

2. Logical Memory Task (Fig. A.3)

The examiner says to the subject: 'The second test is much the same as the first but this time we are going to use different cards. Once again you have to remember where each one goes.' Proceed as before. Most intact subjects of normal intellectual ability, and patients with a 'hippocampal' version of the general amnesic syndrome, will usually succeed in four trials or less. Patients with an amnesia of alcoholic aetiology may not succeed despite a large number of trials. Discontinue after ten trials. This test also proves difficult for the pre-Korsakoff patient (see Ch. 2) and even for many so-called social drinkers. Ready success, on the other hand, strongly raises the possibility of pathology other than that related to alcohol.

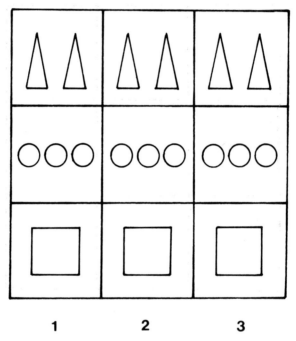

1   2   3

Fig. A.3   Lhermitte and Signoret Logical Arrangement Task. Stimuli in column 1 are blue, column 2 red and column 3 yellow.

3. Code Learning

Coloured counters are used. (Blue, red, yellow and green). The subject must discover the rule being used in the serial presentation of the counters. Begin with two counters (G, Y). 'I am going to show you coloured counters in a certain order according to a rule I have in my mind. I want you to find out what the order is by guessing which colour I am going to show next. Let us begin with just two colours. The colours we will use in each case will be on the desk.' Place a green and yellow counter on the desk. Present the colours one at a time in your closed hand, opening it to disclose the counter as soon as the subject guesses.

After the subject has recognized the order by correctly guessing four consecutive counters, proceed to (2) B,B,R; (3) BYRY; (4) GYYRG. In each case make sure that the subject knows that the counters are being presented in a predetermined order and not just at random. Discontinue after ten trials.

Once again alcoholic patients have significant difficulty with this task which is mastered readily by most normal subjects though a small number of the latter have difficulty with item (3). Success on this task would weigh heavily against an alcoholic aetiology.

These three tests are also 'clinical' in the sense that there are, as yet, no adequate normative data, but they have proved useful in the detection of sub-clinical syndromes and early disruption of frontal lobe function from whatever cause.

The Naylor-Harwood Adult Intelligence Scale (Naylor & Harwood, 1972)

This scale is an Australian adaptation of the Wechsler Adult Intelligence Scale. Though inadequately standardized it provides fresh content while employing the same subtests and scoring methods as the WAIS. Clinical use over a decade suggests that it can reliably substitute for the WAIS where the patient has been exposed to that test on one or more occasions.

The Porteus Maze Test (Porteus 1959, 1965)

This consists of a number of pencil and paper maze problems graded in difficulty from year III to adult problems. It is the oldest mental test of a standard form still in use, having been first used by Porteus in 1914. There are several suitable parallel forms which differ slightly in their level of difficulty at comparable age levels.

Rey Auditory Verbal Learning Test (Rey 1964)

This is a verbal serial learning task using 15 common nouns. The subject is asked to repeat as many of the list as possible after each trial and after attempting one recall of an interpolated second list. Finally the subject is shown or reads a passage of prose in which the first 15 words and distracter nouns are embedded, and asked to indicate the words from the first list. The test is popular since it provides systematic data for evaluation of the patient's learning abilities, susceptibility to interference and other neuropsychological data.

Rey Figure (Rey 1941, Osterrieth 1944)

This test consists of two components: (1) copying the complex geometric figure, and (2) drawing it from memory after a delay. It thus offers an opportunity to study the graphic component as well as to study recall. We follow the original author in asking the patient to change coloured pencils from time to time during the copy, thus allowing a permanent record of the sequential organization, or lack thereof, in the drawing. The sequence of colours is indicated in the figures in the text by the degree of break-up of the lines from solid through a series of dashes to a dotted line. We test recall after three minutes which we fill with some other interpolated task, e.g. the instruction and 90 second execution of a substitution task fill three minutes nicely. We also administer this test at a distance from other tests of memory and do not indicate that the patient will be called on to recall it subsequently. This hopefully allows an examination of 'incidental' memory, i.e. that where the subject has made no definite intention to remember.

L.B. Taylor of the Montreal Neurological Institute devised an alternative form of the Rey Figure which is useful for repeated testing (see Weiskrantz 1968, fig 11-18, p 338).

Trail Making Test

This simple test has been in use since its incorporation into the US Army Individual Test during the Second World War and has formed part of test batteries, particularly the Halstead–Reitan battery, whose users have generated a wealth of data in a great variety of groups and conditions. It consists of two parts. Part A consists of a series of circles each enclosing a number from 1 to 25, scattered at random on the page. The subject's task is to join the circles in numerical order as quickly as possible. Part B has both numbers and letters disposed in random order. The subject must draw a line in the order 1 to A to 2 to B to 3 to C etc.

Apart from its general use as a speeded visuomotor tracking task, we have noted that patients with frontal lobe lesions, particularly those with basomedial damage, have difficulty with the flexible control of inhibition needed for the task so that they are differentially slower on Part B or continue on with one of the series, either numerical or alphabetical. For example:

Subject 1. 1—A—2—B—C—D.
Subject 2. 1—A—2—B—3—4—5.

The normative data provided in Russell et al (1970) are extremely useful.

Verbal Fluency

There are a number of verbal fluency measures in use. We favour the form of spoken fluency used in the aphasia test of Spreen & Benton (1969). The subject is asked to name in sixty seconds as many words as possible beginning with a letter of the alphabet, excluding proper nouns and the same stem with a different suffix. The three letters in this version are F,A,S. The score is the total of the three one-minute trials. The Spreen-Benton version is valuable since it provides adjustment formulae for sex, age and years of education. Perhaps more important are the qualitative features outlined in Chapter 5.

Wechsler Scales

The intelligence and memory scales are discussed at length in Lezak (1983).

Wisconsin Card Sorting Test

This test of concept attainment and conceptual shifting was devised by Grant & Berg (1948). The subject is given a pack of cards, each bearing one to four symbols (circle, triangle, cross or star) in one of four colours. The object is to sort the cards, one at a time, under four key cards: one red triangle, two green stars, three yellow crosses and four blue circles. To do this, the subject must work out, from the examiner's verbal responses, the principle by which the cards should be sorted. This principle changes to a second and third concept that the patient must also attain in the course of the test. In the original version, these changes are made without informing the patient. We prefer the briefer, unambiguous modification by Nelson (1976), as we found, as he did, that many patients became totally confused with the earlier version. The test is very sensitive to frontal lobe involvement, particularly on the left side. These subjects may have difficulty attaining the concepts or have trouble in shifting to a new one (perseveration), or they may inexplicably return to an earlier incorrect mode of responding, as in Case BC (Ch. 1).

APPENDIX REFERENCES

Arthur G 1947 A point scale of performance tests. Psychological Corporation, New York
Barker R G 1931 The stepping-stone maze: a directly visible space-problem apparatus. Journal of General Psychology 5: 280–285
Gates G R, Gregson R A M, Hammond E M 1983 Performance on the Austin maze: a hard look at normative data. In : Stanley G V, Walsh K W (eds) Brain Impairment. Proceedings of the 1982 Brain Impairment workshop. Department of Psychology, University of Melbourne
Goldstein K, Scheerer M 1941 Abstract and concrete behaviour: an experimental study with special tests. Psychological Monographs 43: 1–151
Grant A D, Berg E A 1948 A behavioral analysis of degree of reinforcement and ease of shifting to new responses in a Weigl-type card sorting. Journal of Experimental Psychology 38: 404–411
Lezak M D 1983 Neuropsychological assessment, 2nd edn. Oxford University Press, New York
Lhermitte F, Signoret J L 1972 Analyse neuropsychologique et différenciation des syndromes amnésiques. Revue Neurologique 126: 161–178
Luria A R 1973 The working brain. Allen Lane Penguin Press, London
McElwain D W, Kearney G E 1970 The Queensland Test. Australian Council for Educational Research, Melbourne
Milner B 1965 Visually-guided maze learning in man: effects of bilateral hippocampal, bilateral frontal and unilateral cerebral lesion. Neuropsychologia 3: 317–338
Naylor G F D, Harwood E 1972 Manual of the Naylor–Harwood Adult Intelligence Scale. Australian Council for Educational Research, Melbourne
Nelson H E 1976 A modified card-sorting test sensitive to frontal lobe defects. Cortex 12: 313–324
Osterrieth P A 1944 Le test de copie d'une figure complexe. Archives de Psychologie 30: 206–356
Porteus S D 1959 Recent Maze Test studies. British Journal of Medical Psychology 32: 38–43
Porteus S D 1965 Porteus Maze Test: fifty years' application. Pacific, Palo Alto, California
Rey A 1941 L'examen psychologique dans les cas d'encéphalopathie traumatique. Archives de Psychologie 28 (112): 286–340
Rey A 1964 L'examen clinique en psychologie. Presses Universitaires de France, Paris
Russell E W, Neuringer C, Goldstein G 1970 Assessment of brain damage: a neuropsychological key approach. Wiley, New York
Spreen O, Benton A L 1969 Neurosensory Centre comprehension examination for aphasia. Neuropsychology Laboratory, University of Victoria, Canada
Weiskrantz L (ed) 1968 Analysis of behavioral change. Harper and Row, New York

Index

Ability, premorbid, 6
Abulia, 211, 222
Adaptive behaviour, *see* frontal lobes
Adynamia, 179, 211–212, 237
Alcoholism
  adaptive behaviour, 44–45, 52
  cognitive change, 44–49, 51–52
    hypotheses, 49–52
    intellectual change, 44–47
    memory and learning, 45–46
    recovery, 53
  neuropathology, 42–44
  right hemisphere hypothesis, 49–50
Alexia, pure, 215–216
Alzheimer's disease
  clinical features, 80–83
  pathology, 81–82
Amnesia
  axial (general), 41
  frontal, 181–182
  hysterical, 129–130
  Korsakoff, *see* Korsakoff psychosis
  posterior cerebral artery, 212–213, 216–218
  psychogenic, 128–129
  transient global, 216–218
Aneurysm, 222
Arteries, cerebral
  anterior, 210–213
  middle, 213
  posterior, 214–218
Arteriovenous malformation (AVM), 222
Atherosclerosis, 222

Battery, neuropsychological, 3–4
Blindness, cortical, 215
Blood supply, anatomy, 210–216
  see also Arteries, cerebral

Cerebrovascular disorders
  dementia and, 84–86
  pathology, 207–208
  haemorrhage, cerebral, 221–222
  infarction, 208–209, 222
  surgery for, 220

Confabulation, 40
Contusion, cerebral, 168–170
Conversion reactions, conversion hysteria, 119–120

Dementia
  cerebrovascular, 84–86
  CT scan, 94–96
  diagnosis, 79–80
  multi-infarct, 84–86
  neuropathology, 81–87
  non-Alzheimer, 83–84
  pseudo-, 87–94
    depressive, 88–90
    psychological testing, 88–93
  rating scales, 99
Depression
  dementia, pseudodementia, 88–90
  test performance
    memory and learning, 90–92
    intelligence, 92
  psychological testing, 96–98
Disinhibition, 176–178
Dissociation of function
  congruent, 26
  double, 23–27
  homologous, 25–26
  non-homologous, 26–27

Embolism, 222
Error utilization, 172–173

Fluency, verbal, 180–181, 286
Frontal lobes
  adaptive behaviour, 170
  adynamia, 179, 211–212
  akinetic mutism, 211
  conceptual behaviour, 173–174
  contusion, 168–170
  cortex, basal, 176–178
    dorsolateral, 170–176
    medial, 179
  dementia and, 83–84

Frontal lobes *(contd)*
  disinhibition, 176–178
  laterality, 179–181
  learning, imperfect, 172–173
  personality change, 178
  planning, 171–173
  problem solving, 174–176

Ganser syndrome, 122–123
Ganser symptoms, 122–123

Haemorrhage, cerebral, *see* cerebrovascular disorders
Head indury
  intellectual recovery, 166–167
  outcome
    scales, 167
  pathology, 168–170
  psychological deficit, 170–182
  severity measures, 163–164
Hydrocephalus
  normal pressure, 86–87
Hysteria
  as communication, 121–122
  malingering, and 123–125
  personality and, 120
  psychoanalytic theory, 120–121
  symptoms, 120

Infarct, 222
Infarction, *see* cerebrovascular disorders
Ischaemia, cerebral, 222

Korsakoff psychosis
  see Wernicke-Korsakoff syndrome

Lacunes (lacunar state), 218–219

Malingering, 123–125

Plaque, 222
Premorbid ability, 6
Pseudodementia, 87–94
  depression, 88–90
Pseudoneurological disorders
  assessment, 130–133
  circumscribed, 127
  definition, 119

Role
  concept, 125
  enactment, 125–126
  entrapment, 126
  shaping, 126
  theory, 125
Roles, neuropsychological, 227–234

Stenosis, arterial, 222
Stroke, 222
Syndrome
  concept of neuropsychological, 18–22
  Ganser, 122–123
  sub-, 21–22

Test battery, *see* battery
Testing methods
  fixed vs. flexible, 4–10
  hypothesis, 8–10
Tests
  depression and, 90–92
  organicity, 1
  scores, cut-off, 6–7
  validity, 116–17
Tests, named
  arithmetical problems, 282
  Austin Maze, 279–281
  Colour-Form Sorting, 281
  Knox Cubes, 282
  Lhermitte and Signoret, 282–285
  Naylor-Harwood Adult Intelligence Scale, 285
  National Adult Reading Test, 98–99
  Porteus Maze, 285
  Rey Auditory Verbal Learning, 285
  Rey Figure (complex figure of Rey), 285–286
  Trail Making, 286
  Verbal Fluency, 286
  Wisconsin Card Sorting, 287
Thrombosis, thromboembolism, 222
Transient global amnesia (TGA), 216–218
Transient ischaemia attacks, 219–220

Verbal fluency, 180–181
Vertebrobasilar insufficiency, 218

Wernicke-Korsakoff syndrome
  clinical features, 38–40
  history, 37–38
  neuropathology, 38
  psychometric features, 40–41